Brief Interventions for Psychosis

Basant Pradhan • Narsimha Pinninti
Shanaya Rathod
Editors

Brief Interventions for Psychosis

A Clinical Compendium

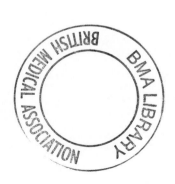

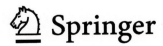

Editors
Basant Pradhan
Cooper University Hospital
Department of Psychiatry
Camden
New Jersey
USA

Shanaya Rathod
Antelope House
Southern Health NHS Foundation Trust
Southampton
UK

Narsimha Pinninti
Rowan University SOM
Department of Psychiatry
Cherry Hill
New Jersey
USA

ISBN 978-3-319-30519-6   ISBN 978-3-319-30521-9   (eBook)
DOI 10.1007/978-3-319-30521-9

Library of Congress Control Number: 2016940090

Printed on acid-free paper

This Springer imprint is published by Springer Nature
The registered company is Springer International Publishing AG Switzerland

Foreword

Treatment of psychotic disorders is undergoing significant change with more importance and focus being given to psychosocial interventions. In this context, the authors of this book, *Brief Interventions for Psychosis: A Clinical Compendium*, present information that is important, timely and fills a wide knowledge gap. Addressing this knowledge gap is critical in helping us update the existing systems of care because many health service systems are currently not set up to provide comprehensive and integrated clinical care to persons with psychotic disorders. Fortunately, more recently many societies are attempting to provide earlier, comprehensive and more effective interventions as the best hope for improving outcomes in psychotic illnesses. Clinical care of persons developing a psychotic disorder can be very effective with early detection, but the duration of untreated psychosis is still measured in years for most cases. There are several evidence-based treatments to implement, but most patients are not treated in settings with a coordinated therapeutic team trained and experienced in delivering these services. A significant chunk of clinical work is based on addressing current needs in each individual without empirical guidance on all available approaches. In addition, the available psychosocial interventions are labor as well as resources intensive and would be out of reach of many needy individuals with psychosis. This is where creating solutions such as evidence-based interventions provided in a brief format could narrow the gap between the needs of individuals with psychosis and the limited resources available to systems of care.

The editors of this book have an outstanding group of authors who clarify the clinical and social issues and then present information about a broad range of brief therapeutic interventions ranging from those supported by high-quality evidence for effectiveness to interventions that are promising. In addition, interventions that are relevant to different cultures and systems of care are addressed. Evidence for each intervention is critically reviewed. But what is most impressive is the user friendly methodology and the clinical situations in which the fundamental elements of each brief intervention are presented so that clinicians can incorporate some of these approaches in their own practice. The readers are offered a strong orientation to the concepts in the beginning chapters followed by descriptions of specific brief therapies with the strongest evidence followed by a chance to learn about recently introduced approaches such as motivational interviewing and *avatar* treatment for auditory hallucinations. Finally, perspectives on the economics and policy implementations that will facilitate wide-spread application of these interventions are discussed.

This textbook can have a broad range of users that include, but are not limited to, practicing psychiatrists, primary care physicians, psychologists, psychiatric nurse specialists, social workers, counselors, case managers, peer specialists, family therapists, researchers as well as health care administrators. This book provides a unique source of information for them and opens up new vistas of thought and praxis for brief interventions in the realm of psychosis.

William T. Carpenter Jr, MD
University of Maryland School of Medicine
Baltimore, MD, USA

Preface

The ever-growing gap between the psychiatric needs of the clients and the limited resources available to provide evidence-based treatments has inspired many academics and researchers to come up with innovative ways of providing good quality, efficient care. One such way is to take existing practices and adapt them to be delivered in a brief format. Brief therapeutic interventions differ from other types of psychotherapeutic interventions primarily in two aspects: these interventions emphasize a focus on a specific problem and are more targeted, thereby expediting and personalizing care. These interventions are of special relevance for the psychiatrists in their medication monitoring visits, by incorporating psychotherapeutic interventions without the burden of significantly adding to their visit time. Not only psychiatrists but also general physicians can find these interventions handy to incorporate into their practice. Even though there is controversy about the definition of brief therapy based on factors such as duration of sessions, number of sessions, or the focus on interventions, the consensus is that brief interventions are beneficial and can very well be part of every physician's repertoire in addressing situational crises and handling both recent onset clinical problems and chronic or long-standing issues. Often, brief and personalized interventions that are timely may have a greater impact on outcomes and experience.

At the present time, in the management of psychotic disorders, a confluence of four different forces is bringing psychotherapeutic and psychosocial interventions to the forefront. The first set of forces are clinical and evidence-based guidelines that recognize the limitation of psychotropic medications in helping clients achieve meaningful life goals and shed light on the critical role of psychosocial treatments for both augmenting the medications and improving meaningful client outcomes. The second set of forces, exemplified by the recovery movement, not only question the existing paradigm of having low expectations for psychotic disorders in the form of achieving just symptom relief but instead set the bar high, i.e., at recovery and rehabilitation. The third set of forces is the increasingly strong voice of individuals with lived experience who are influencing the agenda both in the development and delivery of mental health services. In the final set, there is a general recognition that clients, their families, and communities prefer psychosocial interventions to medication-based interventions while having fewer opportunities to access this kind of services. One important result of these forces is an enormous demand on the existing limited mental health resources; this further necessitates the development of innovative ways to cater this huge need.

There are two pragmatic ways that can work hand in glove to narrow this huge gap between the need and resources. One way is to utilize the existing therapeutic modalities in a brief format by integrating the effective interventions into routine clinical interactions while building the evidence base for the same. Toward this end, this book brings in experts from a variety of psychotherapeutic modalities to focus on adapting their particular modality to fit and enrich the existing system of care delivery. A second way to extend the availability of brief interventions is to utilize the network of providers as well as the social circle of the individuals and delineate interventions that the various members can provide in a coordinated and complimentary manner. This would mean interventions that can be provided by psychiatrists, psychologists, clinical social workers, case managers, peer support specialists, and other providers on one hand, and the family members, friends, and social and religious entities on the other. Organized literature in a book format that bridges across the various brief interventions and their applications in psychosis is really meager and directly necessitates a clinical guide book like this one. This book, through its 13 chapters, aims to shed light on the four areas mentioned earlier. The authors of these chapters are world-class experts in their respective domains whose experience spans the developing as well as the developed world. To provide its readers with a smooth flow, we provide a brief narrative of the individual chapters:

In Chap. 1, authors provide its readers a bird's eye view of psychosis, outline some of the important issues that our field is facing in this context, and suggest some broad directions to address some of these. They make a case for looking at the entire spectrum of psychosis in a continuum and draw attention to the *normal* psychotic experiences (such as spiritual experiences) that are at times difficult to distinguish from psychotic symptoms and, more often than not, are misinterpreted. Drawing the information from many different sources, they leave the readers with the message that broader and combined approaches that include both psychosocial interventions and medications are necessary in the treatment of psychosis.

In Chap. 2, the experienced authors candidly cite rich literature that diligently distinguishes between the psychotic experiences, normal versus pathological. They provide compelling information from many different sources that make the readers rethink and possibly challenge the long-held (mis-)concept that psychotic symptoms are always pathological and/or dangerous. Adapting from the concepts of evidenced-based integrated pathways that have been used successfully in stroke and cardiovascular illnesses, these authors make a case for *integrated pathways of care for psychosis* which provides a standardized framework for good clinical practice that include but not limited to reducing the wide variations and heterogeneity in care, providing timely access to the interventions, and paving the way for achieving improved outcomes for individuals suffering from psychosis.

In Chap. 3, the readers see an eloquent description of the need for and succinct description of the *brief cognitive therapy for psychosis* (brief CBTp). In their pioneering work, these authors also present a review and data on the efficacy of the brief CBTp. In addition, they present pilot data on efficacy of a culturally adapted model of the brief CBTp for clients in the low- and middle-income countries (LAMIC) where resources are even more meager. Importantly, they emphasize on the need for future research to shed more light on a still unresolved question on the dose-response relationship in psychotherapy.

Chap. 4 introduces its readers to the rationale, methodology, and logistics of *Avatar* therapy which is a new generation of translational and technologically sophisticated therapy attempt to deal with hallucinations. This innovative therapy not only establishes better coping mechanisms in the client but also attempts to change the client's personal relationship with auditory hallucinations. In keeping with a continuum view of psychosis, it attempts to change the meanings and the pathological factors that maintain the positive symptoms. In their pioneering work, the authors provide a road map about how *Avatar* therapy can be used to bring normalcy in the clients with refractory auditory hallucinations.

In Chap. 5, readers are introduced to the rationale, roadmap, and logistics of the *Yoga and mindfulness based cognitive therapy for psychosis* (*Y-MBCTp©*) which is a newer evidence-based translational mindfulness therapy designed by the authors. This self-exploratory and client-centered therapy combines together the pragmatism and methodology of brief CBT for psychosis with the scriptural philosophies and techniques of Yoga and mindfulness that are described in sage Patanjali's *Eight-limbed Yoga* (Sanskrit: *Ashtanga Yoga*) and Buddha's mindfulness meditation (Pali. *Satipathana*). This chap. also provides pilot data on efficacy of the *Y-MBCTp©* as a brief therapy model for clients with psychosis and suggests some directions for its future developments.

Drawing from his extensive clinical and scholarly work, in Chap. 6, its author succinctly narrates how a *developmentally informed psychoanalytic treatment approach* can be used in brief format for individuals with psychosis. In his masterly strokes, he elucidates how this approach nurtures the process of development itself and can be used with children, adolescents, and adults, including the ones who are overwhelmed with a psychotic process.

In Chap. 7, its author brings new insights into the application of principles and techniques of *motivational interviewing* strategies for individuals with psychotic disorders, a population for which its use is relatively new. The author makes a strong case that further brain-storming on use of motivational interviewing for individuals with psychotic disorders is particularly important because its different elements have enormous therapeutic potential to enhance the quality and efficacy of the existing interventions and to facilitate readiness of the clients/service users toward making efforts to improve the various aspects of life impacted by psychosis.

In Chap. 8, the author provides a historical context and brief summary of the extensive evidence base for *family interventions in psychosis* and succinctly describes how these can be used as brief interventions as well. In an elaborate and methodical way, this chap. takes its readers, step-by-step on a journey that covers the entire gamut of these brief collaborative systemic interventions for individuals with psychosis. Importantly, the author reflects that therapeutic interventions need not be ritualistic/dogmatic in their styles of implementation. Instead, they need to make the clinician feel more secure and hopeful, and only then regeneration of these feelings in their clients is possible which can lead to better outcomes.

In Chap. 9, its author describes the *recovery-related brief interventions for psychosis* and provide some new ideas. Putting his finger on the pulse of the latest body of research, he makes a strong case that it is rather premature to assume that the most effective way to improve long-term outcomes in psychosis is simply through the administration of symptom-oriented treatments: medical or psychological. He persuasively presents information which advocates to combine traditional treatments with more social models of care in order to improve outcomes.

In Chap. 10, its experienced author informs the readers about the ways in which *support with employment* can be a part of a personal recovery journey for many more people than it is today. It also focuses on interventions that can be provided by the various services to improve the support that clients with psychosis receive in order to gain and retain employment.

Drawing from his extensive clinical and scholarly work and his rich hand-on and lived experiences in cultural psychiatry, in Chap. 11, its author eloquently elaborates upon the *role of cultural factors in the treatment of psychosis*, both from the stand points of medications and psychosocial interventions. He explains that culture provides the belief system and explanatory model which forms the matrix for the psychotic features to play out in its various forms. He urges the readers to distinguish the normal psychosis experience from true indicators of serious psychopathology and cautions against overinterpretation and pathologization of them so that inappropriate treatments are avoided whereas adequate treatments are promptly instituted for those individuals who are in true need for them.

In Chap. 12, its authors describe the limited brief intervention models for psychosis that have begun emerging in the low- and middle-income countries (LAMIC). Focusing on the scenarios mostly from Asia and Africa, they point out that the epidemiological data there are scarce, the treatment strategies are rather at a preliminary stage, and focus is on mostly psychopharmacological or somatic interventions rather than on the psychosocial interventions. They illuminate the readers that in LAMIC, the burden of psychosis is huge, there are many barriers to promote psychosocial interventions, and one way these might be overcome is by implementing there the culturally adapted forms of brief interventions for psychosis.

Finally, in Chap. 13, the authors describe the scenarios on the treatment psychosis in general, and on brief interventions in particular at a broader (macro) level. By contrasting and comparing at the various systems of care that exist globally, they examine the current limitations and wisely recognize that despite the existing wide diversity, these systems share the same common goals of providing effective evidence-based interventions for most people in the most efficient way. In addition, they suggest some steps to be taken in the future endeavors that may include but not limited to improvement of policies, work force, service organization, training, and also further research that may help bring better treatment models for individuals with psychosis.

Rich discussions on the need for cultural and disorder-specific adaptations of the effective therapies are not new. However, through the tireless work of these authors over the years, we have been able to take a large step forward toward actualization of such adaptations in form of brief interventions. These are indeed very timely considering the huge public burden of psychosis, meager therapeutic resources, and a dire need for interdisciplinary integration of effective modalities. We hope that clients, clinicians, and researchers across the globe will benefit from reading this book and by adapting their stance in therapy. The editors truly believe that this is truly an intellectual and experiential journey to improve the therapeutic experience and outcomes for our clients. We invite all readers to be part of this journey by sharing with us their thoughts and opinions about this book.

With best wishes, humility, and gratitude,

Basant Pradhan, MD
Narsimha Pinninti, MD
Shanaya Rathod, MD

Contents

About the Author

Basant Pradhan is a child and adult psychiatrist, educator, researcher, and author. Currently he is an assistant professor of psychiatry and pediatrics and serves as the founding director of the *Yoga and Mindfulness Based Cognitive Therapy* (YMBCT) and the trans-cranial magnetic stimulation (TMS) treatment programs at the Cooper University Health System, Camden, NJ, USA. Pradhan had a few years of monastic training before he entered a career in neuropsychology and neuropsychiatry. His clinical and research work since 1993 has revolved around his pioneering work on child psychiatry epidemiology, translational Yoga and mindfulness research, neuropsychological functioning of bipolar disorder and schizophrenia, and development of new models of treatments that combine cutting-edge psychopharmacology with culturally adapted models of evidence-based psychotherapy. He has developed seven translational YMBCT models among which the prototype model is called TIMBER© (*Trauma Interventions using Mindfulness Based Extinction and Reconsolidation* of trauma memories) which has been successfully used for treatment of chronic and refractory PTSD. For exploring this further and to examine biomarker of response to ketamine and TIMBER©, he has been awarded with a grant support from the National Institute on Aging (NIA/NIH) and the Brain and Behavior Research Foundation, USA. He has authored or coauthored over 30 peer-reviewed articles, editorials, books, and book chapters and has presented his research over 70 conferences at regional, national and international levels.

Narsimha R. Pinninti is a professor of psychiatry at Rowan, School of Osteopathic Medicine in New Jersey, and also medical director of Oaks integrated care in NJ. Dr. Pinninti works at the interface of research and clinical practice and focuses on adapting cognitive behavior therapy and Yoga mindfulness based cognitive therapy (YMBCT) interventions in real-world clinical situations. He provides psychiatric services including CBT and YMBCT for individuals from different ethnic backgrounds in assertive community treatment team and day hospitalization programs. He is the course director for CBT training for psychiatric residents and has trained assertive community team and case managers in CBT. He has authored a number of papers in peer-reviewed journals, book chapters, and books. He has been an invited speaker nationally and internationally.

Shanaya Rathod is a consultant psychiatrist and director of research at the Southern health NHS Foundation Trust in the UK. She is the mental health clinical lead for the Wessex Academic Health Sciences Network and Clinical Research Network. She has been a fellow of the National Institute for Health and Care Excellence, UK. She has a particular interest in developing effective care pathways for psychosis to improve patient outcomes and experience and the cultural and religious aspects of psychopathology of mental illness. She has received grants to explore these areas further to develop a psychosis pathway and culturally sensitive cognitive behavior therapy for psychosis. She has authored a number of papers in peer-reviewed journals, book chapters, and books. She has been an invited speaker nationally and internationally.

Andy Bell is deputy chief executive of the Centre for Mental Health, an independent UK charity that seeks a fairer chance in life for people with mental health problems and aims to find ways of improving people's life chances and breaking down barriers by putting high-quality research into policy and practice.

Frank Burbach is a consultant clinical psychologist of the Somerset Partnership NHS Foundation Trust. He is the head of Clinical Psychology & Psychological Therapies services and lead for the Triangle of Care and Early Intervention in Psychosis. He has a diploma in marital and family therapy and is also a registered cognitive-behavioral psychotherapist. He is a member of the Triangle of Care national steering group, is the South West Early Intervention Lead, and is also a member of the Editorial Board of the *Journal of Family Therapy*. Dr Burbach has a PhD from Plymouth University on developing systemically oriented mental health services and has published numerous papers and book chapters describing the development of family inclusive practice and specialist family interventions in Somerset since 1995.

Tom Craig is professor of social and community psychiatry at King's College London, Institute of Psychiatry, Psychology and Neuroscience, and a consultant psychiatrist with the South London and Maudsley Foundation Trust. His clinical research focuses on evaluating community-based psychiatric services including alternatives to the hospital asylum, specialized services for homeless mentally ill people, supported employment, and services for first episode psychosis, and he is the chief investigator for the current clinical trial of the AVATAR therapy for the treatment of auditory hallucinations. He has published over 300 papers and is the president of the World Association of Social Psychiatry and an associate editor of the *Journal of Mental Health*.

Fallon was trained at the Yale Child Study Center, Western New England Institute for Psychoanalysis, and the Psychoanalytic Center of Philadelphia, and has been involved with numerous research projects and has numerous publications. His recent publication *Disordered Thought and Development: From Chaos to Organization in the Moment* is an outgrowth of his psychoanalytic research and clinical work with psychotic individuals and children in the autistic spectrum. This work has opened up a new paradigm to explore the inner worlds of adults as well as children and adolescents.

Theodore Fallon has a full-time private practice in child and adult psychoanalysis and psychotherapy in a suburb of Philadelphia, Pennsylvania. He is former chair of the Child Psychoanalytic Training Programs at the Psychoanalytic Center of Philadelphia and is associate clinical professor at Drexel College of Medicine. He teaches and supervises medical students, residents, fellows, and psychotherapy students and candidates.

Muhammad Irfan is currently working as head of the Department of Psychiatry and Behavioural Sciences, Peshawar Medical College, Peshawar, Pakistan. His professional interests include public mental health and nonpharmacological interventions in psychiatry. He is the provincial chap. chief of Pakistan Psychiatric Society and also serves as general secretary of the Pakistan Association of Cognitive Therapists (PACT). He has been the senior managing editor of the *Journal of Postgraduate Medical Institute*, Peshawar, since 2009. He is the elected council member of Committee on Publication Ethics (COPE) which is the main representative international organization on publication ethics. He is one of the founding member of the Institutional Review and Ethics Board, Postgraduate Medical Institute, Peshawar. He has regularly been involved in capacity building activities in the fields of mental health, research, and publication ethics.

David Kingdon is professor of Mental Health Care Delivery at the University of Southampton, UK, and honorary consultant adult psychiatrist for Southern Health NHS Trust. He has previously worked as medical director for Nottingham Health Care Trust and senior medical officer in the UK Department of Health. He now does policy and implementation work for NHS England and is editor of their mental health websites. He chaired the Expert Working Group leading to the Council of Europe's Recommendation 2004 on Psychiatry and Human Rights (1996–2003). His research interests are in cognitive therapy of severe mental health conditions and mental health service development on which he has published over 150 papers, chapters, and five books translated into languages including Mandarin, Japanese, Greek, Italian, and French. He has given invited lectures and workshops in the USA, Canada, Brazil, Mexico, Europe, China, Pakistan, Japan, and Korea. He received the Aaron T. Beck award for exceptional cognitive therapy in 2015.

Farooq Naeem is an associate professor of Psychiatry at Queens University, Kingston, Canada. His research interest are CBT, psychosis, culture, and digital media. Farooq is acknowledged as a leader in global mental health. He is a pioneer in culturally adapting CBT. His model of cultural adaptation of CBT is currently being replicated in Middle East, Morocco, and China. During the last 10 years he has promoted CBT in low- and middle-income countries. He has published nearly ten RCTs in this area along with colleagues from the University of Manchester, UK.

He founded the national CBT organization during his 3 years stay in Pakistan in 2006 (Pakistan Association of Cognitive Therapists, PACT). The PACT has so far organized five international conferences and has trained numerous professionals locally and from neighboring countries. He has nearly 80 publications in peer-reviewed journals. He has contributed to 12 books (4 as editor).

Andres J. Pumariega is professor and chair of the Department of Psychiatry at the Cooper Medical School of Rowan University and Cooper University Health System, Camden, NJ. Over his career, he has headed two other departments of psychiatry, three divisions of child and adolescent psychiatry, and two pediatric psychiatry consultation services. He is distinguished life fellow of the American Psychiatric, distinguished fellow of the American Academy of Child and Adolescent Psychiatry (AACAP), and fellow of the American College of Psychiatrists. His main research interests are in cross-cultural psychiatry, particularly work with underserved minority populations, and community systems of care, particularly in children's mental health. He has published over 200 peer-refereed scientific articles and book chapters, edited two books, and three special journal issues. He serves on the editorial boards of *Adolescent Psychiatry*, *Community Mental Health Journal*, and the *Journal of Family Studies*. He has served as associate editor of the *American Journal of Orthopsychiatry* and *Journal of Family Studies*. He has received many honors over his career, including the Simon Bolivar Award in Hispanic Psychiatry from the American Psychiatric Association and Jeanne Spurlock Award for Diversity and Culture from the AACAP.

Rubenstein is associate vice-president for Student Wellness and director of Counseling & Psychological Services at Rowan University. He is also adjunct clinical professor at the Philadelphia College of Osteopathic Medicine and adjunct clinical associate professor of Psychiatry and Psychology at Drexel University College of Medicine. Dr. Rubenstein interests are in the areas of outpatient psychotherapy, supervision, mental health and substance abuse, HIV/AIDS, and leadership. He is coauthor of book chapters and journal publications and has presented workshops at the local, regional, national, and international levels.

Geoff Shepherd is currently a senior consultant for a national program aimed at supporting the recovery of people using mental health services through a process of organizational change (ImROC). This is based in the Centre for Mental Health in London. He also holds a visiting chair position at the Institute of Psychiatry. He trained originally as a clinical psychologist and has worked in public mental health services all his career as both a clinician and a senior manager. His current research interests are in the evaluation of "co-produced" services (peer support, Recovery Colleges, etc.) and the implementation of evidence-based employment programs. He has served on several government committees advising on the development of mental health services in England and has consulted widely on service developments internationally, including in Ireland, mainland Europe, Japan, and Australia.

Brief Interventions for Psychosis: Overview and Future Directions

Basant Pradhan and Narsimha Pinninti

1.1   Introduction

Psychosis (etymology: Gk. *psyche* + *osis,* condition) as defined in the Merriam-Webster dictionary (http://www.merriam-webster.com/dictionary/psychosis) is a mental and behavioral disorder due to fundamental derangement of the mind (as in schizophrenia) and is characterized by defective or lost contact with reality especially as evidenced by delusions, hallucinations, and disorganized speech and behavior. This causes gross distortion or disorganization of a person's mental capacity, affective response, and capacity to recognize reality, communicate, and relate to others to the degree of interfering with that person's capacity to cope with the ordinary demands of everyday life. The word *psychosis* has become a part of the vocabulary of general population including the media and is extremely stigmatizing. For many in general public, psychosis is synonymous with schizophrenia and is associated with dangerousness and negative stereotypy, often leading to social distancing, discrimination, and even victimization (Diefenbach 1996; Wood et al. 2014). Societal stigma combined with self-stigma leads to diminished opportunities, demoralization, and impaired recovery process for individuals with schizophrenia and other psychotic illnesses (Corrigan and Wassel 2008; Horsfall et al. 2010). Also, mental health practice until very recently was guided by the belief that individuals with serious mental illnesses like psychosis do not recover. The course of

B. Pradhan, MD (✉)
Department of Psychiatry, Cooper University Hospital,
401Haddon Avenue, Camden, NJ 08103, USA
e-mail: Pradhan-Basant@Cooperhealth.edu

N. Pinninti, MD
Department of Psychiatry, Rowan University SOM,
Suite 100, 2250 Chapel Avenue East, Cherry Hill, NJ 08034, USA
e-mail: Narsimha.Pinninti@twinoakscs.org; narsimhanrp@gmail.com

© Springer International Publishing Switzerland 2016
B. Pradhan et al. (eds.), *Brief Interventions for Psychosis:
A Clinical Compendium*, DOI 10.1007/978-3-319-30521-9_1

their illness was either seen pessimistically, as deteriorative, or optimistically, as a maintenance course (Harding and Zahniser 1994). The pessimistic outlook goes hand in hand with biomedical conceptualization of psychosis that neglects environmental risk factors (Mizrahi 2015). While the biomedical hypothesis is a driver of pharmacological research and current practice, meta-analyses of first person accounts of mental illness show that there are a variety of opinions about the cause of psychosis. Different individuals view the cause of their condition as spiritual crisis, environmental cause, and political, biological, or specific trauma (Farkas 2007). Psychosis can be attributed to one or other medical illnesses (most importantly neurologic or endocrine), and determination of a cause-effect relationship between a medical illness and psychosis is not always easy. Importantly, the disconnect between the opinion of professionals and individuals extends to the focus of treatment. While professionals have been focused on symptom remission and reduction in hospitalization, people with psychosis are more focused on regaining life roles and improvement in quality of their life. In fact, a recent report of the state of mental health systems in the USA has concluded that mental health care in America fails a wide variety of individuals but particularly fails those with serious mental illnesses (IOM 2006) because it is "not oriented to the single most important goal of the people it serves, that of recovery" (The President's New Freedom Commission on Mental Health 2003). An objective look at the outcomes for psychosis shows that contrary to prevailing professional opinion, there is evidence from several studies that a sizable proportion of individuals with psychotic disorders have good outcomes. For example, in a 15–25-year follow-up of individuals with psychotic disorders in 18 different countries, it has been revealed that the majority (56 %) showed recovery. A sixth of them were completely recovered to the point of not requiring any treatment (Harrison et al. 2001). In addition, people with serious mental illnesses have themselves published accounts of their own recovery as well as advocated for the development of recovery promoting services (Farkas 2007). All the above point to an urgent need for us in the profession of behavioral health to rethink how we conceptualize, label, and treat psychotic disorders. We need to look at our existing services, how they are delivered, and their focus to make them align with the goals of individuals who are suffering with these disorders, their families and communities supporting them.

1.2   Epidemiology

Psychotic experiences are fairly common, with 15 % of normal subjects reporting them at some point in their life. In most individuals these experiences are either transient or do not cause functional impairment and require no treatment (Balaratnasingam and Janca 2015). The distinction between psychotic experience and psychotic symptom is not clear, and the two terms are used interchangeably. As a result all psychotic experiences are considered pathological and may lead to unnecessary use of antipsychotic medication. Even though schizophrenia is considered a prototype of psychotic disorder, psychotic symptoms are trans-diagnostic and seen in all serious mental illnesses and also in some personality disorders. For example, in borderline personality disorder, psychotic symptoms that at times are persistent are seen in 25–50 % of individuals and may indicate the severity of the disorder. Traditionally psychotic symptoms are viewed in categorical terms and always considered to be pathological. This categorical view contributes to the stigma, discrimination, and isolation of individuals with psychotic disorders. However, a paradigm shift is necessary to have a more comprehensive and nuanced approach to psychotic symptoms. The shift should include a distinction between psychotic experiences that are transient and psychotic symptoms and a recognition that some psychotic experiences are described part of spiritual experiences and may be self-enhancing. Secondly, the psychotic symptoms should be viewed dimensionally on a continuum from normal to pathological instead of the current categorical approach (Balaratnasingam and Janca 2015). This is a key premise of cognitive models of psychosis wherein the presence of voices in isolation is not sufficient to determine the transition to clinical psychosis (i.e., "need for care"). Put simply the way in which individuals make sense of, and respond to, their hearing experiences can determine whether voices remain benign (even life enhancing) or alternatively result in distress, impairment, and a need for clinical care (Garety et al. 2001). Thirdly, there should be recognition that the long-held biomedical hypotheses of the cause of psychosis are inadequate as there is evidence for the role of environmental factors in causation and maintenance of psychotic symptoms (Bebbington et al. 1993; Mizrahi 2015).

1.3   Spiritual and Psychotic Experiences

Religion, spirituality, and psychosis intersect and it is difficult to disentangle them. A model has been proposed to distinguish spiritual experiences from psychotic symptoms. Spiritual experience is described as a positively evaluated psychotic experience, which enables the subject to transcend their normal limitations and accomplish more than what he or she normally does, but these distinctions are not always clear. However, there is lack of quality studies that help us distinguish spiritual from psychotic experiences (Menezes and Moreira-Almeida 2010; Moreira-Almeida 2012). In clinical practice it is important to be aware of and understand the religious and spiritual background of individuals so that these resources are utilized for supporting hope, buffering stress, and possibly activating psychosomatic processes that promote health (Griffith 2012). In a normal community sample of individuals, the spiritual emergencies and psychotic symptoms are highly correlated, and some authors suggest that the two concepts are one and the same and all psychotic experiences should be treated as spiritual emergencies (Goretzki et al. 2009). There are individual case examples of psychotic symptoms conceptualized as spiritual emergencies and treated with psychological approaches particularly transpersonal psychotherapy (Lukoff 2005). However, there are no controlled studies to evaluate the effectiveness of transpersonal psychotherapy, and treating psychosis as a spiritual emergency can reduce the stigma associated with it but may lead to the unintended consequence of increasing the duration of untreated psychosis.

1.4   Continuum of Psychotic Process

It is helpful to keep the entire spectrum of psychotic process – from vulnerabilities at one end to recovery and reintegration at other end – in devising systems of care that facilitate phase appropriate interventions.

1.5   High Risk for Psychosis

The risk for psychosis is explained by the stress vulnerability model described by Zubin and Spring (1977) and further elaborated by Neucterlein et al. (2008). It emphasizes the interaction between life events, circumstances, and individual genetic, physiological, psychological, and social predispositions which lead to variation in vulnerability. Meta-analysis of risk factors identified age, sex, minority or migrant status, income, education, employment, marital status, alcohol use, cannabis or other drug use, stress, trauma, living in urban areas, and family history of mental illness as important predictors of psychotic experiences (PE). Of those who report PE, ~20 % go on to experience persistent PE, whereas for ~80 %, PE remit over time. Of those with baseline PE, 7.4 % develop a psychotic disorder outcome (Linscott and van Os 2013). An interesting recent finding is that the degree of psychotic symptoms at baseline does not distinguish individuals who go on to develop a psychotic disorder (Addington and Heinssen 2012). The factors that are likely to determine the long-term outcome of psychotic experiences are resilience, support systems available, individual and family perspective of the experiences, and the type of interventions that were utilized. Study of individuals who develop psychotic experiences but do not develop disorders is likely to provide clues for better treatment of psychotic disorders akin to study of individuals who are HIV infected but remain asymptomatic.

Psychosis has classically five dimensions (positive, negative, affective, cognitive, and disorganization).

The DSM-IV description of psychotic disorders had several limitations including a categorical approach to diagnosis that lent itself to enhancing stigma, questions about the validity of various diagnoses, and lack of clinical utility of some of the subtypes of illnesses. The work group on psychotic disorders for DSM-5 had to juggle multiple challenges of improving validity, reliability, and clinical utility. At the same time, they had to ensure simplicity and easy applicability. This was a huge challenge, and the expectation that there will be a paradigm shift in DSM-5 to a dimensional diagnostic system did not materialize. According to the work group on psychosis, the reason for the same was a lack of adequate research data to support this shift (Tandon 2013; Heckers et al. 2013). However, within the established categorical system, an effort was made to capture the underlying dimensional structure of psychosis. To that end, the terms domains, gradients, and dimensions are introduced. There are five domains of psychopathology that define psychotic disorders. The level of psychosis, the number of symptoms, and the duration of psychosis are the gradients that have been used to demarcate psychotic disorders from each other and continue to be used for the same purpose in DSM-5 (Heckers et al. 2013).

In the dimensional approach in the nosological system, schizophrenia, the prototype of all psychotic disorders, has been conceptualized to consist of five clusters of symptoms, and these are *positive symptoms* (delusions, hallucinations, and disorganization in thoughts, speech, and behavior), *negative symptoms* (social withdrawal, lack of motivations), *cognitive symptoms* (sustained attention, memory, and language), h*ostility and excitement symptoms* (includes impulse dys-control and violent behavior), and *affective symptoms* (includes depression or anxiety symptoms) (DSM-5, 2013). The *International Classification of Diseases* 10th edition (ICD-10) and the *Diagnostic and Statistical Manual of Mental Disorders* 4th edition (DSM-IV) both describe paranoid, hebephrenic, undifferentiated, catatonic, and residual group of schizophrenia. The problems with the subgroups are the instability of diagnosis over time and lack of predictive validity (Deister and Marneros 1994), and hence the subgroups have not been widely used clinically nor in research. The DSM-5 dispenses with these categories and catatonia becomes a different group. Efforts to find more homogenous subgroup of schizophrenia are ongoing. One such effort comes from two researchers working on the effectiveness of CBT for schizophrenia and other severe mental illnesses. Kingdon and Turkington (2005) propose that schizophrenia is a group of disorders and can be distinguished into four categories: (a) stress sensitivity psychosis (20 %), (b) drug-induced psychosis (20 %), (c) traumatic psychosis (49 %), and (d) anxiety psychosis (10 %) (Kingdon and Turkington 2005). A diagnostic instrument developed to distinguish these subtypes is shown to have good psychometric properties (Kinoshita et al. 2012). The categorization of schizophrenia into the above categories has implications for choice of psychosocial interventions based on the particular category. For example, as described in Chap. 5, the *Yoga and Mindfulness-Based Cognitive Therapy for Psychosis* (Y-MBCTp) shows efficacy in traumatic psychosis, in addition to its other benefits.

1.6 Expectation from the Interventions Done for Psychotic Disorders

Interventions for psychotic disorders should look at the entire spectrum from high-risk individuals to those who are in recovery and devise services that are based on their (a) phase of illness, (b) view of illness and receptivity to available interventions, (c) available mental health systems, and (d) mobilizing existing support systems. Services should ideally be provided for an indefinite period of time to reduce the fragmentation and help the individual smoothly transition through the various phases of their illness. Interventions are broadly biological and psychosocial, and the choices of interventions are based on our understanding of the etiology of psychotic disorders. These interventions should match the psychotic spectrum. As Fig. 1.1 illustrates, the first step in the spectrum is to identify individuals who are vulnerable and provide them with educational services to help them mitigate

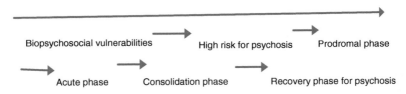

Fig. 1.1 Psychosis Spectrum

vulnerabilities. Next are ultra-high-risk (UHR) individuals for psychosis, and interventions are needed to address this group. Childhood trauma is prevalent in 86.6 % of individuals with UHR and is related to UHR status (Kraan et al. 2015). Interventions for those at UHR are to educate communities about risk for psychosis, identify individuals at risk for psychosis, and provide supportive and therapeutic services to prevent conversion to full-blown psychosis. These services are currently being evaluated on experimental basis and not integrated into the service provision model in most countries. Individuals with prodromal symptoms are usually not detected during this stage, and a diagnosis of prodrome is made in retrospective. Even when individuals develop psychotic symptoms, there is a significant delay in accessing treatment. At the back end of psychosis, rehabilitation and vocational services such as supported employment are not available for most individuals in maintenance phase of treatment. Currently our services are focused on the acute middle (narrow) end of spectrum, and a redesign of services that spans entire spectrum is necessary.

1.7 The Need for Evidence-Based Models Which Are Pragmatic and Client Centered as Well

Individuals who are functioning at a high level despite a diagnosis of psychotic disorder, describe the importance of a trusting relationship with a professional as critical in providing connection and containment during crises. In addition such relationship provides high degree of autonomy in personal decisions during periods of stability and thereby promote recovery and personal growth (Saks 2007). However, a long-term relationship over a period of years is a rare exception due to fragmented nature of the mental health-care provision. Fragmentation is such that an individual may see five different psychiatrists during the course of one acute episode. The closest one that comes to providing a long-term treatment team is the assertive community treatment (ACT) model. An ACT team in the USA is a multidisciplinary team (including psychiatrist, nursing staff, and individuals with lived experience of illness) available 24 h a day 7 days a week providing integrated coordinated care on a long-term basis (Schmidt et al. 2013). However, there are a limited number of ACT teams in the USA, and they focus on the most serious of the mentally ill and transfer individuals when more stable to a less-intensive treatment setting. This is a far cry from a system that is comprehensive enough to address the entire spectrum from identifying and dealing UHR individuals to those that are in recovery. The Affordable Care Act is shifting the focus of care provision from acute treatment to more broad prevention, from individual care to population health and systems of are called Accountable Care Organizations are being developed to help provide this degree of care.

More recently another integrated approach by the National Institute of Mental Health (NIMH) has made waves in the USA. This approach, called *Recovery After an Initial Schizophrenia Episode* (RAISE, detailed in Azrin et al. 2015), tries to catch the clients with first episode psychosis quite early in the course of illness. As the name suggests, RAISE was designed to help specifically the individuals who have experienced an initial psychotic episode. Geared toward reducing the duration of untreated psychosis (DUP) and fostering the recovery process quite early in the course of psychosis and thus attempting to reduce subsequent the disability, these evidence-based interventions integrated the many therapeutic components discussed on the various chapters of this book. These interventions are typically delivered by a clinical team specialized in early psychosis, and the services offered include but not limited to psychiatric treatment, medication management, help with finding a job or returning to school, substance abuse treatment, family education and support, and other support services as needed.

1.8 Mobilizing the Client's Existing Support Systems: The Spirits of Collaborative Empiricism

An unintended consequence of deinstitutionalization in the 1950s is that the burden of caring for individuals with serious mental illnesses shifted from institutions to family members (Solomon 1995). While the burden on families has increased, the importance of appropriate family involvement cannot be understated. A third of individuals with first episode psychosis disengage from services, and family involvement is one of the factors that facilitate engagement (Doyle et al. 2014). Similar to family, the size of an individual's social network and satisfaction with the network are shown to be positively correlated with recovery from SMI (Corrigan and Phelan 2004). A proactive and planned method of evaluating social support and engaging appropriate members of the individuals' social support is shown to aid recovery (Perry and Pescosolido 2015). Families can also have a deleterious effect on individuals as evidenced by increased risk of relapse in individuals whose families have high EE. On the other, intervention to lower the EE is shown to reduce risk of relapse (Butzlaff and Hooley 1998). The three issues family members have to deal with are (a) Maintaining an appropriate emotional distance from the loved ones (b) dealing with feelings of shame, fear, guilt, and powerlessness in the face of a socially stigmatized illness and (c) finally the frustration of navigating the complex network of bureaucracies that govern the mental health system (Karp 2001). In addition, if a family member is the primary caregiver for the individual with mental illness, he/she has to deal with additional issues of financial expenses, higher demands on their personal time for care-giving activities, and being more involved in dealing crises that arise (Lohrer et al. 2007). The burden of care on relatives of mentally ill is considerable, and to the extent their well-being and mental health is seriously impaired (Maurin and Boyd 1990). However, any system of care that is recovery oriented needs to have a family-centered approach. Involving family members fits in with the model of recovery as strengthening an existing support aids in recovery. The core tenets of family-centered approach are (a) non-blaming attitude, (b) developing and maintaining collaborative working relationship with family members, (c) empowering families through choice and control, and (d) an emphasis on strengths and goal of enhancing functioning.

1.9   Conclusions and Future Directions

The ever-growing gap between the needs of the clients with psychosis and the limited therapeutic resources available to them have inspired the innovators in our field not only to develop pragmatic and need-based models of treatment but also have propelled to integrate these with the strength-based and evidence-based models of care. Brief therapeutic interventions probably germinated in those contexts and have proliferated cross-culturally at this time, thereby expediting and personalizing the care for the needy and at the same time not losing their evidence-based foundations. This book amply highlights the current limitations in the care provided for individuals with psychotic disorders, integrates the various evidence-based psychotherapies or psychosocial interventions, and aims to bridge the current gaps in the health-care provision. Care is best provided when we have a longitudinal view of the entire spectrum of psychotic process and devise various interventions appropriate for each stage. We begin by making a case for integrated care pathways for psychosis in Chap. 2, which is followed by chapters on different evidence-based interventions in brief formats.

References

Addington J, Heinssen R (2012) Prediction and prevention of psychosis in youth at clinical high risk. Annu Rev Clin Psychol 8:269–289
Azrin ST, Goldstein AB, Heinssen RK (2015) Early intervention for psychosis: the Recovery After an Initial Schizophrenia Episode (RAISE) project. Psychiatr Ann 45(11):548–553
Balaratnasingam S, Janca A (2015) Normal personality, personality disorder and psychosis: current views and future perspectives. Curr Opin Psychiatry 28(1):30–34. doi:10.1097/YCO.0000000000000124
Bebbington P, Wilkins S, Jones P et al (1993) Life events and psychosis. Initial results from the Camberwell Collaborative Psychosis Study. Br J Psychiatry 162:72–79
Butzlaff RL, Hooley JM (1998) Expressed emotion and psychiatric relapse: a meta-analysis. Arch Gen Psychiatry 55(6):547–552
Corrigan PW et al (2008) Principles and practice of psychiatric rehabilitation: an empirical approach. New York, The Guildford Press

Corrigan PW, Phelan SM (2004) Social support and recovery in people with serious mental illnesses. Community Ment Health J 40(6):513–523

Deister A, Marneros A (1994) Prognostic value of initial subtype in schizophrenic disorders. Schizophr Res 12:145–157

Diefenbach DL (1996) The creation of a reality: the portrayal of mental illness and violent crime on television. US, ProQuest Information & Learning 57:0496–0496

Doyle R, Turner N, Fanning F, Brennan D, Renwick L, Lawlor E, Clarke M (2014) First-episode psychosis and disengagement from treatment: a systematic review. Psychiatr Serv 65(5): 603–611. doi:10.1176/appi.ps.201200570

Farkas M (2007) The vision of recovery today: what it is and what it means for services. World Psychiatry 6(2):68–74

Garety PA, Kuipers E, Fowler D, Freeman D, Bebbington PE (2001) A cognitive model of the positive symptoms of psychosis. Psychol Med 31(02):189–195, http://doi.org/10.1017/S0033291701003312

Goretzki M, Thalbourne MA, Storm L (2009) The questionnaire measurement of spiritual emergency. J Transpers Psychol 41(1):81–97

Griffith JL (2012) Psychiatry and mental health treatment. In: Cobb M, Puchalski CM, Rumbold B, Cobb M, Puchalski CM, Rumbold B (eds) Oxford textbook of spirituality in healthcare. Oxford University Press, New York, pp 227–233

Harding CM, Zahniser J (1994) Empirical correction of seven myths about schizophrenia with implications for treatment. Acta Psychiatr Scand 90:140–146

Harrison G, Hopper K, Craig T, Laska E, Siegel C, Wanderling J, Dube KC, Ganev K, Giel R, an der Heiden W, Holmberg SK, Janca A, Lee PW, León CA, Malhotra S, Marsella AJ, Nakane Y, Sartorius N, Shen Y, Skoda C, Thara R, Tsirkin SJ, Varma VK, Walsh D, Wiersma D (2001) Recovery from psychotic illness: a 15- and 25-year international follow-up study. Br J Psychiatry 178:506–517

Heckers S, Barch DM, Bustillo J, Gaebel W, Gur R, Malaspina D, Owen MJ, Schultz S, Tandon R, Tsuang M, Van Os J, Carpenter W (2013) Structure of the psychotic disorders classification in DSM-5. Schizophr Res 150(1):11–14. doi:10.1016/j.schres.2013.04.039

Horsfall J, Cleary M, Hunt GE (2010) Stigma in mental health: clients and professionals. Issues Ment Health Nurs 31(7):450–455. doi:10.3109/01612840903537167

IOM (2006) Improving the quality of health care for, mental and substance-use conditions. Committee on Crossing the Quality Chasm: Adaptation to Mental Health and Addictive Disorders, Board on Health Care Services, Institute of Medicine, Washington, DC, Retrieved from Washington, DC. National Academies Press: http://www.nap.edu/catalog/11470.html

Karp DA (2001) The burden of sympathy: how families cope with mental illness. Oxford University Press, New York

Kingdon D, Turkington D (2005) Cognitive therapy of schizophrenia. The Guildford Press, New York

Kinoshita Y, Kingdon D, Kinoshita K, Sarafudheen S, Umadi D, Dayson D, Hansen L, Rathod S, Ibbotson RB, Turkington D, Furukawa TA (2012) A semi-structured clinical interview for psychosis sub-groups (SCIPS): development and psychometric properties. Soc Psychiatry Psychiatr Epidemiol 47(4):563–580. doi:10.1007/s00127-011-0357-9

Kraan T, Velthorst E, Smit F, de Haan L, van der Gaag M (2015) Trauma and recent life events in individuals at ultra high risk for psychosis: review and meta-analysis. Schizophr Res 161 (2–3):143–149. doi:10.1016/j.schres.2014.11.026

Linscott RJ, van Os J (2013) An updated and conservative systematic review and meta-analysis of epidemiological evidence on psychotic experiences in children and adults: on the pathway from proneness to persistence to dimensional expression across mental disorders. Psychol Med 43(6):1133–1149

Lohrer SP, Lukens EP, Thorning H (2007) Economic expenditures associated with instrumental caregiving roles of adult siblings of persons with severe mental illness. Community Ment Health J 43(2):129–151. doi:10.1007/s10597-005-9026-3

Lukoff D (2005) Spiritual and transpersonal approaches to psychotic disorders. In: Mijares SG, Khalsa GS, Mijares SG, Khalsa GS (eds) The psychospiritual clinician's handbook: alternative methods for understanding and treating mental disorders. Haworth Press, New York, pp 233–257

Maurin JT, Boyd CB (1990) Burden of mental illness on the family: a critical review. Arch Psychiatr Nurs 4(2):99–107

Menezes A Jr, Moreira-Almeida A (2010) Religion, spirituality, and psychosis. Curr Psychiatry Rep 12(3):174–179. doi:10.1007/s11920-010-0117-7

Mizrahi R (2015) Social stress and psychosis risk: common neuro-chemical substrates? Neuropsychopharmacology. doi:10.1038/npp.2015.274

Moreira-Almeida A (2012) Assessing clinical implications of spiritual experiences. Asian J Psychiatry 5(4):344–346. doi:10.1016/j.ajp.2012.09.018

Nuechterlein KH, Subotnik KL, Turner LR, Ventura J, Becker DR, Drake RE (2008) Individual placement and support for individuals with recent-onset schizophrenia: integrating supported education and supported employment. J Psychiatr Rehab 31(4):340–349

Perry BL, Pescosolido BA (2015) Social network activation: the role of health discussion partners in recovery from mental illness. Soc Sci Med 125:116–128. doi:10.1016/j.socscimed.2013.12.033

Saks ER (2007) The center cannot hold: my journey through madness. Hyperion, New York

Schmidt LT, Pinninti NR, Garfinkle B, Solomon P (2013) Assertive community treatment teams. In: Yeager KR, Cutler DL, Svendsen D, Sills GM (eds) Modern community mental health: an interdisciplinary approach. Oxford University Press, New York, pp 293–303

Solomon P, Draine J (1995) Subjective burden among family members of mentally ill adults: relation to stress, coping, and adaptation. Am J Orthopsychiatry 65(3):419–427

Tandon R (2013) Definition of psychotic disorders in the DSM-5 too radical, too conservative, or just right! Schizophr Res 150(1):1–2. doi:10.1016/j.schres.2013.08.002

The President's New Freedom Commission on Mental Health (2003) Achieving the promise: transforming the mental health care in America. U.S. Department of Health and Human Service, Substance Abuse and Mental Health Services Administration, Center for Mental Health Services, Rockville, Retrieved from http://www.mentalhealthcommission.gov/reports/finalreport/fullreport.htm)

Wood L, Birtel M, Alsawy S, Pyle M, Morrison A (2014) Public perceptions of stigma towards people with schizophrenia, depression, and anxiety. Psychiatry Res 220(1–2):604–608

Zubin J, Spring B (1977) Vulnerability–a new view of schizophrenia. J Abnorm Psychol 86(2):103–126

Integrated Pathways of Care for Psychosis: An Overview

2

Shanaya Rathod and Narsimha Pinninti

2.1 Introduction

Psychiatry has reached a crossroads with respect to the way we understand and treat psychotic symptoms. In the past, psychotic symptoms have been mainly studied in clinical situations and as a result, we have viewed them as pathological entities that more often than not result in psychiatric evaluation and treatment. In addition to that, individuals with mental illnesses have been portrayed, by the media, as unpredictable and violent. This leads to the perception in the general public that individuals with psychosis are violent (Athanasopoulou et al. 2015) and cannot recover or lead meaningful lives. These misrepresentations have not improved with time (Clement and Foster 2008). However, as described in Chap. 1 and elaborated upon below, information from many different sources make us rethink and possibly challenge this long held conceptualization of psychotic symptoms as pathological or leading to violence.

The first source is a strong voice using the growing influence of people with lived experiences who advocate that we look at psychotic symptoms from a much broader perspective than the current illness prism. Ignored for a long time, the viewpoint of individuals who experienced psychosis is now rightly being increasingly considered in the delivery of mental health services.

The second is the study of psychotic experiences in normal populations also highlighted in Chapter 1. Psychotic experiences (PE), i.e., delusions and hallucinations,

S. Rathod, MD (✉)
Antelope House, Southern Health NHS Foundation Trust,
Southampton, SO14 0YG, UK
e-mail: Shanaya.rathod@southernhealth.nhs.uk; shanayarathod@nhs.net

N. Pinninti, MD
Department of Psychiatry, Rowan University SOM,
Suite 100, 2250 Chapel Avenue East, Cherry Hill, NJ 08034, USA
e-mail: Narsimha.Pinninti@twinoakscs.org; narsimhanrp@gmail.com

© Springer International Publishing Switzerland 2016
B. Pradhan et al. (eds.), *Brief Interventions for Psychosis:
A Clinical Compendium*, DOI 10.1007/978-3-319-30521-9_2

are seen in about 15 % of the normal population at some point in their lives (Balaratnasingam and Janca 2015). Many of these individuals are not in treatment and do function normally. Of those who report PE, only 20 % go on to experience persistent PE, whereas for 80 %, PE reduces over time. Of those with baseline PE, 7.4 % develop a persistent psychotic disorder outcome. Another compelling finding is that the severity of psychotic symptoms is not correlated that well with the level of functioning, and individuals with same degree of psychotic symptoms have been shown to have quite different levels of functioning (Linscott and van Os 2013). There is also evidence that psychotic symptoms are on a continuum with normal experiences (Johns and van Os 2001). This means that our existing paradigm that psychotic syptoms are qualitatively different from normal experiences and pathological need to be reexamined.

The third source of information is from spiritual literature wherein experiences that are phenomenologically similar to psychosis are described in normal populations and in advanced spiritual practitioners (Rolland 1929; Epstein 1990). There have been attempts to distinguish spiritual from psychotic experiences. Some features that distinguish spiritual from psychotic experiences are lack of distress, lack of impairments in social and occupational functioning, compatibility with the patient's cultural background and recognition by others, absence of psychiatric comorbidities, control over the experience, presence of good level of insight, and personal growth over time (Wilber et al. 1986, 2013). We have also discussed this in Chap. 1.

The study of normal psychotic experiences supports a more benign view and the need for adopting a *wait and see approach* to the psychotic experiences. On the other hand, study of people with recurrent episodes or persistent psychosis shows that a key predictor of recovery in psychosis is the duration of untreated psychosis (DUP), which is the time between the onset of psychotic symptoms and the start of treatment. The longer the duration of untreated psychosis, the worse the outlook can be (McGorry et al. 1996). DUP is considered to be the strongest predictor of symptom severity and outcome (Drake et al. 2000). Delayed treatment can lead to significant impairments in social functioning and recovery which become increasingly difficult to repair (Birchwood et al. 1998). Evidence from transcultural and international research suggests that DUP ranges between 364 and 721 days (McGlashan 1999; Marshall et al. 2005), and therefore reducing DUP is of imminent interest internationally (WHO 2001). Hence, the treatment goals in psychosis are to identify the illness as early as possible, treat the symptoms, provide education and skills to individuals and their families, maintain the improvement over a period of time, prevent relapses, and promote recovery (Rossler et al. 2005).

Reconciling the two ends of the spectrum from the wait and watch approach of psychotic experiences to reducing DUP in persistent psychosis can be a clinical conundrum. Since the mid-1990s, individuals have been considered to be at ultrahigh risk (UHR) for psychosis if they met at least one of three criteria: the presence of attenuated psychotic symptoms (APS); the presence of positive symptoms at full psychotic intensity for brief, limited time points (known as BLIPS); and/or a combination of genetic risk or schizotypal personality disorder accompanied by functional decline (known as genetic risk and decline syndrome [GRD]) (Fusar-Poli et al. 2015). However, the risk of psychosis of these different groups has remained unknown, and only recently, Paolo Fusar-Poli and colleagues (2015) analyzed the outcomes of 33 independent studies in a meta-analysis, including over 4,000 UHR individuals monitored for psychosis progression. The authors found that people with BLIPS had the highest risk of conversion to psychosis (39 % after 24 months), followed by APS (19 %) and GRD (3 %). They concluded that in addition, patients who had both APS and GRD had a similar risk of conversion to psychosis as those with only APS across all time points studied—suggesting GRD may not be a valid component of the UHR profile. Based on the information above, medically treating all psychotic experiences in order to reduce the duration of untreated psychosis may include people whose symptoms naturally resolve or are spiritual in nature. In these situations, we can accept a much broader understanding of psychotic experiences that views them as a variation in normal human experience and one that need not be medicalized. On the other hand, there is a risk that this approach can discourage people with persistent psychotic symptoms to seek helpful treatment, lengthening the duration of untreated psychosis and worsening the outcome.

What is required is an acknowledgment that our understanding of psychotic experiences is evolving and needs further research. On one hand, we do not know enough about the resilience of individuals who have these experiences and are able to integrate them into their life and function at a higher level. On the other hand, diagnoses such as schizophrenia are reliable, but their validity is being increasingly questioned (Johns and Van Os 2001). So the discourse at the level of the community should be changed from an assumption that psychotic symptoms are necessarily pathological to one that they could have a range of outcomes with psychological growth, spiritual progress, and higher level of functioning and progression at one end to persistent psychosis that requires ongoing monitoring and treatment at the other.

In the last two decades, evidence has built on the effectiveness of psychological therapies such as cognitive behavior therapy and family interventions for schizophrenia and other psychotic disorders (NICE 2014). There are therapies that target symptom dimensions such as positive symptoms as well as those targeting individual symptoms such as auditory hallucinations (Thomas et al. 2014). While most of the studies of psychological interventions have been conducted in people who are on antipsychotic medication, there is some evidence to suggest that people who do not want to take medication can still be helped by cognitive behavior therapy interventions (Morrison et al. 2014) and a proportion of individuals can be engaged with services if they are given the option to accept psychosocial interventions without medication. Other novel interventions that optimize recovery and aim to improve an individual's resilience through utilizing the entire social network of that individual using a "dialogical approach" to understanding psychotic experiences have shown that almost two thirds of individuals with psychosis could be managed without medication or on very small doses for brief periods of time and more importantly the duration of untreated psychosis in that community decreased to 3 weeks (Seikkula et al. 2011). While the idea of network therapy has originally come from the USA, managed care has limited its applicability (Seikkula et al. 2011) and similar discussions would be encountered in the NHS without changes to the current model (Razzaque and Wood 2015) of delivery of care.

There is a need to develop services that subscribe to this broad approach toward psychosis while making all medication and psychosocial interventions available to individuals at different stages of their experiences. The individual and their families and clinician decide on the best treatment approach for them at that particular stage of their experiences. This way the treatment is highly individualized and has the person with the psychotic experience at the center of decision-making. This type of individualized approach helps people engage with services, reduces stigma, and optimizes the use of limited resources.

2.2   Duration of Untreated Psychosis

The duration of untreated psychosis (DUP) remains high in most countries and is correlated with poor outcomes such as higher degree of positive symptoms, reduced overall functioning, and quality of life. Patients with a long DUP are significantly less likely to achieve remission (Drake et al. 2000; Marshall et al. 2005). In the USA, the duration of untreated psychosis in a community sample was found to be 74 weeks with 68 % of individuals with DUP greater than 6 months. Correlates of longer DUP included earlier age at first psychotic symptoms, substance use disorder, positive and general symptom severity, poorer functioning, and referral from outpatient treatment settings (Addington et al. 2015). Early intervention programs were developed in some countries to address the long duration of untreated psychosis and have been shown to reduce the DUP when first introduced. However, this effect was not sustained and for established early intervention centers did not reduce the duration of untreated psychosis (Marshall et al. 2014).

Longer durations of untreated psychosis can occur due to client-related factors or service-related factors. Client-related factors could be due to an inability to recognize early symptoms or due to the illness itself such as poor insight and social and emotional withdrawal (Connor et al. 2014) or due to cultural values systems like attributions to illness and help-seeking pathways into care (Rathod et al. 2015a). In people with first episode of psychosis, carers and families play a key role in determining and facilitating help-seeking behaviors (Logan and King 2001; Connor et al. 2014).

Community education and awareness campaigns have been tried to identify symptoms early with limited success (Lloyd-Evans et al. 2011). Educating general practitioners to reduce delays in referrals to secondary care services has had limited impact (Lester et al. 2009a) in increasing the number of referrals. Delays within secondary care mental health services have been found to be of most significance in the care pathways of those with long DUP (Birchwood et al. 2013; Norman et al. 2001). Paradoxically, Birchwood and colleagues (2013) found that first contact with an "acute service" (crisis team, home treatment, or admission) predicted shorter subsequent treatment delays within the mental health service and DUP overall. Similar trends have been reported through international research (Platz et al. 2006) and highlight the pressures on services that cope with routine referrals. Anderson and colleagues conducted a systematic review of international studies and concluded that a common theme is the need to understand the barriers faced when seeking help for psychosis, especially the response of service providers (2010). The Finnish open dialogue long-term studies show promise in addressing several of the barriers existing in other systems and facilitate help-seeking behaviors in individuals with and without psychosis while giving them as much say in decision-making as possible. The method consists of training entire staff in a geographical region and involving the networks of individuals who develop psychosis in the process of treatment. This approach has shown that the crises are detected early and the population is more trained in responding appropriately to crises leading to quicker resolution of psychosis and reduced incidence of new cases of schizophrenia. If these findings are replicated in other settings, it will have profound implications for models of services in psychiatry (Seikkula et al. 2011).

2.3 Current Service Models for Individuals with Psychosis

As currently delivered, there is a considerable unmet need in the way individuals with psychosis can access services and receive evidence-based treatments as prescribed by the National Institute for Health and Care Excellence (NICE) (2014) in a timely fashion. Early intervention in psychosis (EIP) teams had been set up in many countries like Australia and the UK for first-episode psychosis to improve access to services and interventions with limited impact on DUP (Lester et al. 2009b). The remit of the early intervention in psychosis teams had been to raise awareness in communities, education in schools and community programmers, and early identification and engagement with people who have early psychosis with a view to providing a range of interventions that include psychotropic medication and psychosocial therapies including family work and skills on relapse prevention. However, due to budgetary constraints, most EIP services, especially in the UK, have lost resources and many have been dissolved into community teams, thereby loosing quality (Rethink Mental Illness 2014; Rathod et al. 2014).

If the EIP services worked to their desired specification and therefore reduced the likelihood of relapse, or rates of detention under the Mental Health Act, in the UK alone, they could potentially save the NHS £44 million each year through reduced use of hospital beds (Rethink Mental Illness 2014) and reduce the risk of suicide from up to 15–1 % (Melle et al. 2006). Above all, it is difficult to put a price tag on the reduction in burden of illness for individuals and families.

In the USA as well, Mueser and colleagues (2015) replicated this comprehensive model of care called NAVIGATE that included four core interventions: individualized medication management, family psychoeducation, resilience-focused individual therapy, and supported employment and education. The model was delivered at community-based clinics to mirror real-world settings and demonstrated that the patients in the intervention arm experienced greater improvement in quality of life and psychopathology and experienced greater involvement in work and school compared with patients in community care. The study also confirmed that NAVIGATE participants with duration of untreated psychosis of less than 74 weeks had greater improvement in quality of life and psychopathology compared with those with longer duration of untreated psychosis and those in community care.

For people who have a relapsing and remitting psychotic illness, multiple admissions, and some disengagement from services, assertive community teams or assertive outreach teams have been set up in many countries like the USA and UK. Assertive community treatment teams are designed to be self-contained multidisciplinary teams that address all medical and psychosocial needs of the consumers by providing services that are round the clock, across different settings, and for an indefinite period of time (Schmidt et al. 2013). The remit of these teams had been to provide intensive support, assertive engagement, and work on relapse prevention. While the organization of community care around fidelity to a recognized model had developed in the USA and enabled the use of extensive research in comparing and refining service configurations or interventions, unfortunately the commissioning of assertive outreach services has not been closely defined in the UK, and many opportunities have been missed (Wharne 2013). Therefore, in the UK, with the redesigns, remodeling, and constant changes in community services, the majority of assertive outreach teams have been dismantled, with some functions integrated into community mental health teams (Firn et al. 2013; Rathod et al. 2014).

In addition to these specific psychosis services, in the UK, crisis resolution home treatment teams have been created that care for people when they are in crisis or require hospital admission but may benefit from intensive support at home rather than in the hospital (Johnson 2013). While the vision with the number of different teams that care for a person is aimed at reducing hospital admissions, it does cause fragmentation of care as people are cared for by a number of staff and therefore continuity of care can become an issue.

Some countries like the Netherlands developed the flexible assertive community team (FACT) model that is a variant on the original ACT model. Although designated teams do exist in the Netherlands, mostly in urban areas, about 70 % of teams providing services to people with psychosis are FAC teams. These combine functions that, in the UK context, would be provided by a variety of services, including assertive outreach, crisis resolution, recovery, and rehabilitation. The variety of need is met by providing two distinct levels of service within a single team: one which is high intensity, following the classic assertive outreach shared caseload approach, and the other offering low intensity, which is more like individual case management. Patients move easily between these levels depending on need, but the staff group remains the same, ensuring continuity of care (Van Veldhuizen 2007).

The Schizophrenia Commission Report (2012) and National Audit of Schizophrenia (2012) in the UK have highlighted deficiencies in psychopharmacological and psychological care and recommended changes to the way care is provided to people with schizophrenia. Spending is currently skewed toward the more expensive parts of the system, at £350 average cost per day for inpatient care compared with £13 average cost per day in community settings (Knapp et al. 2014). People from some minority communities are often overrepresented in the more intense and coercive forms of care, and this can be attributed to their nonengagement with services until a point of crisis (Mental Health Bulletin 2009) making a case for cultural adaptation of services and interventions (Rathod et al. 2015a, b).

Therefore, it would be reasonable to conclude that due to a lack of guidance and prescription around when interventions should be available to people who suffer with psychosis, the variations in the DUP and the length of time people have to wait before receiving interventions impact on poor prognosis.

In order to begin to address these issues and reduce the DUP, the Access and Waiting Time Standard (NHS England 2015) for first-episode psychosis has been established in the UK. This standard also aspires to address the issue of psychotic experiences in individuals that may never become persistent by prescribing a NICE concordant package of care for people with "at-risk mental state" (ARMS). The main modality of treatment in this group is nonmedical, but should they need to, they can be progressed to first-episode psychosis pathway. This new standard may catalyze the reformation of EIP teams in the nation. However, the introduction of targets and policy is not enough. A social movement and cultural change are required to ensure that people who suffer with psychosis receive the right interventions in a timely manner and lead fulfilling lives. Integrated pathways that define time frames for delivery of treatments and a range of interventions personalized to an individual's needs and provide holistic care are key to this.

2.4   Case for Integrated Pathways

Evidenced-based integrated pathways have been used successfully in stroke and cardiovascular illness. They provide a standardized framework for good clinical practice, reduce variation in care, and have improved outcomes for patients through providing timely access and intervention. Standardized pathways improve quality by improving multidisciplinary communication with different care agencies and care planning and improve patient satisfaction (Campbell et al. 1998). While currently there are pathways and guidance available for psychosis care in some countries such as the UK (NICE 2014), they do not provide prescriptive time frames to improve access to care and interventions. In order to improve the DUP and outcomes for people who suffer with psychosis, there is a need for defined pathways prescribing key stages, timelines, and a range of evidence-based interventions matched to the diversity of presentations that occur with psychosis, e.g., comorbidity with substance misuse and trauma, which will improve access to evidence-based services and interventions and support recovery. It is also fundamental to improving the physical health and reducing premature mortality in people with psychosis as currently the average lifespan of people who suffer with psychosis is shortened by 15–20 years compared with the general population (Brown et al. 2010). Integrated pathways can ensure delivery of appropriate health promotion and prevention at key stages, e.g., weight gain from antipsychotic medication is especially pronounced in the first 8 weeks of administration, but it is rare that specific support is offered at this stage. Similarly, smoking cessation support and employment support can be built in at critical periods, e.g., on admission to hospital. In those countries where independent, unbiased, and expert guidance is not available from one source, creation of such an entity should be a priority (Vissers and Beech 2005) or a global approach to guidance can be considered.

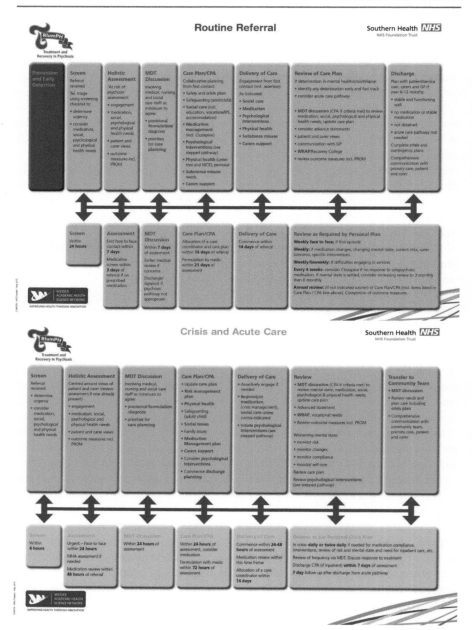

Fig. 2.1 Treatment and Recovery In PsycHosis (TRIumPH) pathway

For the first time in the history of mental health, an integrated care pathway called TRIumPH (Treatment and Recovery In PsycHosis) (Fig. 2.1)—that prescribes time frames around access and clinical interventions—has been developed and evaluated in the United Kingdom (Rathod and Psychosis Pathway Steering

Group 2015). The work has used a similar approach to that taken to improve stroke care, where there has been a demonstrable improvement in outcomes for patients and carers. The new psychosis pathway aims to reduce the impact of disease and promote recovery by ensuring that every individual gets the best evidence-based care at the right time and in the right place.

In developing the pathway, a multipronged approach has been used, using (i) research and data, (ii) coproduction with individuals with lived experience of mental illness and their carers, and (iii) engagement with clinicians and other stakeholders including commissioners, primary care, and third sector organizations (Rathod et al. 2015b). The approach has used a robust methodology which can be adapted and adopted nationally and internationally.

2.5   Delivery of Care: Treatment and Therapy Options

Traditionally, treatment in psychosis has meant the use of psychotropic medications which for very long time have been considered to be critical in the early treatment of psychosis. Chlorpromazine, introduced in 1952, was the first antipsychotic agent shown to have significant efficacy in the treatment of positive psychotic symptoms. It contributed to the reduction of inpatient population from its peak in 1950 to its current low in the USA. Antipsychotic medications range from the first-generation typical drugs like Chlorpromazine and Haloperidol to second-generation atypical medications like Olanzapine, Risperidone, and Aripiprazole. All antipsychotics block dopamine receptor pathways, but atypicals also tend to act on Serotonin receptors in addition. Neuromodulatory treatments for a very long time were limited to electroconvulsive treatment but now include transcranial magnetic stimulation (TMS) and transcranial direct current stimulation (TDCS). We now have evidence for the effectiveness of TMS in schizophrenia while the data is not yet adequate on TDCS (Cole et al. 2015).

Psychosocial interventions for psychosis can be classified as evidence-based or promising practices according to the extent to which efficacy is supported by meta-analyses, randomized controlled trials (RCTs), and best practice guidelines, e.g., NICE (2014). The best evidenced therapies for people with psychosis are currently cognitive behavior therapy (CBT) (Dixon et al. 2009; Wykes et al. 2008; Turner et al. 2014; NICE 2014), family interventions (FI) (Pharoah et al. 2010), and supported employment for psychosis (Dixon et al. 2009). Evidence is building for cognitive remediation therapy (CRT) although literature suggests that it is more effective when patients are clinically stable and stronger effects have been found when CRT has been combined with adjunctive rehabilitation (Wykes et al. 2011).

Promising psychosocial interventions include cognitive adaptive therapy, healthy lifestyle interventions, peer support services, physical disease management, prodromal stage intervention, social cognition training, supported education, and supported housing (Mueser et al. 2013). There are some innovative approaches, such as Finnish open dialogue and Avatar therapy (Leff et al. 2013; Seikkula 2002), and a new Yoga Mindfulness based cognitive therapy (Y-MBCT) for individuals with psychosis and significant trauma (Please see Chap. 5), currently under evaluation. Most of these interventions are delivered in individual format. However, group CBT has shown promising value (Gledhill et al. 1998; Wykes et al. 1999) in psychosis (Kumari et al. 2011) and has the added benefit of maximizing the available resources.

It is very tempting to suggest standard interventions in the name of uniformity of care. However, individuals vary very significantly in their symptoms, their coping skills, their cultural and familial background, and their resilience, and therefore, standards across the board interventions are not very helpful to everyone. Instead, people would benefit from a personalized approach to psychosocial interventions. Often, psychoeducation that is nonstigmatizing and hope engendering complimented with low-intensity interventions based on CBT principles of identifying and strengthening existing coping strategies or mindfulness (Walker et al. 2013) is helpful in meeting people at the level they are in and keeps them engaged in treatment. Any intervention should be person centered and needs-led. With this philosophy in mind, Rathod and colleagues (2015a, b) recommend a stepped care model and approach to providing psychological therapies as described below. Such an approach ensures that people who suffer with psychosis have access to interventions that are needs-led and cost-effective. A stepped care approach requires clinicians to work with patients based on a collaboratively agreed plan and helps patients prepare for further interventions like intensive CBT in the future. These are described below (Fig. 2.2).

2.5.1   Phase 1 Interventions

Current literature indicates a modest but growing evidence base for the following interventions:

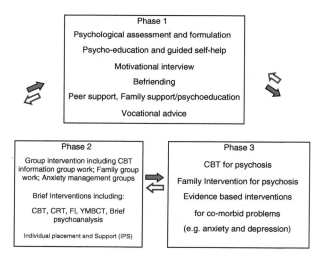

Fig. 2.2 Stepped care approach to psychosocial interventions (Ref: Adapted from Rathod and psychosis pathway steering group, 2015)

2.5.1.1 Psychoeducation and Guided Self-Help

Symptoms of psychosis can be frightening to many and, especially in the first episode, difficult to comprehend and understand. Psychoeducation and self-management help to improve the person's understanding of their experiences, mental health needs, treatment options, and self-management skills. Psychoeducation should include the broad perspective of the psychotic experiences having very different outcomes and an acknowledgment that the understanding of the field about these experiences is still evolving. It is important to give examples of individuals who are diagnosed with psychotic symptoms and functioning at a high level. For many, the aim of psychoeducation is to improve understanding and functioning, reduce risk of relapse, and improve medication concordance (Gellatly et al. 2007; Xia et al. 2011). Psychoeducation should reduce stigma, provide a broad understanding of the symptoms and the available options, and empower individuals to make treatment choices that are consistent with their world view and belief systems. This would also mean that some individuals and families make a decision to delay pharmacotherapy and opt for more psychosocial interventions. Friends and family of all people who suffer with psychosis also benefit immensely through this package (NICE 2014) as it helps them understand the symptoms, mental health needs of the person they care for, and how to support recovery.

2.5.1.2 Peer Support

There is growing evidence that peer support may improve mental health, coping skills, use of inpatient services, and quality of life (Davidson et al. 1999, 2012). Furthermore, literature suggests that peer support can have a beneficial impact on people's social networks (Castelein et al. 2008). In a review, the Centre for Mental Health analyzed six empirical studies to examine the economic case for peer support workers in mental health settings. The value of bed-days saved per peer support worker ranged from £42,653 to £146,330 over 6 months and from £44,578 to £245,515 over 12 months. Using a weighted average across all studies, the report concluded that £4.76 would be saved for every £1 invested (Trachtenberg et al. 2013).

The aim of peer support is to provide credible support from someone who has also experienced psychosis. This can include personal advice about living with psychosis and recovery (NICE 2014). One of the difficulties with psychosis is navigating a mental health system that is complex, fragmented, and not always client centered. A peer can be a navigator of the complex health system in addition to their role of providing mentorship, support and advice about recovery. A system of care where every individual with psychosis is paired with a peer navigator can go a long way in helping individuals work through their psychotic experiences.

2.5.1.3 Befriending

There is some evidence that befriending may be effective in reducing relapse and hospitalization (Buckley et al. 2007—Cochrane review). This intervention may also reduce depression (Mead et al. 2010) and implicitly challenge delusional beliefs (Samarasekera et al. 2007). Befriending involves the facilitation of longer-term friendships for social and emotional support, thereby providing an informal and flexible approach in supporting people.

2.5.1.4 Vocational Advice

Evidence suggests that educational and vocational support promote recovery (Killackey et al. 2008; Nuechterlein et al. 2008, 2013). There is a relationship between employment and severe mental illness like psychosis. People with mental health problems, especially psychosis, are much less likely than average to be in paid employment (Rinaldi et al. 2011) although they often wish to be. Vocational advice can include a number of different options like:

- Information gathering (NICE 2014) and identification of occupational short-/long-term goals
- Motivational interviewing regarding education and work
- Assessment of skill set
- Support with contacting job center
- Support with CV, forms, and interviews
- Support with return to work
- Coping strategies
- Individual placement support

2.5.2   Phase Two: Brief Interventions in Psychosis

The rest of the book will focus on this aspect of care for people with psychosis. The chapters that follow will focus on evidence-based interventions and discuss the evidence and feasibility of providing the interventions in a brief format. These interventions not only include psychological therapies but also social interventions like employment support. Each one of the chapters is written by experts or a group of experts in that particular intervention with the expressed idea of adapting it to the limitations of time and resources that we all have to work under. The brief interventions are essentially a solution to the current resource constraints that deprive people from receiving evidence-based care. So, for example, if a client is being monitored for medications, brief family intervention is integrated into the medication visit for someone with family conflicts. Alternately, if substance abuse is an issue, motivational interview is incorporated into the medication monitoring visit. The same goes to other interventions including cognitive behavior therapy, supported employment, etc. This allows practitioners to define treatment goals and work with clients in a more meaningful way.

In the case of some individuals, they may choose not to engage in intensive CBT and therefore, brief interventions like motivational interviewing and recovery-focused sessions may help engage them and prepare them for future CBT. The brief interventions per se may not be adequate for a number of people, and in those instances, the phase three interventions of a full course of CBT or family therapy would be incorporated into the treatment of the clients. As the reader goes through Chaps. 3, 4, 5, 6, 7, 8, 9, 10, 11, and 12, they would be approaching them from a perspective of taking the brief interventions that can be incorporated into their regular practice settings.

Conclusion

It is time now that we review the way we provide care for people who suffer with psychosis. Evidence is emerging that a number of treatment modalities can be helpful to people in dealing with their symptoms and supporting them to achieve recovery so that they can lead meaningful lives.

Acknowledgments Dr. Rathod (SR) would like to acknowledge the support of all patients, carers, clinicians, and partners from other agencies who have supported and contributed to the development of TRIumPH (Treatment and Recovery In PsycHosis) through coproduction workshops and engagement events. SR's organization received support from the Wessex Academic Health Sciences Network and grants from NHS England (Regional Innovation Fund) and the Royal College of Psychiatrists General Adult Faculty for this work.

Psychosis Pathway Steering Group: Alison Griffiths, Carolyn Asher, Chris Woodfine, Christie Garner, Claire Morrish, David Butler, David Kingdon, Dawn Pease, Deborah Tee, Jason Hope, Jeremy Rowland, Katherine Newman-Taylor, Lars Hansen, Michael James, Nicola Abba, Paul Tabraham, Pippa North, Kerry Elliott and Rob Kurn.

References

Addington J, Heinssen RK, Robinson DG, Schooler NR, Marcy P, Brunette MF, Correll CU, Estroff S, Mueser KT, Penn D, Robinson JA, Rosenheck RA, Azrin ST, Goldstein AB, Severe J, Kane JM (2015) Duration of untreated psychosis in community treatment settings in the United States. Psychiatr Serv 66(7):753–756, PMID:25588418, http://www.ncbi.nlm.nih.gov/pubmed/?term=25588418

Anderson K, Fuhrer R, Malla K (2010) The pathways to mental health care of first-episode psychosis patients: a systematic review. Psychol Med 40:1585–1597

Athanasopoulou C et al (2015) Attitudes towards schizophrenia on YouTube: a content analysis of Finnish and Greek videos. Inform Health Soc Care 1–18. DOI: 10.3109/17538157.2015.1008485

Balaratnasingam S, Janca A (2015) Normal personality, personality disorder and psychosis: current views and future perspectives. Curr Opin Psychiatry 28(1):30–34. doi:10.1097/YCO.0000000000000124

Birchwood, Todd P, Jackson C (1998) Early intervention in psychosis. The critical period hypothesis. Br J Psychiatry 172(suppl 33):53–59

Birchwood M, Connor C, Lester H et al (2013) Reducing DUP in first-episode psychosis: care pathways to early intervention in psychosis teams. Br J Psychiatry 202:1–7

Brown S, Kim M, Mitchell C, Inskip H (2010) Twenty-five year mortality of a community cohort with schizophrenia. Br J Psychiatry 196(2):116–121. doi:10.1192/bjp.bp.109.067512

Buckley LA, Pettit TA, Adams CE (2007) Supportive therapy for schizophrenia. The Cochrane Library Syst Rev. 18(3):CD004716.

Campbell et al (1998) Integrated care pathways. Br Med J 316:133, http://dx.doi.org/10.1136/bmj.316.7125.133 (Published 10 January 1998)

Castelein S, Bruggeman R, van Busschbach JT, van der Gaag M, Stant AD, Knegtering H, Wiersma D (2008) The effectiveness of peer support groups in psychosis: a randomized controlled trial. Acta Psychiatr Scand 118:64–72

Clement S, Foster N (2008) Newspaper reporting on schizophrenia: a content analysis of five national newspapers at two time points. Schizophr Res 98(1–3):178–183

Cole JC et al (2015) Efficacy of Transcranial Magnetic Stimulation (TMS) in the treatment of schizophrenia: a review of the literature to date. Innov Clin Neurosci 12(7–8):12–19

Connor C, Greenfield S, Lester H, et al (2014) Seeking help for first-episode psychosis: a family narrative. Early Interv Psychiatry. doi: 10.1111/eip.12177

Davidson L, Chinman M, Kloos B, Weingarten R, Stayner D, Tebes JK (1999) Peer support among individuals with severe mental illness: a review of the evidence. Clin Psychol Sci Pract 6(2):165–187

Davidson L, Bellamy C, Guy K, Miller R (2012) Peer support among persons with severe mental illnesses: a review of evidence and experience. World Psychiatry 11(2):123–128

Dixon B, Dickerson F, Bellack S, Bennett M, Dickinson D, Goldberg W, Lehman A, Tenhula N, Calmes C, Pasillas M, Peer J, Kreyenbuhl J, Schizophrenia Patient Outcomes Research Team (PORT) (2009). The 2009 schizophrenia PORT psychosocial treatment recommendations and summary statements. Schizophr Bull 36(1):48–70. doi:10.1093/schbul/sbp115

Drake R, Haley C, Akhtar S, Lewis S (2000) Causes and consequences of duration of untreated psychosis in schizophrenia. Br J Psychiatry 177(6):511–515. doi:10.1192/bjp.177.6.511

Epstein, M. (1990). Beyond the Oceanic Feeling: Psychoanalytic Study of Buddhist Meditation. International Review of Psycho-Analysis, 17, 159–165.

Firn M, Hindhaugh K, Hubbeling D, Davies G, Jones B, White J (2013) A dismantling study of assertive outreach services: comparing activity and outcomes following replacement with the FACT model. Soc Psychiatry Psychiatr Epidemiol 48(6):997–1003. doi:10.1007/s00127-012-0602-x

Gellatly J, Bower P, Hennessy S, Richards D, Gilbody S, Lovell K (2007) What makes self-help interventions effective in the management of depressive symptoms? Meta-analysis and meta-regression. Psychol Med 37:1217–1228

Gledhill A, Lobban F, Sellwood W (1998) Group CBT for people with schizophrenia: a preliminary evaluation. Behav Cogn Psychother 26:63–76

Johns LC, van Os J (2001) The continuity of psychotic experiences in the general population. Clin Psychol Rev 21(8):1125–1141

Johnson, S. (2013). Crisis resolution and home treatment teams: An evolving model. Advances in Psychiatric Treatment 19(2):115–123.

Knapp M, Andrew A, McDaid D et al (2014) Investing in recovery. Rethink, London

Killackey E, Jackson HJ, McGorry PD (2008) Vocational intervention in first-episode psychosis: individual placement and support v. treatment as usual. Br J Psychiatry 193(2):114–120

Kumari V, et al (2011) Neural changes following cognitive behaviour therapy for psychosis: a longitudinal study. Brain. http://dx.doi.org/10.1093/brain/awr1542396-2407

Leff J, Williams G, Huckvale A et al (2013) Avatar therapy for persecutory auditory hallucinations: what is it and how does it work? Psychosis. Published online 4 March 2013

Lester E, Birchwood M, Freemantle N, Michail M, Tait L (2009a) REDIRECT: cluster randomised controlled trial of GP training in first-episode psychosis. Br J Gen Pract 59:183–190

Lester H, Birchwood M, Bryan S, England E, Rogers H, Sirvastava N (2009b) Development and implementation of early intervention services for young people with psychosis: case study. Br J Psychiatry 194:446–450

Linscott RJ, van Os J (2013) An updated and conservative systematic review and meta-analysis of epidemiological evidence on psychotic experiences in children and adults: on the pathway from proneness to persistence to dimensional expression across mental disorders. Psychol Med 43(6):1133–1149

Logan E, King A (2001) Parental facilitation of adolescent mental health service utilization: a conceptual and empirical review. Clin Psychol Sci Pract 8:319–340

Lloyd-Evans B, Crosby M, Stockton S, Pilling S, Hobbs L, Hinton M et al (2011) Initiatives to shorten duration of untreated psychosis: systematic review. Br J Psychiatry 198:256–263

Marshall M, Lewis S, Lockwood A, Drake R, Jones P, Croudace T (2005) Association between duration of untreated psychosis and outcome in cohorts of first-episode patients. A systematic review. Arch Gen Psychiatry 62:975–983

Marshall M, Husain N, Bork N, Chaudhry IB, Lester H, Everard L et al (2014) Impact of early intervention services on duration of untreated psychosis: data from the National EDEN prospective cohort study. Schizophr Res 159(1):1–6

McGorry PD, Edwards J, Mihalopoulos C et al (1996) EPPIC: an evolving system of early detection and optimal management. Schizophr Bull 22:305–326

McGlashan H (1999) Duration of untreated psychosis in first-episode schizophrenia: marker or determinant of course? Biol Psychiatry 46:899–907

Mead N, Lester H, Chew-Graham C, Gask L, Bower P (2010) Effects of befriending on depressive symptoms and distress: systematic review and meta-analysis. Br J Psychiatry 196(2):96–101

Melle I, Johannesen O, Friis S, Haahr U, Joa I, Larsen K et al (2006) Early detection of the first episode of schizophrenia and suicidal behaviour. Am J Psych 163:800–804. doi:10.1176/appi.ajp.163.5.800

Mental Health Bulletin (2009) Third report from Mental Health Minimum Dataset (MHMDS) annual returns, 2004–2009. The NHS Information Centre, Mental Health and Community Care Team, London

Morrison AP et al (2014) Cognitive therapy for people with schizophrenia spectrum disorders not taking antipsychotic drugs: a single-blind randomised controlled trial. Lancet 383(9926):1395–1403

Mueser KT, Deavers F, Penn DL, Cassisi JE (2013) Psychosocial treatments for schizophrenia. Annu Rev Clin Psychol 9:465–497. doi:10.1146/annurev-clinpsy-050212-185620

Mueser K, Penn L, Addington J, Brunette F et al (2015) The NAVIGATE program for first-episode psychosis: rationale, overview, and description of psychosocial components. Psychiatr Serv 66(7):680–690. doi:10.1176/appi.ps.201400413

National Institute for Health and Care Excellence (2014) Service user experience in adult mental health: improving the experience of care for people using adult NHS mental health services (Clinical guideline 136)

NHS England (2015) Guidance to support the introduction of access and waiting time standards for mental health services. NHS E, London.

Norman M, Malla K (2001) Duration of untreated psychosis: a critical examination of the concept and its importance. Psychol Med 31:381–400

Nuechterlein KH, Subotnik KL, Turner LR, Ventura J, Becker DR, Drake RE (2008) Individual placement and support for individuals with recent-onset schizophrenia: integrating supported education and supported employment. Psychiatr Rehabil J 31(4):340–349

Nuechterlein KH, Subotnik KL, Ventura J, Turner LR, Gitlin MJ, Gretchen-Doorly D, Becker DR, Drake RE, Wallace CJ, Liberman RP (2013) Successful return to work or school after a first episode of schizophrenia: the UCLA RCT of individual placement and support and workplace fundamentals module training. Manuscript submitted for publication

Fusar-Poli P et al (2015) Heterogeneity of psychosis risk within individuals at clinical high risk. A meta-analytical stratification. JAMA Psychiatry. doi:10.1001/jamapsychiatry.2015.2324, Published online December 30, 2015

Pharoah et al (2010) Family intervention for schizophrenia. Cochrane Database Syst Rev (12):CD000088

Platz C, Umbricht S, Cattapan-Ludewig K, Dvorsky D, Arbach D, Brenner D et al (2006) Help-seeking pathways in early psychosis. Soc Psychiatry Psychiatr Epidemiol 41:967–974

Rathod S, Lloyd A, Asher C et al (2014) Lessons from an evaluation of major change in adult mental health services: effects on quality. J Ment Health 23(5):271–275

Rathod S, Kingdon D, Pinninti N, Turkington D, Phiri P (2015a) Cultural adaptation of CBT for serious mental illness: a guide for training and practice. Wiley – Blackwell, Chichester, West Sussex, UK.

Rathod S, Griffiths A, Kingdon D, Tiplady B, Jones T (2015b) Pathways to recovery: a case for adoption of systematic pathways in psychosis. Jointly produced by Imperial College Health Partners and Wessex Academic Health Science Network; Supported by the Royal College of Psychiatrists and Rethink Mental Illness, London.

Rathod S, Psychosis Pathway Steering Group (2015) TRIumPH: psychosis care pathway and narrative. Wessex Academic Health Sciences Network, Southampton, Wessex.

Rethink Mental Illness (2014) Lost generation: protecting early intervention in psychosis services. London

Razzaque R, Wood L (2015) Open dialogue and its relevance to the NHS: opinions of NHS staff and service users. Community Ment Health J 51(8):931-8. doi: 10.1007/s10597-015-9849-5.

Rinaldi M, Montibeller T, Perkins R (2011) Increasing the employment rate for people with longer-term mental health problems. Psychiatrist 35:339–343

Rolland, R. (1929). The Life of Ramakrishna. Calcutta, India: Vedanta Press.

Rössler W, Salize HJ, Van Os J, Riecher-Rössler A (2005) Size of burden of schizophrenia and psychotic disorders. Eur Neuropsy 15:399–409

Royal College of Psychiatrists (2012) Report of the National Audit of Schizophrenia (NAS) 2012. Healthcare Quality Improvement Partnership, London

Schmidt, L. T., et al. (2013). Assertive Community Treatment teams. Modern community mental health: An interdisciplinary approach. K. R. Yeager, D. L. Cutler, D. Svendsen and G. M. Sills. New York, NY, US, Oxford University Press: 293–303

Seikkula, J. (2002). Open dialogues with good and poor outcomes for psychotic crises: examples from families with violence. J Marital Fam Ther 28(3):263–274

Seikkula J et al (2011) The comprehensive open-dialogue approach in Western Lapland: II. Long-term stability of acute psychosis outcomes in advanced community care. Psychosis: Psychol Soc Integr Approaches 3(3):192–204

Samarasekera N, Kingdon D, Siddle R, O'Carroll M, Scott JL, Sensky T, Barnes TR, Turkington D (2007) Befriending patients with medication-resistant schizophrenia: can psychotic symptoms predict treatment response? Psychol Psychother Theory Res Pract 80(1):97–106

Schizophrenia Commission (2012) The abandoned illness: a report from the Schizophrenia Commission. Rethink Mental Illness, London.

Thomas N et al (2014) Psychological therapies for auditory hallucinations (voices): current status and key directions for future research. Schizophr Bull 40(Suppl 4):S202–S212

Trachtenberg M, Parsonage M, Shepherd G, Boardman J (2013) Peer support in mental health care: is it good value for money? The Sainsbury Centre for Mental Health, London

Turner D, Gaag M, Karyotaki E, Cuijpers P (2014) Psychological interventions for psychosis: a meta-analysis of comparative outcome studies. Am J Psychiatry. doi:10.1176/appi.ajp.2013.13081159

Van Veldhuizen R (2007) FACT: a Dutch version of ACT. Community Ment Health J 43(4):421–433

Vissers J, Beech R (2005) Health operations management: patient flow statistics in health care. Routledge, Taylor & Francis Group Publishers, New York, p 3

Walker H, Tulloch L, Ramm M, Drysdale E, Steel A, Martin C, MacPherson G, Connaughton J (2013) A randomised controlled trial to explore insight into psychosis; effects of a psycho-education programme on insight in a forensic population. J Forensic Psychiatry Psychol 24(6):756–771

Wilber, K., Engler, J. & Brown, D.P. (1986). Transformations of Consciousness: Conventional and Contemplative Perspectives on Development. Boston, MA: Shambhala Publications, Inc.

World Health Organization (2001) The World Health report 2001. Mental health: new understanding, new hope. WHO, Geneva

Wharne S (2013) Whatever happened to Assertive outreach? http://www.hsj.co.uk/comment/whatever-happened-to-assertive-outreach/5064403.article

Wheeler C, Lloyd-Evans B, Churchard A, Fitzgerald C, Fullarton K, Mosse L et al (2015) Implementation of the crisis resolution team model in adult mental health settings: a systematic review. BMC Psychiatry 15:74

Wykes T, Parr AM, Landau S (1999) Group treatment of auditory hallucinations. Exploratory study of effectiveness. Br J Psychiatry 175:180–185

Wykes T, Steel C, Everitt B, Tarrier N (2008) Cognitive behaviour therapy for schizophrenia: effect sizes, clinical models, and methodological rigor. Schizophr Bull 34(3):523–537

Wykes T, Huddy V, Cellard C, McGurk SR, Czobor P (2011) A meta-analysis of cognitive remediation for schizophrenia: methodology and effect sizes. Am J Psychiatry 168(5):472–485

Xia J, Merinder B, Belgamwar R (2011) Psychoeducation for schizophrenia. Cochrane Database Syst Rev 15(6):CD002831

Brief Cognitive Behavior Therapy for Psychosis

3

Farooq Naeem and David Kingdon

3.1 Introduction

Cognitive behavior therapy for psychosis (CBTp) was developed in the post-institution era. Despite the case studies by Beck (1952) and Shapiro and Ravenette (1959) in the 1950s, specific symptom interventions for schizophrenia did not appear until much later. The first controlled studies on cognitive behavior therapy for psychosis (CBTp) emerged in the early 1990s in the UK. It was felt that traditional therapies and antipsychotics at that time were not able to help patients with psychosis who needed more support with managing their distress, dealing with psychotic symptoms, and in improving their functioning in the community. Theoretical underpinnings such as the stress vulnerability models were developed to understand not only the development of the disorder but also its maintenance. These also began to be informed by research on expressed emotion (Butzlaff and Hooley 1998; Vaughn and Leff 1981) and so began to include social and psychological markers as well as biological ones. The difficulty in identifying rigorous and unambiguous psychosocial markers for psychosis may have hampered further development of this area initially, but the identification of ethnicity, deprivation, trauma, and drug misuse as key factors in its etiology and relapse has subsequently influenced interventions.

The 1990s was also the time when public pressure following some notorious scandals in the UK led to major changes in the health system, including the rise of clinical governance, need for evidence-based practice, and better coordination of care through the Care Programme Approach. Cognitive behavior therapy for anxiety

F. Naeem, MSc Research Methods, MRCPsych, PhD (✉)
Queens University, Kingston, ON, Canada
e-mail: farooqnaeem7@gmail.com

D. Kingdon, MRCPsych, MD
Southampton University, Southampton, England

and depression was recommended by the National Guideline development bodies (e.g., the UK National Institute for Health and Clinical Excellence, now called the National Institute for Health and Care Excellence), and during this time CBT also increased its theoretical research base. It was inevitable that eventually some of the developed techniques would be used for people with a diagnosis of schizophrenia. Since the emergence of the first controlled studies on cognitive behavior therapy for psychosis (CBTp) in the early 1990s in the UK, this treatment has developed further and included some of the theoretical underpinnings of CBT from other disorders. However, unlike CBT for other disorders which generally have its roots in the USA and particularly the Beck Institute in Philadelphia, CBTp developed predominantly in the UK (Wykes et al. 2008), and Beck himself was very supportive of it. Reviews of studies of CBTp have suggested that they are useful for the treatment of schizophrenia. Twelve to twenty sessions of CBT for psychosis (CBTp) is now recognized as an effective intervention for schizophrenia in clinical guidelines in the UK and the USA (Dixon et al. 2010; NICE 2014). There is evidence from meta-analyses, too, that it is effective. For example, Wykes and colleagues (2008) reported overall beneficial effects of the target symptom (33 studies; effect size 0.40 [95 % confidence interval) as well as significant effects on positive symptoms (32 studies), negative symptoms (23 studies), functioning (15 studies), mood (13 studies), and social anxiety (2 studies) with effect sizes ranging from 0.35 to 0.44.

3.2   What Happens in Cognitive Behavior Therapy for Psychosis

The cognitive theory proposes that through the examination of thought processes and by evaluating their accuracy, many negative emotional reactions due to inaccurate or distorted thinking could be reduced or extinguished (Beck and Emery 1979). The key elements of CBT for depression and anxiety include engaging the patient, collaboratively developing a problem list, and deciding on a clear goal for the therapy session (Beck et al. 1979). Homework assignments are agreed between the patient and the therapist. The aim of homework is to help the person become their own therapist and practically link behavior with thoughts and emotions. This essentially means that the patient uses self-help, and the therapist guides the patient during a session while the patient works as his own therapist during the period between two sessions. Regular feedback from the therapist and from the patient with regular summaries is also a crucial element. This therapy structure relies on collaborative working with the patient within an empirical methodology. The overall style of therapy is underpinned by a problem-solving approach that is grounded in reality. The patient is trained to think like a scientist looking for evidence, testing hypotheses, and exploring the reality of their thoughts and perceptions. A formulation is jointly generated to make sense of the emergence and maintenance of the problem at hand (Tai and Turkington 2009). The therapist uses guided discovery and Socratic questioning to identify distortions in the thinking style of the patient.

Communication in CBT uses a Socratic dialogue rather than therapist interpretation of thoughts, feelings, and behaviors. Beck et al. (1979) proposed that this method can be used to examine thoughts and beliefs for their accuracy. He demonstrated the usefulness of the Socratic questioning technique to encourage the probing of evidence, reason, and rationale. For example, a patient who believed that he was under surveillance would be asked to give a rationale for his belief. Other useful techniques include reality testing where a patient will be encouraged to actively find evidence to test the reality base of a belief or assumption. This is a process which is done in collaboration with the therapist, and behavioral experiments whereby a scientific experiment can be set up to test a specific prediction. For example, a person who believes that his next-door neighbor is constantly talking about him can be asked to record the conversation.

Cognitive behavior therapy for psychosis (CBTp) is based on these above principles. In particular, it heavily relies on the use of Socratic dialogue, guided discovery, reality testing, and behavioral experiments. It also uses work on improving coping (Tarrier and Calam 2002), building social and independent living skills, and increasing compliance using behavioral strategies such as linking medication taking to another activity. Similarly, negative symptoms were targeted by providing graded activity programs (Meichenbaum and Cameron 1973) and understanding them as protective and providing alternative strategies for them. These approaches have continued to be applied where deficit symptoms of schizophrenia and improving functional outcomes are the main focus of intervention. According to the cognitive model, hallucinations and delusions can occur when anomalous experiences that are common to the majority of the population are misattributed in a way that has extreme and threatening personal meaning (Garety et al. 2001; Morrison 2001). These models specify the role of faulty beliefs, increased attention to threat-related stimuli, biased information processing of confirmatory evidence, and safety behaviors (i.e., avoidance of specific situations) in the experience of positive symptoms. The emphasis is in the distress resulting not necessarily from difficult experiences, but the *meaning* placed on those very experiences. Cognitive theory is based on the notion that the cognitive processes implicated in mood and anxiety disorders occur transdiagnostically. Research findings support the notion that psychotic symptoms can be conceptualized with reference to normal psychological processes, whereby the content of symptoms is understandable and amenable to CBT (Allison Harvey 2004; Haddock and Slade 1996).

It was recognized that CBT for disorders such as anxiety and depression could be applied in schizophrenia with some key adjustments (Tai and Turkington 2009). Stigma was addressed by identifying the negative beliefs and assumptions people held about the diagnosis and prognosis of schizophrenia and then providing evidence that some of these experiences are actually fairly common in the general population, i.e., normalizing. In addition, the therapist provided alternative explanations, such as explaining the role of stress, that provided more optimistic and hopeful perspectives (Harrison et al. 2001) promoting beliefs in the potential for recovery. Compared with CBT for other disorders, the sessions were often shorter in length and much more flexible, and homework was simplified. The role of sleep disturbance, affect, and safety behaviors (e.g., behaviors such as avoidance that maintained faulty beliefs) was identified to produce mini-formulations of positive symptom maintenance (Morrison 2001). Cognitive biases are directly addressed by

CBT predominantly through focusing on the content of thoughts and styles of thinking. These include the jumping to conclusions error and biases in styles of judgment found in individuals with unusual beliefs (delusions) and the biases in attributional styles and attentional processing associated with hallucinations. In CBT, it is the individual's personal meaning, understanding, and coping with symptoms that are the focus of treatment. For example, individuals are facilitated in testing out the location of the hallucinations (internal vs external), carefully examining the appearance and behavior of suspected persecutors, and attempting homework that is pertinent to their stated goals (Tai and Turkington 2009).

3.3   Need for the Development of Brief CBTp

In spite of a strong evidence base, availability of CBTp remains an issue. *This is especially true for the North America compared to the UK.* It has been suggested that potential factors contributing to this difference include greater skepticism about the benefits of psychotherapy for persons with severe mental illness, overoptimism concerning the clinical benefits of polypharmacy, and the traditional separation between psychology and psychiatry in the USA as compared to the UK (Mueser and Noordsy 2005). A recently conducted survey of training directors in US psychiatry residency and clinical psychology doctoral programs to characterize the penetration of CBTp training and to assess their familiarity with basic CBTp facts reported that directors displayed limited knowledge of CBTp effectiveness, with only 50 % of psychiatry and 40 % of psychology directors believing that CBTp is efficacious. Only 10 % of psychiatry and 30 % of psychology directors were aware that the CBTp evidence base is based on meta-analyses (Kimhy et al. 2013). There are, however, limitations in availability of CBTp even in the UK, and the current evidence suggests that at most 50 % of those suffering from schizophrenia in the UK have access to CBTp (D. Kingdon and Kirschen 2006). This has led the UK government to introduce an "access and waiting standard" requiring services to offer CBT and family intervention within 2 weeks from referral for assessment of psychosis, beginning from April 2015.

Some approaches to increase the efficiency of CBT treatments include adapting individual treatments to a group format, self-help materials, bibliotherapy, and eMedia-assisted therapy programs. Other options might include training frontline staff in CBT interventions and utilizing families or peers in providing CBT interventions. The most common approach for enhancing efficiency, however, is to abbreviate existing CBT treatments by reducing the number of treatment sessions. There is evidence from research that brief CBT for psychosis can be delivered by community mental health nurses (Turkington et al. 2006). Brevity has many clear advantages. Increased cost-effectiveness could make treatment accessible to more individuals in need of assistance. Patients enjoy rapid treatment gains, and this may also improve the credibility of the treatment and increase the motivation for further change (Hazlett-Stevens and Dryden 2005). These efficient ways of delivering therapy have the potential to substantially reduce the gap if the effectiveness of a brief CBT can be demonstrated.

3.4   What Is Brief CBT for Psychosis

Currently there is more literature on brief CBT for depression and anxiety disorders than for schizophrenia. Standard CBT for depression is considered by most to be delivered between 10 and 20 sessions, but there is no agreement as to how many sessions should be included in brief CBT for depression (Bond and Dryden 2005). Churchill et al. (2001) described brief psychological interventions for depression to be delivered in 20 or fewer sessions, while Cully (2008) described brief CBT for depression to be delivered in between four and eight sessions. The Improving Access to Psychological Treatment (IAPT) services which exist across England offer a "low-intensity" range of treatments which are CBT based and meant for their use in the initial referrals with anxiety and depression; only if these are not successful, patients are offered standard CBT. In a recent Cochrane review, we have suggested that the standard CBT for psychosis (CBTp) involves around 16 sessions (12–20 sessions) over 4–6 months, while brief CBTp involves around 6–10 sessions in less than 4 months (Naeem et al. 2014a). This cutoff was based on the observation that current standard CBTp treatments typically span 12–20 sessions over 4–6 months (NICE 2014). We located empirical studies of the efficacy of brief CBTp by asking experts in a variety of areas about available research and by searches of Psychological Abstracts. In the absence of a clear definition for brief CBT for schizophrenia, we adopted our definition after a careful review of the literature on brief CBT for depression.

Although there is no difference in terms of theory or technical application of brief therapy compared with normal CBT, brief CBT focuses on more intensive work. Therefore, it might not be suitable for every patient with psychosis. There might also be differences in therapy when delivered by expert therapists compared with nonexperts. Brief CBT puts a greater burden on the patient to engage actively in treatment both during and between sessions. It can be argued that in psychotic disorders, especially with symptoms such as severe auditory hallucinations and high conviction delusions, brief therapy may not work as engaging patients and overcoming psychotic phenomenon may need a prolonged and intensive treatment approach. It is also possible that brief therapy may leave patients more confused and could prove harmful. However, the literature on the use of brief CBT for psychotic disorders does not seem to substantiate these apprehensions. There is some evidence to suggest that brief therapies are effective for clients with psychosis, but the research in this area needs to address the fundamental issue of the dose-effect relationship in CBT. We have described the three major trials of brief CBTp in the next section to give the reader a better understanding of these brief therapies.

3.5   Evidence from Research

In a recent review of the literature, we identified nine papers (covering seven studies) that included 1,207 participants, 636 in CBTp arm and 571 in the comparison arms. Brief CBTp showed moderate effect sizes (Hedge's g = 0.43) (Naeem et al. in press).

In this review we used our previously suggested criteria flexibly. We will briefly describe four studies, which fully fulfill the criteria for brief CBTp that we have proposed.

3.6   Description of Studies That Fulfill the Criteria for Brief CBTp

There are three randomized controlled studies of brief, six-session CBT currently published which are modularized but with different approaches. The Insight study (Malik et al. 2009; Rathod et al. 2005; Turkington et al. 2002, 2006) used the approaches described for CBT for psychosis but reduced the number of sessions to six and included three sessions with carers, where the client agreed to this. The other study reported a culturally adapted CBT for psychosis from Pakistan that delivered six sessions of therapy (Naeem et al. 2015). The Worry Intervention Trial (WIT) (Freeman et al. 2015) for paranoia involved an assessment of the current state and symptoms but then focused directly on worry and used techniques to address this specific issue. Each will be described and then proposals for a phased approach to the use of brief and standard CBT for psychosis described. The fourth study reported a group CBTp approach for hallucinations (Wykes et al. 2005).

3.7   Insight Study

The Insight study was a multicenter randomized controlled trial which compared a brief CBT intervention and carer sessions with treatment as usual. It had wide inclusion criteria: anyone with a diagnosis of schizophrenia, schizoaffective, or delusional disorders and relatively narrow exclusions: unable to communicate in English and substance dependence (use did not lead to exclusion). Four hundred twenty-two patients were recruited and 357 completed the study. The therapists were psychiatric nurses who were provided with 2–3 weeks therapy training and then weekly supervision. They were not experienced in using CBT and did not have CBT accreditation.

The results at 3 months (end of therapy) were a significant improvement in overall symptoms, insight, and depressive symptoms compared to treatment as usual. At 1 year, there were continuing positive effects on insight and depression and for negative symptoms. The effects on insight were for treatment and symptoms, but not into being ill at 3 months: the acceptance of the need for treatment was still present at 1 year. There were distinct effects on different cultural groups with those from black minority ethnic populations not doing as well which has led to a series of studies seeking to address this (Rathod et al. 2005). Further analysis established that those with mild-to-moderate drug misuse did no worse than others (Naeem et al. 2005) and that anxiety symptoms also improved (Naeem et al. 2006). Predictors of good outcome were higher levels of positive symptoms and insight (Naeem et al. 2008).

The therapy was adapted from that described in standard approaches involving 16–20 sessions. The initial phase involved assessment and engagement, followed by formulation using a "Making Sense" approach. This assembled information on current problems were identified with the client and then predisposing, precipitating, perpetuating, and protective factors (explained as what happened before and what happened when you became unwell, what's kept it going, and what can stop it) were explored. Relevant connections between current and past issues and between the thoughts, feelings, and behavior were then made with consideration of relevant social circumstances and physical symptoms/illnesses.

Once these were established, the next phase was to work directly with the problems elicited using the formulation to make sense of them and then move to problem-solving. This usually involved direct work with voices, delusions, and negative symptoms. Work with voices would involve understanding and reattribution with normalizing to reduce fear and self-stigmatization. Coping strategies that were helpful were reinforced and further developed. Content of voices were discussed and debated such that, in some instances, clients could begin to enter into a constructive dialogue with their voices, reducing distress and working toward a correction of the power imbalance they experienced.

Delusions were explored with a focus on when the belief emerged allowing for a supported reassessment of the prevailing circumstances and events. Discussion included seeking relevant information about the focus of delusions, e.g., satellites or the Internet if these were considered to be causing concern. This process generally improved engagement and often led to behavioral changes, e.g., increased socialization. Changes in beliefs themselves were less likely within the short timescale of therapy but sometimes followed.

Work with negative symptoms accompanied approaches with other symptoms as simply equipping clients with an understanding of voices or paranoia, e.g., delusions of reference, and these interventions led to increased motivation and interaction with others. Specific long-term goals were discussed to instill hope and provide direction. Short-term goals were usually quite simple and readily achievable to build confidence and to instill a sense of self-efficacy.

Carer work was acceptable to many clients when an explanation of the reason for it was given – to help the carer understand and cope better – and agreement made about what should and should not be disclosed. It was usually agreed that the formulation could be shared – often with the client present – and then work on coping with specific symptoms and situations usually proceeded. Occasionally it involved negotiation between client and carer about specific issues but generally consisted of a sharing of information and problem-solving areas of uncertainty. Three sessions over the 3-month period of intervention was assessed as very valuable by carers and seen as sufficient by most. Clients were asked about how sufficient they found six sessions over 20 weeks, and while around 40 % were satisfied, a majority expressed that they would have liked more number of sessions.

3.8 Worry Intervention Trial (WIT) for Paranoia

The WIT trial randomized 150 patients in two centers to an assessment and then four sessions of a worry intervention (Freeman et al. 2015). The clients were included if they met criteria for paranoid delusions and worry. Very few patients referred with paranoia failed to reach the threshold for worry. Exclusion criteria included substance dependence. The therapists were clinical psychologists who had a brief training and weekly supervision in the use of the intervention.

The results were that the WIT group improved significantly in terms of worry, well-being, and delusional conviction compared to treatment as usual. The reduction in worry was a mediator of the effect on delusions.

The intervention is based on that used in generalized anxiety disorder which was found in a pilot study to be effective in paranoia. The theoretical basis for this had been well established by Daniel Freeman (Foster et al. 2010) but required substantive evaluation in a fully powered RCT. The therapy included six modules covering the following: assessment of the situation and symptoms, then focus on worry – whatever has happened, worrying about it is certainly not helping – let's see if we can do something about that. Psychoeducation about worry was provided with review of positive and negative beliefs about worry. An increased awareness of the initiation of worry was developed with the identification of individual triggers. The client was encouraged to learn to "let go" of worry with the use of worry periods. Problem-solving was substituted for worry and clients were encouraged to use relaxation exercises. A simple individualized formulation of each person's worry was developed and homework between sessions was agreed. Written information was provided in the form of leaflets about relevant issues, e.g., "winning against worry."

The therapy was remarkably well accepted by patients, and recruitment to the study was straightforward with the recruitment target reached within the required timescale. Dropout rates were very low – less than 5 % – and results were similar in both centers, Oxford and Southampton (UK). It therefore seems to be an intervention which is generalizable and applicable in clinical practice.

3.9   Brief Culturally Adapted CBT for Psychosis

In this study brief culturally adapted CBT for psychosis (CaCBTp) (Naeem et al. 2014b, 2015) was adapted on the basis of qualitative work with service users, professionals, and carers. The intervention was targeted at symptoms of schizophrenia for outpatients from these groups compared to treatment as usual (TAU). A total of 116 participants with schizophrenia who were recruited from two hospitals in Karachi, Pakistan, and randomized into two groups with 1:1 allocation (CaCBTp plus TAU = 59, TAU = 57). A brief version of CaCBTp (six individual sessions with the involvement of main carer, plus one session for the family) was provided over 4 months. Psychopathology was measured using the Positive and Negative Syndrome Scale (PANSS) of schizophrenia, the Psychotic Symptom Rating Scales (PSYRATS), and the Schedule for Assessment of Insight (SAI) at baseline and end of therapy. Participants in treatment group showed statistically significant improvement in all measures of psychopathology at the end of the study compared with control group. Participants in treatment group showed statistically significant improvement in positive symptoms (PANSS, Positive Symptoms Subscale; $p = 0.000$), negative symptoms (PANSS, Negative Symptoms Subscale; $p = 0.000$), delusions (PSYRATS, Delusions Subscale; $p = 0.000$), hallucinations (PSYRATS, Hallucination Subscale; $p = 0.000$), and insight (SAI; $p = 0.007$). The results suggest that brief, culturally adapted CBT for psychosis can be an effective treatment when provided in combination with TAU, for patients with schizophrenia in a low- and middle-income country (LAMIC) setting. This is the first trial of CBT for psychosis from outside the Western world. These findings need replicating in other low- and middle-income countries.

Therapy was provided according to a manualized treatment protocol (Kingdon and Turkington 2002). Therapists were three psychology graduates with more than 5 years experience of working in mental health, who were trained by Farooq Naeem (FN). An important part of cultural adaptation of the CBT for psychosis is the involvement of the family member (Naeem 2013). Families are heavily involved in patient's care and serve as the main caregivers to psychiatric patients in Pakistan, and, through our experience of adaptation of CBT for Pakistan, we understand that their involvement can enhance the acceptability of treatment. Therefore, this brief version consisted of six sessions for participant plus one session for the family. Every participant was accompanied by a carer who acted as co-therapist. Although therapy was provided flexibly, the sessions typically focused on the following:

1. Formulation and psychoeducation
2. Normalization and introduction to stress vulnerability model
3. Working with hallucinations
4. Working with delusions
5. Working with negative symptoms
6. Termination work and relapse prevention

Therapy was delivered using guidelines developed for cultural adaptation in Pakistan. These guidelines were developed in our preliminary work, in which CBTp was adapted using a series of qualitative studies similar to those we used for cultural adaptation of CBT for depression. During this preliminary work to adapt CaCBTp for use in Pakistan, we explored the views of patients, their carers, and the health professionals in this area. A total of 92 interviews was conducted by three psychologists. We conducted qualitative interviews with mental health professionals ($n = 29$) and patients ($n = 33$) and their carers ($n = 30$). The results of the mentioned studies highlighted the barriers in therapy (e.g., lack of awareness of therapy, family's involvement, traveling distance and expenses, and uncooperative family caregivers) as well as strengths while working with this patient group. Patients and their carers in Pakistan use a bio-psycho-spirituo-social model of illness. They seek help from various sources, including faith healers. Therapists did make minor adjustments in therapy.

In addition to one additional session for the whole family and the involvement of a carer throughout the therapy, other salient cultural adaptations that we incorporated in the CBT manual were the following:

- A spiritual dimension was included in the formulation, understanding, and in planning the therapy.

- Urdu equivalents of CBT jargons were used in the therapy.
- Culturally appropriate homework assignments were selected, and participants were encouraged to attend even if they were unable to complete their homework.
- Folk stories and examples relevant to the religious beliefs of the local population were used to clarify issues.

3.10   Group CBT for Voices

Wykes et al. (2005) conducted a study of group CBT for voices that was delivered in seven sessions. The therapists who carried out this therapy were drawn from local services and then trained in group CBT techniques. Many but not all were experienced in providing individual CBT. Group CBT for the positive symptoms of psychosis provided the four key elements of CBT: engagement, collaborative discussion about an agreed model, cognitive restructuring of delusional beliefs, and reducing negative self-evaluation. Group CBT for voices used a manualized therapy for seven sessions each having a specific goal. The sessions included (i) engagement and sharing of information about the voices, (ii) exploring models of psychosis, (iii) exploring beliefs about hallucinations, (iv) developing effective coping strategies, (v) how to improve self-esteem, (vi) developing an overall model of coping with voices, and (vii) following up session.

Participants were included in this study, only if they had a diagnosis of schizophrenia and experienced distressing auditory hallucinations (rated on the PANSS). They were randomly allocated to group CBT ($n=45$) or a control group who received treatment as usual ($n=40$). The two main outcomes were social functioning as measured by the Social Behavior Schedule and the severity of hallucinations as measured by the total score on the Hallucinations Scale of PSYRATS. Assessments were carried out at baseline, 10 weeks (post therapy) and 36 weeks (6 months following therapy).

Results: Mixed random effects models revealed significant improvement in social functioning (effect size 0.63 six months after the end of therapy). There was no general effect of group CBT on the severity of hallucinations. However, there was a large cluster effect of therapy group on the severity of hallucinations, such that they were reduced in some but not all of the therapy groups. Improvement in hallucinations was associated with receiving therapy early in the trial and having very experienced therapists (extensive CBT training which included expert supervision for a series of individual cases for at least a year following initial training).

3.11   Summary

To summarize, there is now some evidence to suggest that brief CBT for psychosis can be effective in treating symptoms of schizophrenia. These interventions can form the basis for establishing an evidence-based treatment strategy for CBT for psychosis to assist in meeting implementation targets, e.g., the English "access and waiting standard" of treatment for psychosis within 14 days of presentation (https://www.gov.uk/government/uploads/system/uploads/attachment_data/file/361648/mental-health-access.pdf). They can form the first phase of intervention using trained mental health practitioners (Insight) and clinical psychologists (WIT, culturally adapted CBT). Whether WIT can be delivered successfully by other trained practitioners has yet to be demonstrated, although proposals for such a study have been prepared for submission for funding. Delivery of CBTp using a stepped-care approach is in line with the current model of service delivery and is a major development in delivering CBTp for a very deserving population.

Conclusion

Brief CBT for psychosis is a developing area. Furthermore, research needs to be done to compare brief with standard CBTp. There is also a need to further explore the possibility of delivering CBTp using self-help, guided self-help, and eMedia. One important area in which brief interventions can be tried is case management, where frontline workers can be easily trained to deliver therapy. This has enormous implications for service delivery, reduction of distress and disability in clients with psychosis, and, above all, in terms of costs. Ideally CBTp should be provided in a variety of formats, with the dose of therapy being increased for those who do not respond to low-intensity approach.

References

Allison Harvey EW (2004) Cognitive behavioural processes across psychological disorders: a transdiagnostic approach to research and treatment. Retrieved March 25, 2015, from https://www.escholar.manchester.ac.uk/uk-ac-man-scw:4d87

Beck A (1952) Successful outpatient psychotherapy of a chronic schizophrenic with a delusion based on borrowed guilt. Retrieved 18 Oct 2015. From http://www.tandfonline.com/doi/abs/10.1521/00332747.1952.11022883?journalCode=upsy20#.ViPb_Wur_IU

Beck AT, Emery G (1979). Cognitive therapy of depression (1st Edition). The Guilford Press. New York, USA

Bond FW, Dryden W (2005) Handbook of brief cognitive behaviour therapy. Wiley, Chichester, West Sussex, England

Butzlaff RL, Hooley JM (1998) Expressed emotion and psychiatric relapse: a meta-analysis. Arch Gen Psychiatry 55(6):547–552

Churchill R (2001) Systematic review of controlled trials of the effectiveness and cost-effectiveness of brief psychological treatments for depression. Retrieved 27 Mar 2015. From http://scholar.google.ca/scholar?q=Churchill+R%2C+Hunot+V%2C+Corney+R%2C+Knapp+M%2C+McGuire+H%2C+Tylee+A%2C+Wessely+S.+A+systematic+review+of+controlled+trials+of+the+effectiveness+and+cost-effectiveness+of+brief+psychological+treatments+for+depression.+&btnG=&hl=en&as_sdt=0%2C5

Cully (2008) A therapist's guide to brief cognitive behavioral therapy. Retrieved 27 Mar 2015. From https://www.scribd.com/doc/115070925/A-Therapist-s-Guide-to-Brief-Cognitive-Behavioral-Therapy

Dixon LB, Dickerson F, Bellack AS, Bennett M, Dickinson D, Goldberg RW, Lehman A, Tenhula WN, Calmes C, Pasillas RM, Peer J, Kreyenbuhl J (2010) The 2009 schizophrenia PORT psychosocial treatment recommendations and summary statements. Schizophr Bull 36(1):48–70. http://doi.org/10.1093/schbul/sbp115

Foster C, Startup H, Potts L, Freeman D (2010) A randomised controlled trial of a worry intervention for individuals with persistent persecutory delusions. J Behav Ther Exp Psychiatry 41(1):45–51, http://doi.org/10.1016/j.jbtep.2009.09.001

Freeman D, Dunn G, Startup H, Pugh K, Cordwell J, Mander H, Černis E, Wingham G, Shirvell K, Kingdon D (2015) Effects of cognitive behaviour therapy for worry on persecutory delusions in patients with psychosis (WIT): a parallel, single-blind, randomised controlled trial with a mediation analysis. Lancet Psychiatry 2(4):305–313. http://doi.org/10.1016/S2215-0366(15)00039-5

Garety PA, Kuipers E, Fowler D, Freeman D, Bebbington PE (2001) A cognitive model of the positive symptoms of psychosis. Psychol Med 31(02):189–195, http://doi.org/10.1017/S0033291701003312

Haddock G, Slade PD (1996) Cognitive-behavioural interventions with psychotic disorders. Psychology Press. New York, USA

Harrison G, Hopper K, Craig T, Laska E, Siegel C, Wanderling J, Dube KC, Ganev K, Giel R, an der Heiden W, Holmberg SK, Janca A, Lee PW, León CA, Malhotra S, Marsella AJ, Nakane Y, Sartorius N, Shen Y, Skoda C, Thara R, Tsirkin SJ, Varma VK, Walsh D, Wiersma D (2001) Recovery from psychotic illness: a 15- and 25-year international follow-up study. Br J Psychiatry. 178(6):506–517. http://doi.org/10.1192/bjp.178.6.506

Hazlett-Stevens HCM, Dryden W (2005) Brief cognitive-behavioral therapy: definition and scientific foundations. In: Handbook of brief cognitive behaviour therapy. Wiley. New York, USA

Kimhy D, Tarrier N, Essock S, Malaspina D, Cabannis D, Beck AT (2013) Cognitive behavioral therapy for psychosis – training practices and dissemination in the United States. Psychosis 5(3):296–305, http://doi.org/10.1080/17522439.2012.704932

Kingdon D, Kirschen H (2006) Special section: a memorial tribute: who does not get cognitive-behavioral therapy for schizophrenia when therapy is readily available? Psychiatr Serv 57(12):1792–1794, http://doi.org/10.1176/appi.ps.57.12.1792

Kingdon DG, Turkington D (2002) Cognitive-behavioral therapy of schizophrenia. Guilford Publications, New York, USA

Malik N, Kingdon D, Pelton J, Mehta R, Turkington D (2009) Effectiveness of brief cognitive-behavioral therapy for schizophrenia delivered by mental health nurses: relapse and recovery at 24 months. J Clin Psychiatry 70(2):201–207

Meichenbaum D, Cameron R (1973) Training schizophrenics to talk to themselves: a means of developing attentional controls. Behav Ther 4(4):515–534, http://doi.org/10.1016/S0005-7894(73)80003-6

Morrison AP (2001) The interpretation of intrusions in psychosis: an integrative cognitive approach to hallucinations and delusions. Behav Cogn Psychother 29(03):257–276, http://doi.org/10.1017/S1352465801003010

Mueser KT, Noordsy DL (2005) Cognitive behavior therapy for psychosis: a call to action. Clin Psychol: Sci Pract 12(1):68–71, http://doi.org/10.1093/clipsy.bpi008

Naeem F (2013) Culturally adapted CBT (CaCBT) for depression, therapy manual for use with South Asian Muslims [Kindle Edition]. Pakistan Association of Cognitive Therapists, Lahore, Pakistan

Naeem F, Kingdon D, Turkington D (2005). Cognitive behaviour therapy for schizophrenia in patients with mild to moderate substance misuse problems. Cognitive Behaviour Therapy, 34(4):207–215.

Naeem F, Kingdon D, Turkington D (2006). Cognitive behaviour therapy for schizophrenia: Relationship between anxiety symptoms and therapy. Psychology and Psychotherapy: Theory, Research and Practice, 79(2):153–164

Naeem F, Kingdon D, Turkington D (2008). Predictors of response to cognitive behaviour therapy in the treatment of schizophrenia: A comparison of brief and standard interventions. Cognitive Therapy and Research, 32(5):651–656

Naeem F, Farooq S, Kingdon D (2014) Cognitive behavioral therapy (brief versus standard duration) for schizophrenia. Cochrane Database Syst Rev (4):CD010646. http://doi.org/10.1002/14651858.CD010646.pub2

Naeem F, Habib N, Gul M, Khalid M, Saeed S, Farooq S, Munshi T, Gobbi M, Husain N, Ayub M, Kingdon D (2014) A qualitative study to explore patients', carers' and health professionals' views to culturally adapt CBT for psychosis (CBTp) in Pakistan. Behav Cogn Psychother 1–13. http://doi.org/10.1017/S1352465814000332

Naeem F, Saeed S, Irfan M, Kiran T, Mehmood N, Gul M, , Munshi T, Ahmad S, Kazmi A, Husain N, Farooq S, Ayub M, Kingdon D (2015) Brief culturally adapted CBT for psychosis (CaCBTp): a randomized controlled trial from a low income country. Schizophr Res 0(0). http://doi.org/10.1016/j.schres.2015.02.015

National Institute for Health and Care Excellence (2014) Psychosis and schizophrenia: treatment and management (Clinical guideline 178). http://guidance.nice.org.uk/CG178

Rathod S, Kingdon D, Smith P, Turkington D (2005) Insight into schizophrenia: the effects of cognitive behavioural therapy on the components of insight and association with sociodemographics – data on a previously published randomised controlled trial. Schizophr Res 74(2–3): 211–219, http://doi.org/10.1016/j.schres.2004.07.003

Shapiro MB, Ravenette AT (1959) A preliminary experiment on paranoid delusions. Br J Psychiatry 105(439):295–312, http://doi.org/10.1192/bjp.105.439.295

Tai S, Turkington D (2009) The evolution of cognitive behavior therapy for schizophrenia: current practice and recent developments. Schizophr Bull 35(5):865–873, http://doi.org/10.1093/schbul/sbp080

Tarrier N, Calam R (2002) New developments in cognitive-behavioural case formulation. Epidemiological, systemic and social context: an integrative approach. Behav Cogn Psychother 30(03):311–328, http://doi.org/10.1017/S1352465802003065

Turkington D, Kingdon D, Turner T, Insight into Schizophrenia Research Group (2002) Effectiveness of a brief cognitive – behavioural therapy intervention in the treatment of schizophrenia. Br J Psychiatry 180(6):523–527, http://doi.org/10.1192/bjp.180.6.523

Turkington D, Kingdon D, Rathod S, Hammond K, Pelton J, Mehta R (2006) Outcomes of an effectiveness trial of cognitive-behavioural intervention by mental health nurses in schizophrenia. Br J Psychiatry: J Mental Sci 189:36–40, http://doi.org/10.1192/bjp.bp.105.010884

Vaughn CE, Leff JP (1981) Patterns of emotional response in relatives of schizophrenic patients. Schizophr Bull 7(1):43–44

Wykes T, Hayward P, Thomas N, Green N, Surguladze S, Fannon D, Landau S (2005) What are the effects of group cognitive behaviour therapy for voices? A randomised control trial. Schizophr Res 77(2–3):201–210, http://doi.org/10.1016/j.schres.2005.03.013

Wykes T, Steel C, Everitt B, Tarrier N (2008) Cognitive behavior therapy for schizophrenia: effect sizes, clinical models, and methodological rigor. Schizophr Bull 34(3):523–537, http://doi.org/10.1093/schbul/sbm114

AVATAR Therapy for Refractory Auditory Hallucinations

4

Tom Craig, Tom Ward, and Mar Rus-Calafell

4.1 Psychological Therapies for Voice Hearing: An Overview

While attempts to understand voice hearing need to acknowledge the complexity and diversity of the experience (Woods et al. 2014), the majority of hearers describe voices that take the form of a characterized "other" with whom a personally meaningful relationship develops (Beavan 2011; McCarthy-Jones et al. 2014). AVATAR therapy is part of a new and exciting wave of therapies which adopt an explicitly relational and dialogic approach to working with the distressing voices. To understand the AVATAR approach, it is important to consider its position in the evolution of psychological interventions for distressing voices.

Developments in psychological approaches to working with voices have been articulated in a recent review by an international collaboration of experts (Thomas et al. 2014). Following an early focus on functional-analytic approaches such as coping strategy enhancement (Tarrier et al. 1993), cognitive conceptualizations of psychosis came to prominence (Garety et al. 2001; Morrison 2001). A key premise of cognitive models, in keeping with a continuum view of psychosis, is that the presence of voices in isolation is not sufficient to determine the transition to clinical psychosis (i.e., "need for care"), a position that is supported by evidence of non-distressing voices in the general population (de Leede-Smith and Barkus 2013; Johns et al. 2014). Instead, cognitive models propose that beliefs and appraisals play a central role in the development and persistence of positive symptoms of psychosis (Garety et al. 2007). Put simply the way in which individuals make sense of, and respond to, their voices can determine whether voices remain benign (even

T. Craig (✉) • T. Ward • M. Rus-Calafell
Psychology and Systems Sciences, Kings College London,
Institute of Psychiatry, Psychology and Neuroscience,
Box 33, HSPRD, De Crespigny Park, London SE5 8AF, UK
e-mail: thomas.craig@kcl.ac.uk

© Springer International Publishing Switzerland 2016
B. Pradhan et al. (eds.), *Brief Interventions for Psychosis*:
A Clinical Compendium, DOI 10.1007/978-3-319-30521-9_4

life-enhancing) or alternatively result in distress, impairment, and a need for clinical care. Drawing on work in the field of anxiety disorders, Morrison has conceptualized distressing voices as occurring when "intrusions" into awareness are subject to "culturally unacceptable" misinterpretation, a stage of meaning-making that is influenced by the person's prior life experiences together with beliefs about the self, the world, and others (Morrison 2001). Seminal early work by Paul Chadwick and Max Birchwood has demonstrated that beliefs about voices (specifically regarding identity, power, intention, and control) are key to understanding distress and maladaptive responding in the context of voices (Birchwood and Chadwick 1997; Chadwick and Birchwood 1994). Factors such as mood and physiology, safety behaviors (including hypervigilance), meta-cognitive processes, and faulty self- and social knowledge are viewed as key maintenance processes which fuel distressing appraisals and beliefs about voices (Morrison 2001). Consequently, a range of cognitive-behavioral therapy approaches have been developed, which intervene at the level of individual "meaning-making" (i.e., beliefs and appraisals) and target the key maintenance processes outlined above (Thomas et al. 2014).

In more recent times Birchwood and colleagues (2000, 2004) have integrated their original cognitive model of voices with a "social mentalities" approach which proposes that humans have evolved mechanisms for recognizing dominant-subordinate interactions, i.e., their social rank (Gilbert and Allan 1994; Gilbert et al. 2001). Beliefs about the power of the voice are essentially viewed as a differential judgment the hearer makes regarding their power (or more usually lack of power) in relation to the voice, i.e., a relational judgment. Individuals who have experienced powerlessness and inferiority in social relationships have been found to be more likely to report similar experiences during the voice interaction (Birchwood et al. 2000). It is argued that negative experiences within social relationships establish social schemata that drive the subsequent appraisals of voices and ultimately lead to significant levels of distress and depression (Birchwood et al. 2004). Recent reviews have provided support for the hypothesis that social schema may mediate the appraisal-distress relationship with the implication that therapies could benefit from targeting social and interpersonal variables (Mawson et al. 2010; Paulik 2012). These theoretical developments have informed a specific cognitive therapy for command hallucinations (CTHC; Birchwood et al. 2014; Trower et al. 2004). A randomized controlled trial of this approach (the COMMAND trial; Birchwood et al. 2014) has recently reported a reduction in the rate of compliance behavior to the voices compared with the treatment as usual group (odds ratio 0.45) along with an associated reduction in the specific treatment target (the power difference between the perceived threat of the voice and the hearer's ability to mitigate this threat). Interventions such as CTHC answer an identified need for the development of more targeted therapeutic approaches to specific experiences and symptoms of psychosis and the putative mechanisms of persistence and distress (Garety and Freeman 2013; Thomas et al. 2014).

The approach of Birchwood and colleagues provides a bridge between early formulation-based approaches centering on intra-psychological (cognitive, affective, and behavioral) processes and a new wave of relational approaches which focus on the interpersonal relationship between the voice-hearer and the voice (Corstens et al. 2012; Hayward et al. 2014; Leff et al. 2013). Relating therapy (Hayward et al. 2009) specifically applies Birtchnell's (1996) interpersonal model to the voice-hearer relationship, identifying key interpersonal dimensions of *power* and *proximity* (Birtchnell 1996). While *interpersonal power* can be viewed as analogous to the social rank characterization of dominant-subordinate interactions, maladaptive relationships along the *proximity* dimension are defined by opposing poles of "withdrawal/self-isolation" versus "over-involvement/intrusiveness" (Hayward et al. 2011). Therapy begins by exploration of similarities between the person's relationship with their voice and other social relationships (in line with the mirroring noted above by Birchwood and colleagues 2000). Following this awareness-building stage, sessions move on to explore different ways of relating to the voice using assertiveness training (including role-play and empty chair work (Chadwick 2006) with the aim (again consistent with CTHC) of increasing the person's appraisal of control within the relationship.

"Talking with voices" (Corstens et al. 2012) is a relational approach which emphasizes the importance of understanding voices (and voice relationships) within the person's biographical context (Longden et al. 2012). Voices are understood as a reflection of conflict within a person's life story, a conflict that becomes manifest in the voice that the person hears. The approach involves a "facilitator" engaging in dialogue with the voice(s), asking direct questions the answers to which are relayed back via the voice-hearer. Rather than seeking to eradicate the experience of voice hearing, or indeed target specific cognitive mechanisms, this approach aims to provide an opportunity to resolve social-emotional dilemmas in order to achieve a sense of acceptance or mastery over previously distressing, disempowering experiences.

4.2   AVATAR Therapy: History, Method, and Evidence So Far

AVATAR therapy (Leff et al. 2013) is a recent *relational approach* which draws on the theoretical and clinical developments outlined above, within the context of a novel therapeutic milieu. Using specially designed computer software, the clients create a visual representation of the entity (human or nonhuman) that they believe is talking to them. Additional software is used to transform the voice of the therapist to match the pitch and tone of the voice heard by the person; the two processes finally being combined to produce a computer simulation (a virtual agent or "avatar") through which the therapist can have a dialogue with the person. In addition to the time taken to create the "AVATAR", therapy comprises approximately 6×45 minutes sessions of which around 15 minutes is spent in dialogue with the avatar. The therapist (sitting in a separate room to the participant and communicating through linked computers) promotes a dialogue between the participant and the avatar, *one goal of which is that the hearer will experience more power and control within the relationship* (Leff et al. 2014). The sessions are audio recorded and provided to the participant on an MP3 player for continued use at home.

AVATAR therapy can be embraced within the generation of virtual reality-based psychological therapies using technology to integrate real-time graphics, sounds, and other sensory inputs to create a computer-generated world with which the user can interact (Gregg and Tarrier 2007). Although AVATAR therapy is not provided in a complex immersive environment, the platform uses virtual reality to create and allow the person to access and visualize the abstract nonphysical information of his/ her voice. One could define it as a *virtual embodiment of the experience*: to give a physical representation to the personified but disembodied voice. This visualization of the voice may facilitate two essential processes in the AVATAR therapy: (a) validation of the experience and (b) the flow of dialogue with the voice through the sessions while modifying the type of relationship between the voice and the participant. This *virtual embodiment* of the experience is achieved by matching the voice of the avatar to the current auditory hallucination and, in early sessions, by the avatar using verbatim statements from the voice, as reported by the voice-hearer. These add realism to the experience and seem to be a key aspect of the therapy.

Morrison and colleagues showed that approximately 75 % of people with psychosis could identify images that occurred spontaneously in relation to their voices (e.g., having an image of the perceived source of a voice when hearing it) (Morrison et al. 2002). They also reported that some of the voice-hearers used their images as evidence to support their beliefs about voices (e.g., believing that a voice is omnipotent, powerful, and omniscient because they have a concurrent image of God or the Devil). They concluded that working with these images, for example, altering the content or meaning of the image, could result in a reduction of the distress associated with them and even increase the sense of control over the images (Morrison 2010). The exposure to the experience of seeing an image and hearing an avatar uttering the same statements as the voice in therapy sessions, along with the modification of the relationship with the voice, may be contributing to the reduction of the voice's associated distress and to the disconfirmation of maladaptive beliefs about the voice. The mechanism of this may be anxiety related: the therapy may be reducing cognitive avoidance of fear-relevant information (i.e., the voice and its content) and also reducing anxiety as a direct consequence of exposure (Foa and Kozak 1986). Re-listening to MP3 recordings of each dialogue between sessions may facilitate this exposure process.

In line with the early theoretical work outlined above, the voicing/characterization of the avatar reflects a detailed understanding of the person's beliefs about the voices (e.g., regarding identity, power, intention, and the consequences of resistance; Chadwick and Birchwood 1994). This includes an assessment of how a person's cultural background influences what participants think are the origin of their voices but also informs how the therapist should enact the avatar in dialogue with the participant. Therapists on the trial have been required to enact spiritual entities located within different systems of beliefs, sometimes in combination (including among others Islamic, Christian, Spiritualist, and region-specific African and Rastafarian beliefs). In addition avatars representing characterized people gain validity when voiced to reflect the cultural norms of the experienced other (this typically proceeds via a synthesis of the therapist's existing cultural competence together with assessment of the beliefs and assumptions of the voice-hearer). A specific example was the enactment (by author TC) of an avatar viewed as a local Rastafarian drug dealer, where it was important that the avatar was voiced from a position reflecting the basic tenets of Rastafarianism, specifically views about cannabis. Differing representations of the self and related beliefs about the reason for persecution (Trower and Chadwick 1995), together with comorbidity of depression and associated negative self-schemata (Vorontsova et al. 2013), also impact on the nature of the dialogue (e.g., assertiveness work and relinquishing of a "victim role" or work on attribution of guilt and self-blame). Within the AVATAR therapy approach, the person's relationship with their voice is fundamentally viewed in the context of their current and previous significant relationships (Birchwood et al. 2000, 2004). The possible role of early trauma is sensitively addressed from the first meeting and in line with the "talking with voices" approach (Corstens et al. 2012); unresolved social and emotional issues that may be relevant to the person's experience of voice hearing are considered throughout the therapy. The nature of the relationship as it varies along dimensions of interpersonal power and proximity (Birtchnell 1996) also influences the evolving dialogue. While all dialogues (particularly early sessions) involve negotiation of a transfer of power and control from voice/avatar to hearer, relationships characterized by "withdrawal" require an initial "turning to face" the previously avoided experience, while "clinging" relationships typically necessitate a process of disengagement (i.e., "not getting drawn in" to what might be termed as the habitual "dance of distress"). Such strategies share some commonalities with an acceptance and commitment therapy approach to working with psychosis (Bach and Hayes 2002; Gaudiano and Herbert 2006) insomuch as relationships characterized by "withdrawal" and "clinging" could be viewed as involving unhelpful levels of *experiential avoidance* and *cognitive fusion*, respectively. Following the initial assertiveness phase, the avatar's character gradually changes to become conciliatory or even helpful. This initiates a second phase which focuses on issues of self-esteem and identity, work that is consistent with other recent approaches emphasizing the importance of self-esteem and self-compassion in working with distressing voices (Mayhew and Gilbert 2008; van der Gaag et al. 2012). Specific work on self-esteem typically includes asking the person to get friends and family to provide a list of their strengths and best qualities which can then be used in dialogue with the avatar. For some people the extent of current social isolation means that it can be difficult to identify someone to provide the list (in such cases it can be obtained from a trusted professional or the therapist may "work up" the list in collaboration with the person). For those who can identify someone to provide a list, the simple act of hearing a positive view from someone else can be a powerful (and surprising) experience. For others the discussion of positive qualities triggers embarrassment and awkwardness, and for some hearing positive qualities spoken aloud can seem an almost aversive experience (reflecting, in our view, the extent of the dissonance between this positive information and the ingrained negative view of the self). Given these potential challenges as in the earliest assertiveness sessions, it can often be necessary to engage in preparatory role-play with the therapist before attempting to raise the topic with the avatar.

The final sessions of AVATAR therapy often involve discussion around hopes for the future and are influenced by consideration of the personal meaning of recovery in the context of the voice hearing experience (Romme et al. 2009).

An abbreviated outline of the evolution of a typical dialogue is given in Fig. 4.1.

In an initial pilot study (Leff et al. 2013), 26 patients were randomized to therapy ($n = 14$) or a waiting list control group ($n = 12$). Therapy was provided for a maximum of seven sessions lasting 30 minutes. While the control group reported no change over time, those receiving AVATAR therapy reported an average reduction of 8.7 points ($p = 0.0003$) in the total score of the PSYRATS-AH rating scale for auditory hallucinations (Haddock et al. 1999) with three participants reporting a complete cessation of voices. Participants in the therapy arm also reported an average 5.9 point ($p = 0.0004$) reduction in scores on the omnipotence and malevolence subscales of the revised Beliefs About Voices Questionnaire (BAVQ-R; Chadwick et al. 2000).

AVATAR therapy is currently being examined in a larger, well-powered methodologically rigorous clinical trial ($n = 142$), in which a comparison is made between the effects of AVATAR therapy and supportive counseling, the control group chosen to take account of nonspecific elements of therapy exposure (ISRCTN: 65314790). Early qualitative impressions from the trial therapy team indicate that the virtual reality aspects of the setup, fostering a sense of "presence," facilitate a dialogue whereby affect is "on line," with participant reports of high ecological validity of the avatar. Some respondents report that the experience with the avatar is "100 % like hearing my troubling voice" potentially conferring benefits over existing helpful techniques such as role-play and "empty chair" work (e.g., Chadwick 2006; Hayward et al. 2009). In order to record and evaluate this reported verisimilitude,

	AVATAR is person's main bullyingvoice. Hostile critical, name-calling ("stupid", "ugly" "piece of shit"). History of significant bullying throughout life. Voice uses same phrases as school bullies (although he had never linked this prior to coming to therapy). N.B this is a composite to reflect typical dialogue within the trial and not a direct transcript.
Phase1 : **Session 1**	*[Session 1 involves highest frequency of direct therapist input; this reduces as sessions progress]:* AV: ' You are an idiot...' 'Piece of shit!' [initial silence in response] AV: "you heard me... you're a piece of shit" Pt: "that's not right, [slightly halting] I don't want to listen to you" Tx: "that's really good [encouragement, reinforcing positive assertiveness and checking in], How did that feel? Pt: "a bit better, still a bit weird" Tx: "you're doing really well..... I want you go even stronger next time he comes in.
Transition: **Session 3**	AV: 'You are a waste of space' Pt: [more forcefully] I won't stand for this, this is bullying and I'm not listening anymore Tx: That's very strong... absolutely right to call it bullying....you sound in control. Well done! AV: "What do you want to say to me today?" Pt: "I want to say that I've had enough of you, You can't push me around anymore" AV: "you do seem different recently...what's changed?" [Avatar conceding] Pt: 'I've changed a lot....I've learnt how to deal with you and you can't get to me now." AV: "I can see you are not the push-over I once took you for" Pt: "that's right...those days are gone....I'm not a victim now" Tx: Well done! Absolutely right. You are not a victim [Therapist reinforcing this key statement] AV: Maybe I have got you wrong, I can see you are no victim anymore, what kind of person are you then? [Avatar continues to concede, begins to cue in subsequent self-esteem work]

Fig. 4.1 Example of a dialogue

Phase 2: **Session 4**	*[Self-esteem discussed between sessions; person has collected list of positive qualities]* AV: "I've been thinking about what you said last time. It seems I may have got you wrong?" Px: "yes… I am a good person…..I don't deserve to be bullied….I'm too strong for you anyway?" AV: "what do other people think about you?" Px- "Well I asked my sister and she said…I am a good person….kind.. caring…strong….. good fun….loyal and a good brother". Av- "Why does she say that do you think?" Px- "Well I helped when she was having problems with her husband….he was not nice you know so I told him to leave her" AV- "Well you know how to deal with bullies…..but I thought you said that people think you are lazy?" Px- "yeah I know…I was shocked when I read the list…I didn't really want to ask her at first…I thought she wouldn't be able to come with anything"
Session 6	AV- "It seems to me you have got used to thinking badly about yourself over the years…. The things I have said to you have also been the things you think about yourself deep down…" [developing link between voice content, previous bullying and low self-esteem] AV- "this is the last time we will be talking together like this" AV- "I have seen so much change in you over the time we have spoken together" Px- "Yes……I feel different….I mean I'm the same person but you know I feel stronger". AV- Yes, you are certainly a strong person….so what now? Px- I still, you know, want to do more, get a job, meet some people, but I feel I can do it. AV- I think you are right…you have shown me you are a good person with lots of qualities. Px- yeah, I'm starting to see that too now [laughs] AV- It is important that you do. As long as you continue to see your own strength and qualities as a person, you can deal with any bullies, just like you have with me and your sister's husband. [generalising from what has worked with the avatar to wider social relationships] Px- Yeah I think so too. AV- Is there anything else you want to say to me? Px- no, just, good-bye and I'm pleased we sorted things out. AV- Good-bye

Fig. 4.1 (continued)

we have incorporated an adapted version of the Sense of Presence Questionnaire (Slater et al. 1994) that evaluates the participant's sense of "hearing the voice" and their perception of the avatar as their "voice talking to me." As we are also interested in the persecutory experience and level of anxiety when confronting the avatar, we have adapted the State Social Paranoia Scale (Freeman et al. 2007) to measure persecutory and positive thoughts about the experience (e.g., "the avatar was trying to irritate me" and "the avatar was friendly towards me"). Visual analogical scales are used to capture reported anxiety and perceived hostility of the avatar at the end of every therapy session.

4.3   Challenges of AVATAR Therapy

For good or bad (or sometimes both) the relationship with the voice often forms a key part of the person's life and in many cases represents the main source of current social relating. As such the meaning and implications of changes in this important relationship require sensitive, open-minded discussion between the voice-hearer and therapist as part of the person's engagement with the therapy. While the pilot study provided evidence of reductions in voice frequency and intensity, AVATAR therapy, in common with other psychological approaches and hearing voice networks, targets the reduction of distress and disruption to the life of the voice-hearer. Ultimately the aim is for the person to begin to experience a sense of power and control within their relationships (with their voice *and* other people) such that they emerge more confident in their ability to navigate their social world and engage with the possibility of a different, more positive future.

As is apparent from all we have said to this point, a key component of therapy is the ability of the therapist to understand the nature and possible purpose of the person's voice and to deliver a "realistic" enactment of this entity during the dialogue. In the initial sessions, the therapist is required to use verbatim statements delivered with the prosodic features (including tone and rhythm) and force that the hearer usually hears from their persecutory voice. This presents a number of immediate challenges. The necessity to speak these typically abusive, threatening, and overtly hostile comments (including racist terms) directly to the person (albeit via a modified voice transform) sits uneasily with all the instincts and training of therapists. Early sessions aim to strike a balance between creating and dialoguing using a realistic representation of the voice experience while ensuring that the person feels sufficiently safe to approach something which may feel frightening and trigger concerns about possible voice retaliation. Getting the balance right can be tricky. On the one hand is the risk that the person is unable to tolerate the session as, for example, the person who terminated a session saying "...I have to put up with this rubbish day and night; this is just too much..." while on the other hand being so mild that the experience is perceived as contrived and unrealistic as, for example, a comment such as "oh, my voice would never speak like that...." In practice such occurrences have been rare, probably because a great deal of effort is put into preparing the participant for the sessions including role-play and rehearsal of responses before the first encounter with the avatar. A related challenge is presented when the voice is experienced with a particular accent where again the immersive reality of the experience is enhanced if the therapist is able do a fair imitation of the accent. Interestingly, when the balance is right, the immersive experience appears remarkably high with several participants commenting that they felt they were really in a dialogue with their voice.

A typical therapy experience for participants who engage with the approach involves some initial (often marked) anxiety (in particular preceding the first confrontation with the avatar) followed, during the first session debrief, by a reported sense of relief, achievement, power, and even liberation. Over time the reported in-session anxiety typically reduces and the participant is able to reflect with the therapist on a significant challenge which has been faced and overcome. For participants who choose not to continue with sessions (to date approximately 20 % of those who attend at least one session), reported reasons for discontinuation are varied (and in some cases simply logistical). Withdrawal factors that are related to the therapy typically involve the person finding early sessions overly stressful (including in rare instances increased hostility, threats, and commands not to continue from voices) or the participant not seeing how the approach could help in terms of their voices. It is worth noting that a similar dropout rate is seen in the supportive counseling control group (approximately 18 %) and is comparable to that seen in several other exposure-based therapies including PTSD (Imel et al. 2013; van den Berg et al. 2015).

One of the most significant challenges for the therapist is the transition from the initial, largely verbatim sessions where the task is mainly to establish a fair simulacrum of the voice hearing experience toward a second more dialogic phase in which the character of the avatar shifts to being less threatening and more considerate of the individual. This dialogic shift has to be appropriately timed, should be in response to changes in the preceding dialogue, and should be based on the therapist's understanding of the participant's key beliefs about the origin, nature, and function of the voice in their life. A key task for the therapist (in keeping with cognitive approaches to working with psychosis more generally) would be to determine whether the evolving dialogue is situated "within the belief" (e.g., someone definitively identifying the voice as caused by an external entity, e.g., a demon, a school bully, or a drug dealer) or whether the dialogue is evolving toward an understanding of the voice experience as having its origin within the self (e.g., the identification of the voice/avatar as representing low self-esteem or "memory echoes" of past bullying/abuse/trauma). In the former case (i.e., "working within") a rationale for the diminishing presence or power of the "other entity" is negotiated, e.g., the bully who accepts the person is now too strong to be pushed around. In the latter case (i.e., a more internal attribution of voice) an understanding that the avatar/voice content represents "the negative things I think about myself" can be developed with the implication that the necessary change is for the person to begin viewing themselves in a more positive and compassionate way (this is framed as a process of change as opposed to a "quick fix" particularly for the many participants in the trial with significant abuse and bullying histories). The therapist aims to avoid "forcing" the dialogue into one direction or the other but rather adapts their approach to connect with the person's evolving understanding of their voice and what would constitute a positive change in the relationship with their voice.

It should be noted that even assuming it is possible to deliver a realistic voice hearing experience, the task of transforming the avatar experience to becoming less hostile and more under the control of the voice-hearer is no guarantee that the actual voice hearing experience will similarly moderate. In cases where the avatar has transitioned, while the day-to-day voice remains hostile, the avatar typically suggests the person tries the strategies that worked in earlier sessions with their day-to-day voices reinforcing key messages that have emerged from the dialogue (e.g., relating to the person's strength, resilience, and positive qualities). Throughout the trial, the therapy team has considered other potential adverse reactions to the therapy including the risk that the avatar voice becomes incorporated in a negative way into the voice-hearer's experience/beliefs or that the avatar computer system is seen as the source of the voice hearing. Neither of these has yet been observed though in one instance a person reported hearing their avatar's voice in a helpful way outside of a session. A number of people have also reported completely new, benign/

reassuring content from their voices by the end of therapy which they view as a positive change. As is customary in any clinical trial of a new therapy, all possible negative outcomes are recorded and monitored and will form a key component of the final report of the trial.

4.4 The Future: Implementing AVATAR Therapy in Routine Care

The current clinical trial is being provided in NHS facilities and the majority of the participants are receiving continuing care from secondary psychiatric services. The number and spacing of sessions are such that the therapy is easily fitted in to the wider care program and is delivered alongside routine case management and medical treatment. At present the delivery system is fairly cumbersome, requiring the fixed installation of two desktop computers that are hardwired, but in fact, the software is capable of running on laptops or tablet computers over the hospital intranet given the appropriate data protection and governance permissions. With such a configuration it would be entirely feasible to incorporate this therapy into routine outpatient clinical settings, and sessions could be tailored to integrate with other components of overall care. This is indeed the future pathway envisaged. A component of the current project led by our colleagues in University College London is the development of a portable multi-platform system, available for future research and ultimately clinical use. This more flexible system should be available in 2016.

The larger potential barrier to routine implementation lies in identifying, training, and supervising clinical staff to deliver the therapy. This represents a major challenge more generally for psychological therapies for psychosis (Haddock et al. 2014; Prytys et al. 2011). All the AVATAR therapy to date has been delivered by very experienced clinicians, all of whom have considerable prior training in psychological therapies, and the group meets regularly for peer supervision, which is essential. Initial training involved each of the therapists working with two patients outside of the clinical trial and was provided by Professor Julian Leff against an outline manual that has subsequently been elaborated as we all gain experience across the trial. All therapists come from a background where the clinical formulation of a person's problems is seen as essential for therapy to proceed and undoubtedly has determined the elaboration of therapy model as we deliver it.

It is difficult to envisage AVATAR therapy being delivered by novice therapists without competency in clinical formulation and familiarity with a variety of psychotherapeutic techniques. On the other hand, our current "homework" task of listening to MP3 recordings of the therapy sessions could certainly be enhanced through the use of more sophisticated tablet-based software that included the visual imagery (e.g., using augmented reality on a smartphone or tablet) and, perhaps in time, also could be programmed as a self-help top-up to practice the use of key assertive phrases in standing up to prespecified content. We are of the opinion that these represent methods of augmenting the standard one-on-one delivery of the therapy rather than offering a separate self-help alternative given the often strong emotional responses and the consequent importance of in-session monitoring and therapeutic work before and after the active dialogue.

In addition to the use of this therapy as a "stand-alone" intervention for people with diagnoses of schizophrenia and other psychoses, our experience suggests that the approach could be easily adapted for voice-hearers with other conditions. We also believe that AVATAR therapy may be a very helpful component of a broader therapeutic approach, included, for example, within a typical 16-session course of CBT where the voices reflect just one component of the individual's experience. For example, during the trial training phase, TW saw an individual for 6 sessions of AVATAR therapy following a period of individual CBTp (approximately 20 sessions), which had taken place around 6 months earlier. The participant and therapist experience suggested that the two approaches operated in a complementary fashion with benefits that generalized from the voices to broader distressing persecutory beliefs.

Another frequently asked question is whether AVATAR could be helpful for people with psychosis who do not want to take medication. The inclusion criteria for the current trial are that participants hear voices despite continuing to take medication. As a result, we have excluded a small number of referrals of young people from early intervention services who were being managed off medication. We believe that this cautious approach is the right one at this stage of development of AVATAR. Should evidence from a number of trials show a low risk of adverse clinical effects, it would be appropriate to move toward a carefully conducted clinical trial as has been implemented for CBTp (Morrison et al. 2015). Another important though rather obvious consequence of the approach is that it provides a unique opportunity for the participant to share the voice hearing experience with the therapist and others – a feature that has been commented upon favorably by several participants, a number of whom have decided to play the sessions to friends and families. Working with and through an avatar provides an opportunity for the therapist to reflect on what living with such hostility on an ongoing basis might actually be like. In this way, empathy is taken from an abstract clinical plane and brought closer to the experience of people living with distressing voices.

Conclusion

AVATAR therapy is part of a new and exciting wave of therapies which adopt an explicitly relational and dialogic approach to working with distressing voices experienced by individuals suffering from psychosis. Although this work needs replication in future trials, initial data on the use of this novel approach offers many opportunities both in terms of the delivery of therapy and in elaborating our understanding of the phenomenology of "voice hearing." Also AVATAR therapy has the potential of being applied to other mental health disorders and conditions which of course require further work and adaptations.

Acknowledgments The AVATAR clinical trial is funded by the Wellcome Trust (FWBC-AVATAR WT098272/Z/12/Z).

References

Bach P, Hayes SC (2002) The use of acceptance and commitment therapy to prevent the rehospitalization of psychotic patients: a randomized controlled trial. J Consult Clin Psychol 70(5):1129–1139. doi:10.1037//0022-006x.70.5.1129

Beavan V (2011) Towards a definition of "hearing voices": a phenomenological approach. Psychosis Psychol Soc Integr Approaches 3(1):63–73. doi:10.1080/17522431003615622

Birchwood M, Chadwick P (1997) The omnipotence of voices: testing the validity of a cognitive model. Psychol Med 27(6):1345–1353. doi:10.1017/S0033291797005552

Birchwood M, Meaden A, Trower P, Gilbert P, Plaistow J (2000) The power and omnipotence of voices: subordination and entrapment by voices and significant others. Psychol Med 30(2):337–344. doi:10.1017/S0033291799001828

Birchwood M, Gilbert P, Gilbert J, Trower P, Meaden A, Hay J, Murray E, Miles JN (2004) Interpersonal and role-related schema influence the relationship with the dominant 'voice' in schizophrenia: a comparison of three models. Psychol Med 34(8):1571–1580

Birchwood M, Michail M, Meaden A, Tarrier N, Lewis S, Wykes T, Davies L, Dunn G, Peters E (2014) Cognitive behaviour therapy to prevent harmful compliance with command hallucinations (COMMAND): a randomised controlled trial. Lancet Psychiatry 1(1):23–33

Birtchnell J (1996) How humans relate: a new interpersonal theory. Psychology Press, Hove

Chadwick P (2006) Person-based cognitive therapy for distressing psychosis. Wiley-Blackwell, Oxford

Chadwick P, Birchwood M (1994) The omnipotence of voices – a cognitive approach to auditory hallucinations. Br J Psychiatry 164:190–201. doi:10.1192/bjp.164.2.190

Chadwick P, Lees S, Birchwood M (2000) The revised Beliefs About Voices Questionnaire (BAVQ-R). Br J Psychiatry 177:229–232. doi:10.1192/bjp.177.3.229

Corstens D, Longden E, May R (2012) Talking with voices: exploring what is expressed by the voices people hear. Psychosis Psychol Soc Integr Approaches 4(2):95–104

de Leede-Smith S, Barkus E (2013) A comprehensive review of auditory verbal hallucinations: lifetime prevalence, correlates and mechanisms in healthy and clinical individuals. Front Hum Neurosci 7:367. doi:10.3389/Fnhum.2013.00367

Foa E, Kozak MJ (1986) Emotional processing of fear: exposure to corrective information. Psychol Bull 99:20–35

Freeman D, Pugh K, Green C, Valmaggia L, Dunn G, Garety P (2007) A measure of state persecutory ideation for experimental studies. J Nerv Ment Dis 195:781–784

Garety PA, Freeman D (2013) The past and future of delusions research: from the inexplicable to the treatable. Br J Psychiatry 203(5):327–333. doi:10.1192/bjp.bp.113.126953

Garety PA, Kuipers E, Fowler D, Freeman D, Bebbington PE (2001) A cognitive model of the positive symptoms of psychosis. Psychol Med 31(2):189–195

Garety PA, Bebbington P, Fowler D, Freeman D, Kuipers E (2007) Implications for neurobiological research of cognitive models of psychosis: a theoretical paper. Psychol Med 37(10):1377–1391. doi:10.1017/S003329170700013x

Gaudiano BA, Herbert JD (2006) Acute treatment of inpatients with psychotic symptoms using Acceptance and Commitment Therapy: pilot results. Behav Res Ther 44(3):415–437. doi:10.1016/j.brat.2005.02.007

Gilbert P, Allan S (1994) Assertiveness, submissive behavior and social-comparison. Br J Psychiatry Clin Psychol 33:295–306

Gilbert P, Birchwood M, Gilbert J, Trower P, Hay J, Murray B, Meaden A, Olsen K, Miles JN (2001) An exploration of evolved mental mechanisms for dominant and subordinate behaviour in relation to auditory hallucinations in schizophrenia and critical thoughts in depression. Psychol Med 31(6):1117–1127

Gregg L, Tarrier N (2007) Virtual reality in mental health: a review of the literature. Soc Psychiatry Psychiatr Epidemiol 42:343–354

Haddock G, McCarron J, Tarrier N, Faragher FB (1999) Scales to measure dimensions of hallucinations and delusions: the psychotic symptom rating scales (PSYRATS). Psychol. Med. 29:879–89. doi: 10.1017/S0033291799008661

Haddock G, Eisner E, Boone C, Davies G, Coogan C, Barrowclough C (2014) An investigation of the implementation of NICE-recommended CBT interventions for people with schizophrenia. J Ment Health 23(4):162–165

Hayward M, Overton J, Dorey T, Denney J (2009) Relating therapy for people who hear voices: a case series. Clin Psychol Psychother 16(3):216–227. doi:10.1002/Cpp.615

Hayward M, Berry K, Ashton A (2011) Applying interpersonal theories to the understanding of and therapy for auditory hallucinations: a review of the literature and directions for further research. Clin Psychol Rev 31(8):1313–1323. doi:10.1016/j.cpr.2011.09.001

Hayward M, Strauss C, Bogen-Johnston L (2014) Relating therapy for voices (the R2V study): study protocol for a pilot randomized controlled trial. Trials 15:325. doi:10.1186/1745-6215-15-325

Imel ZE, Laska K, Jakupcak M, Simpson T (2013) Meta-analysis of dropout in treatments for post-traumatic stress disorder. J Consult Clin Psychol 81:394–404. doi:10.1037/a0031474

Johns LC, Kompus K, Connell M, Humpston C, Lincoln TM, Longden E, Preti A, Alderson-Day B, Badcock JC, Cella M, Fernyhough C, McCarthy-Jones S, Peters E, Raballo A, Scott J, Siddi S, Sommer IE, Laroi F (2014) Auditory verbal hallucinations in persons with and without a need for care. Schizophr Bull 40:S255–S264. doi:10.1093/schbul/sbu005

Leff J, Williams G, Huckvale MA, Arbuthnot M, Leff AP (2013) Computer-assisted therapy for medication-resistant auditory hallucinations: proof-of-concept study. Br J Psychiatry 202:428–433. doi:10.1192/bjp.bp.112.124883

Leff J, Williams G, Huckvale M, Arbuthnot M, Leff AP (2014) Avatar therapy for persecutory auditory hallucinations: what is it and how does it work? Psychosis Psychol Soc Integr Approaches 6(2):166–176. doi:10.1080/17522439.2013.773457

Longden E, Corstens D, Escher S, Romme M (2012) Voice hearing in a biographical context: a model for formulating the relationship between voices and life history. Psychosis Psychol Soc Integr Approaches 4(3):224–234. doi:10.1080/17522439.2011.596566

Mawson A, Cohen K, Berry K (2010) Reviewing evidence for the cognitive model of auditory hallucinations: the relationship between cognitive voice appraisals and distress during psychosis. Clin Psychol Rev 30(2):248–258. doi:10.1016/j.cpr.2009.11.006

Mayhew SL, Gilbert P (2008) Compassionate mind training with people who hear malevolent voices: a case series report. Clin Psychol Psychother 15(2):113–138. doi:10.1002/Cpp.566

McCarthy-Jones S, Thomas N, Strauss C, Dodgson G, Jones N, Woods A, Brewin CR, Hayward M, Stephane M, Barton J, Kingdon D, Sommer IE (2014) Better than mermaids and stray dogs? Subtyping auditory verbal hallucinations and its implications for research and practice. Schizophr Bull 40:S275–S284. doi:10.1093/schbul/sbu018

Morrison AP (2001) The interpretation of intrusions in psychosis: an integrative cognitive approach to hallucinations and delusions. Behav Cogn Psychother 29(3):257–276. doi:10.1017/S1352465801003010

Morrison AP (2010) The use of imagery in cognitive therapy for psychosis: a case example. Memory 12:517–524

Morrison AP, Beck AT, Glentworth D, Dunn H, Reid GS, Larkin W, Williams S (2002) Imagery and psychotic symptoms: a preliminary investigation. Behav Res Ther 40:1063–1072

Morrison AP, Turkington D, Pyle M, Spencer H, Brabban A, Dunn G, Christodoulides T, Dudley R, Chapman N, Callcott P, Grace T, Lumley V, Drage L, Tully S, Irving K, Cummings A, Byrne R, Davies LM, Hutton P (2015) Cognitive therapy for people with schizophrenia spectrum disorders not taking antipsychotic drugs: a single-blind randomised controlled trial. Lancet 383:19–25

Paulik G (2012) The role of social schema in the experience of auditory hallucinations: a systematic review and a proposal for the inclusion of social schema in a cognitive behavioural model of voice hearing. Clin Psychol Psychother 19(6):459–472. doi:10.1002/Cpp.768

Prytys M, Garety PA, Jolley S, Onwumere J, Craig T (2011) Implementing the NICE guideline for schizophrenia recommendations for psychological therapies: a qualitative analysis of the attitudes of CMHT staff. Clin Psychol Psychother 18(1):48–59

Romme M, Escher S, Dillon J, Corstens D, Morris M (2009) Living with voices: 50 stories of recovery. PCCS Books, Ross-on-Wye

Slater M, Usoh M, Steed A (1994) Depth of presence in virtual environments. Presence: Teleoperators Virtual Environ 3:130–144

Tarrier N, Beckett R, Harwood S, Baker A, Yusupoff L, Ugarteburu I (1993) A trial of 2 cognitive behavioral-methods of treating drug-resistant residual psychotic symptoms in schizophrenic-patients. 1. Outcome. Br J Psychiatry 162:524–532. doi:10.1192/bjp.162.4.524

Thomas N, Hayward M, Peters E, van der Gaag M, Bentall RP, Jenner J, Strauss C, Sommer IE, Johns LC, Varese F, García-Montes JM, Waters F, Dodgson G, McCarthy-Jones S (2014) Psychological therapies for auditory hallucinations (voices): current status and key directions for future research. Schizophr Bull 40:S202–S212. doi:10.1093/schbul/sbu037

Trower P, Chadwick P (1995) Pathways to defense of the self – a theory of 2 types of paranoia. Clin Psychol Sci Pract 2(3):263–278

Trower P, Birchwood M, Meaden A, Byrne S, Nelson A, Ross K (2004) Cognitive therapy for command hallucinations: randomised controlled trial. Br J Psychiatry 184:312–320

van den Berg DP, de Bont PA, van der Vleugel BM, de Roos C, de Jongh A, Van Minnen A, van der Gaag M (2015) Prolonged exposure vs eye movement desensitization and reprocessing vs waiting list for posttraumatic stress disorder in patients with a psychotic disorder: a randomized clinical trial. JAMA Psychiatry 72(3):259–267. doi:10.1001/jamapsychiatry.2014.2637

van der Gaag M, van Oosterhout B, Daalman K, Sommer IE, Korrelboom K (2012) Initial evaluation of the effects of competitive memory training (COMET) on depression in schizophrenia-spectrum patients with persistent auditory verbal hallucinations: a randomized controlled trial. Br J Clin Psychol 51:158–171. doi:10.1111/j.2044-8260.2011.02025.x

Vorontsova N, Garety P, Freeman D (2013) Cognitive factors maintaining persecutory delusions in psychosis: the contribution of depression. J Abnorm Psychol 122(4):1121–1131

Woods A, Jones N, Bernini M, Callard F, Alderson-Day B, Badcock JC, Bell V, Cook CC, Csordas T, Humpston C, Krueger J, Larøi F, McCarthy-Jones S, Moseley P, Powell H, Raballo A, Smailes D, Fernyhough C (2014) Interdisciplinary approaches to the phenomenology of auditory verbal hallucinations. Schizophr Bull 40:S246–S254. doi:10.1093/schbul/sbu003

Yoga and Mindfulness-Based Cognitive Therapy for Psychosis (*Y-MBCTp©*): A Pilot Study on Its Efficacy as Brief Therapy

Basant Pradhan and Narsimha R. Pinninti

5.1 Introduction

Psychotic disorders affect 6 % of population, and their optimal management requires integration of pharmacotherapy, effective psychotherapy, and psychosocial management. Schizophrenia is the prototype of the psychotic disorders, and its main symptom clusters are conceptualized in five dimensions, i.e., *positive symptoms* (delusions, hallucinations, and disorganization in thoughts, speech, and behavior), *negative symptoms* (social withdrawal, lack of motivation), *cognitive symptoms* (impairments in sustained attention, memory, and language), *hostility and excitement symptoms* (includes poor impulse control and violent behavior), and the *affective symptoms* (includes depression and anxiety symptoms) (DSM-5 2013). Of note, more than 50 % of patients with schizophrenia suffer from negative and/or cognitive symptoms in the prodromal phase (Seidman et al. 2010), during the phase of florid psychosis in which positive symptoms dominate (Schretlen et al. 2007) and even after the remission of these positive symptoms (Demjaha et al. 2012). Also negative and cognitive symptoms are found to be strong predictors of transition to the phase of florid psychosis in *ultrahigh-risk* samples (Koutsouleris et al. 2012) and are considered as indicators of poor prognosis and worse functional outcomes (Kirkpatrick et al. 2006).

B. Pradhan, MD (✉)
Department of Psychiatry, Cooper University Hospital,
401 Haddon Avenue, Camden, NJ 08103, USA
e-mail: Pradhan-Basant@Cooperhealth.edu

N.R. Pinninti, MD
Department of Psychiatry, Rowan University SOM,
Suite 100, 2250 Chapel Avenue East, Cherry Hill, NJ 08034, USA
e-mail: Narsimha.Pinninti@twinoakscs.org; narsimhanrp@gmail.com

© Springer International Publishing Switzerland 2016
B. Pradhan et al. (eds.), *Brief Interventions for Psychosis: A Clinical Compendium*, DOI 10.1007/978-3-319-30521-9_5

Global burden of psychosis is huge in terms of prevalence, comorbidity, dysfunctions, and healthcare cost. For example, the worldwide prevalence estimate of schizophrenia is around 1 %. Of note, schizophrenia is just one fraction of the whole gamut of psychotic disorders. One bothersome fact is that the persons with psychosis pose a high risk for suicide. Approximately one-third of patients with schizophrenia will attempt suicide, and, eventually, about one out of ten take their own lives (Kirkpatrick et al. 2006). Apart from this, psychotic illnesses pose a high burden on healthcare. For example, a Canadian study done a decade ago found that in schizophrenia, the costs from direct healthcare and non-healthcare when combined with the high unemployment rates due to schizophrenia and the added morbidity, mortality, and the loss of productivity did amount to a total cost estimate of 6.85 billion dollars (Goeree et al. 2005). It is clear from several well-designed studies that the duration of untreated psychosis (DUP) has impact on recovery from psychosis (Thirthalli et al. 2012). In one such longitudinal study (Cehnicki et al. 2014) that involved 20 years of follow-up, the authors noted that the relationship between longer DUP and worse overall treatment outcomes was sustained throughout the 20 years, and a positive correlation between DUP and the severity of psychopathological symptoms was observed over the first 12 years of illness. Taken together, these findings not only highlight the existing burden but also underscore the need for implementing effective interventions early in the course of psychosis so that further damages and dysfunctions could be prevented (Nicholl et al. 2010).

Treatment of psychosis should be comprehensive and include biological (medication) as well as psychosocial interventions. It is a fact that many patients with positive psychotic symptoms respond only partially or not at all (Conley and Buchanan 1997). Also functional improvement does not always follow the symptomatic improvement (Harvey et al. 2004). With emerging new understandings from recent research that examines the effectiveness of the pharmacologic and psychosocial interventions for psychosis and lived experiences of clients based on their stories of recovery from severe illnesses such as schizophrenia, the treatment goals for these clients is changing from symptom control to functional recovery, improved quality of life, and reintegration into the community (Kane 2004; American Psychiatric Association's Work Group on Schizophrenia 2004; Ragins 2012). Unfortunately, despite several therapeutic advancements, the current range of interventions for psychosis are only partially effective, and there are several unmet needs for this population. The unmet needs include the long DUP, trauma associated with psychosis not being addressed effectively, poor functional recovery, reduced longevity, and above all, the enormous burden on individuals, their families, and communities. As Insel (2009) points out, the reasons for premature death in individuals with severe mental illnesses include known consequences of cardiometabolic disease secondary to the use of second-generation antipsychotic agents but also less well-known factors such as trauma and loneliness (i.e., social disconnection), and hence addressing these is likely to have a positive impact on health and probably longevity. Yoga and mindfulness-based cognitive therapy for psychosis (*Y-MBCTp©*) is a newer evidence-based translational mindfulness therapy designed by Pradhan that can be used not only as a brief therapy in most instances to optimize resource utilization but also can be used in its extended format as well depending upon the treatment needs and available resources. This self-exploratory and client-centered therapy combines together the pragmatism and methodology of brief CBT for psychosis with the scriptural philosophies and techniques described in Patanjali's eight-limbed Yoga (Sanskrit: *Ashtanga Yoga*, Satchidananda 1978) and Buddha's mindfulness meditation (Pali. *satipatthana*, Nyanamoli 1975). This model of psychotherapy is our humble attempt to bridge across some of the gaps that exist in the psychotherapeutic realms for individuals with psychosis. In this chapter, we present a conceptual overview and pilot data on efficacy of *Y-MBCTp©* as a brief therapy model for clients with psychosis. In addition, in the various sections, we discuss cultural adaptability, replicability, and training implications of this model.

5.2 Cognitive Behavioral Therapy for Psychosis (*CBTp*)

Despite some remarkable progress in implementation of cognitive behavioral therapy (CBT), more so since 1990s, effective psychotherapeutic options for treatment of schizophrenia are still not at optimal levels and remain a big challenge to our field. Treatment refractory symptoms, stigma associated with mental illness and limited theraputic resources are the main reasons why effective psychotherapeutic interventions are not available for most people with psychosis. Importantly, whatever limited resources are there, many of them may have important issues with respect to their feasibility, affordability, acceptability, and difficulties in matching them in a culturally competent manner with the real-life situations of the individuals with psychosis. CBT, since its initial application by its founder Dr. Aaron Beck (1979) in patients suffering from depression, has come a long way in its applications in other psychiatric disorders including psychosis. It is being increasingly recognized that incorporating the therapeutic techniques into medication monitoring clinics is one way to improve access to therapy for patients with serious mental illnesses. However, despite psychotherapy's benefits, access to it is available only at select centers and thus is extremely limited. In one survey, only 7.3 % of patients with non-affective psychosis received at least "minimally adequate" care (four or more medication visits that did not include psychotherapy) (Wang et al. 2002). Also the duration (and quality) of psychotherapy in the medication clinics varies and usually range from 15- to 45-min sessions (Rector and Beck 2002).

As detailed in Chap. 3 of this book, the *cognitive behavioral therapy for psychosis* (*CBTp*, Kingdon and Turkington 2005) is a form of CBT specialized for individuals with psychotic disorders and teaches these clients about how to establish links between their thoughts, feelings, or actions with respect to current or past symptoms of psychosis and the accompanying dysfunctions. *These* interventions rely on Socratic dialogue, destigmatization and normalization of the psychotic features, building of coping skills, problem-solving, and implementation of behavioral experiments and help the clients to reevaluate/reappraise their perceptions, beliefs, or reasoning pertaining to these clinical symptoms which are the essential targets of these interventions. The first controlled studies on *CBTp* were conducted in the United Kingdom in the 1990s, and since then, emerging data from the various studies inform us that *CBTp* is an effective treatment for psychosis (Bond et al. 2005; Kingdon and Turkington 2005; Wykes et al. 2008; Naeem et al. 2014a, b; Habib et al. 2014) and can be done transculturally as well (Naeem at el. 2014a; Habib et al. 2014). Quite rightly, *CBTp* has been recommended by the national guidelines in both the UK and the USA.

5.3   Need for the Brief Version of *CBTp* (*Brief CBTp*)

Many individuals with psychosis prefer therapy sessions that are shorter and infrequent compared the the traditional one hour a week sessions. In fact, a study by Coursey et al. (1995) which involved 212 patients with schizophrenia, 85 % of the patients preferred psychotherapy sessions less often than once a week and preferred more pragmatic approaches, i.e., to focus on pragmatically solving the problems they encounter in their daily life. Also, the availability of the usual longer version of the CBT remains limited due to a myriad of factors including lack of awareness and lack of trained personnel (Kimhy et al., 2013). Thus, lately there is a trend to modify the usual sessions of CBT to *brief CBT* sessions. Rudd (2012) outlines some of the main differences between the usual version and the brief version of CBT with respect to the technical and process aspects as described below:

(i)   Brief CBT is purposefully brief to accommodate the time demands on the therapist whose resources are limited: this helps to cater more needy clients and also to decrease the waiting time for therapy.
(ii) Brief CBT incorporates all the common and effective elements of usual CBT and, in addition, is more focused on skills development.
(iii) It emphasizes internal self-management and encourages efforts geared toward self-exploratory therapy, mood regulation, and problem-solving skills in the client.
(iv) It provides more effective coping strategies to the client.

As Pinninti et al. (2005) have succinctly identified, the *five key steps* in carrying out the CBT interventions effectively during a therapy session are (i) to *identify* the problem the client wants to work on and to narrow it down; (ii) to *rate* the identified symptom or issue (using a simple 0–10 rating scale); (iii) to *choose and use* an intervention followed by *rating* the target symptoms again and to modify the intervention (if necessary) after getting client's feedback (post-vention); (iv) to *ask* client to write down what is learned on a card or in a notebook; and finally, (v) to encourage the client to have an *assignment at home* to reinforce the learning and generalization of the therapeutic gains. The *brief CBT for psychosis* (*brief CBTp*) incorporates these elements in order to meet some of the unmet clinical needs of the individuals with psychosis and could be an effective way to overcome some of the current barriers present in care of these needy individuals which includes but not limited to reduction in the waiting times for therapy, reduction of DUP, etc. Although there is lack of a clear definition of brief CBTp, empirically researchers have defined it as *an expedited form of CBTp which can be delivered in six to ten sessions conducted over less than 4 months* (Naeem et al. 2014b). Of note, the usual version of CBTp involves around 16 sessions (12–20 sessions), which is about twice the number of sessions needed for brief CBTp. Also these sessions in the usual CBTp are carried out over a longer period, i.e., over 4–6 months as compared to those in the brief CBTp. There are no differences qualitatively between these two versions although the brief version may be more intense nonetheless more targeted in approach. So far preliminary evidence indicates that *brief CBTp* is effective in reducing psychotic symptoms. However, the pioneers in this area opine that efficacy research on *brief CBTp* still has a long way to go, and more importantly, it still needs to address the fundamental issue of the *dose-effect relationship* with respect to its effect on symptoms/dysfunctions (Naeem et al. 2014b; Habib et al. 2014).

5.4 Clarifications on Some Concepts in Yoga and Meditation and Their Use in Healthcare

Yoga and meditation are probably among the most ancient mind-body medicine interventions that have shed light not only on the intricate, complex, and dynamic interplay between the body and mind but also has provided us with clear methods about how one can achieve physical, mental, and spiritual well-being. From ancient times, Yoga and meditation have been advocated not only as techniques but also rich philosophies, as a way of life and as a kind of psychosomatic preparation for spiritual elevation and alleviation of the sufferings of the mankind. Interestingly, health is not the goal, but rather is a by-product of the practice of Yoga and meditation. In the original traditions, maintenance of good health is primarily seen as a preparatory requisite for achieving the higher goals of life that Yoga purports to achieve (Iyengar 2001). Unfortunately, many concepts on Yoga and meditation are rather mystified and add to the existing misconceptions. For example, the terms "Yoga," "meditation," and "mindfulness" are often used interchangeably. It is important to understand that *Yoga, meditation,* and *mindfulness* are conceptually three overarching circles and belong to the broad scheme of Yoga. As proposed originally in the scriptural traditions of ancient India, Yoga used to be conceptualized in more holistic ways than it is generally understood these days. In these ancient spiritual traditions that advocated for the *eight-limbed Yoga* (Sanskrit: *Astanga Yoga*, Satchidananda 1978) in the Vedic traditions or the *Noble Eightfold Path* (Pali. *Atthangika Magga*, Nyanamoli 1975) in the Buddhist traditions, Yoga is all-encompassing and tends to span from one's lifestyle and life views to one's physical aspects that include one's body, breathing, and postures and eventually culminates in liberation of the individual from the sufferings of life by use of meditation (Eliade 1969; Dalai Lama 2009). In these ancient schemes that advocated for use of Yoga *in its entirety, Yoga comprised of eight limbs that include meditation as its sixth and seventh steps* (i.e., concentrative-type meditation [Pali. *samatha*] and mindfulness-type meditation [Pali. *satipatthana* or *vipassana*], respectively) (Nyanamoli 1975; Nyanaponika 1954; Pradhan 2014). Thus, mindfulness is a type of meditation, and Yoga is inclusive of meditation. Technically, Yoga involves balanced lifestyle (*that of moderation rather than of extremes, otherwise called as the Middle Way*, Dalai Lama 2009) and the psychosomatic preparatory stages that make oneself ready for meditation which is considered as the central aspect in the broad scheme of Yoga. *Meditation practice usually begins with cultivation of one's attention and induction of detached and nonjudgmental awareness* in which one learns how *to maintain and shift flexibly one's attention at will onto an object of choice* while disengaging oneself from the elaborative processing of these objects by one's mind. These *object of choice* can be *physical* (such as body parts or various physical objects), *physiological* (such as one's breathing, heart rate, etc.), or *mental* (such as one's thoughts, bodily feelings, emotional experiences, etc.).

One major objective of Yoga is to acquire deep insights into one's inner self which not only includes one's own abilities and coping but also requires one to use one's spiritual strength for well-being. Yoga and meditation interventions can be broadly conceptualized as self-management strategies for gaining insight into the principles of the human mind that explain the nature of its attending thoughts, feelings, and the various experiences. These insights help one realize the ways to reaccess the natural and positive states of mind and to experience sustained calmness regardless of the circumstances one encounters in daily life. As elaborated in the meditative philosophies passed down since millennia, when actions of the individual (Sanskrit: *jiva*) are governed by the meditative insights (which results in *wisdom*) rather than by just the reactionary responses to the underlying impulses, these *wise actions* don't bring *suffering* (Sanskrit: *dukkha*, which means *sadness* as well) (Nyanamoli 1975). Meditation is essentially an ongoing self-reflective cognitive-emotive-reappraisal process that takes place within the individual. It helps the individual to experience the various mind-body phenomena first hand, *directly and without distortion*. This results in increased self-knowledge (*insight*, Pali. *nana*) as well as deeper understanding into these various mind-body phenomena. *This enhanced level of self-knowledge forms the basis for use of meditation as a type of self-exploratory therapy.* The World Health Organization (WHO 2009) defines *health* as *a state of complete physical, mental, and social well-being and not merely the absence of disease or infirmity*. Taking a close look at the original concepts of Yoga, one can realize that the comprehensive view concept of Yoga which includes meditation as part of it has the biopsychosocial elements of health already ingrained in these eight limbs. In these concepts of Yoga and meditation, the prerequisites for achieving good health are already inbuilt. As *self-exploratory therapy and self-help models of care*, Yoga and mindfulness interventions combine humanistic models of treatment with the positive psychology of the client in strength-based ways. They promote the autonomy of the individual which could decrease the burden of care not only in the clients or their caregivers but also in the healthcare providers. Being mother to *Ayurveda* (the herbal medicinal system of ancient India), one can clearly see that Yoga doesn't negate the utility of appropriate pharmacological interventions, rather it supplements them (Frawley 1999). In addition to their utility as self-management techniques that empower the person, other benefits of these interventions are in terms of their low cost and lack of side effects when practiced under a trained teacher (Sanskrit, *Guru*) or drug-drug interactions that are the concerns typically seen with the use of the pharmacological interventions. Contrary to the beliefs that practice of Yoga and meditation is time consuming or difficult, authors of one recent study conducted at the Mayo Clinic (Prasad et al. 2011) note that even 15 min of daily meditation practice could significantly reduce stress and improve quality of life in the healthcare professionals.

Yoga and mindfulness interventions are complex and rather heterogeneous. Mindfulness-based interventions represent a group of cognitive and behavioral interventions using meditation. Historically they represent Buddhist practices to alleviate suffering (Kabat-Zinn et al. 1992; Ludwig and Kabat-Zinn 2008), and in modern days, they have been modified and integrated into present-day therapeutic practices. Like the usual CBT, mindfulness-based cognitive therapy (MBCT) functions on the theory that in pathological conditions such as depression, anxiety, etc., the normal psychological processes of thoughts, feelings, perceptions, etc., lead to either deliberate or automatic processes which are experienced as distressing and lead to dysfunctional behaviors. Mindfulness practice allows the practitioners not only to notice when these deliberate or automatic processes are occurring in them but also enables them to alter their reactions in *reflective* rather than reactive ways (Kristeller 2004; Felder et al. 2012). This is done by teaching participants to observe and acknowledge these processes without judgment and in the process not react to them. These Yoga and mindfulness interventions, as they are being used in psychiatric disorders, can be broadly categorized as two types: (a) nontargeted approaches which, as the name suggests, employ general or nonspecific use of Yoga and meditation, mostly for stress reduction or improving quality of life, and (b) targeted approaches that more specifically address the individual symptoms. The more known targeted approaches are *mindfulness-based cognitive therapy* (MBCT, Segal et al. 2002), *dialectic behavioral therapy* (DBT, Linehan 1993), *acceptance and commitment therapy* (ACT, Hayes et al. 1999), and *trauma interventions using mindfulness-based extinction and reconsolidation* of trauma memories (*TIMBER©*, Pradhan 2014). Despite some methodological difficulties involved in evaluating their efficacy in the various studies, Yoga and mindfulness interventions have been found to be feasible and effective in many mental illnesses, both in adults and children, e.g., schizophrenia (Vancampfort et al. 2012; Gangadhar and Varambally 2012), attention deficit and hyperactivity disorder (ADHD) (Zylowska et al. 2008), posttraumatic stress disorder (PTSD) (Brown and Gerberg 2005; Pradhan et al. 2015a, Pradhan and Sharma 2015), depression (Segal et al. 2002; Ludwig and Kabat-Zinn 2008; Pradhan 2015, Pradhan et al. 2015b), other anxiety and stress-related disorders (Kabat-Zinn et al. 1992), and substance abuse disorders (Brown and Gerberg 2005). Balasubramaniam et al. (2013) have written a comprehensive review on therapeutic utility of these interventions. Another recent study specifically examined efficacy of Yoga in subjects with schizophrenia. In this study, in a sample of 120 subjects with chronic schizophrenia that were stabilized on pharmacological therapy, 1-month training followed by 3 months of home practices of Yoga as an add-on treatment offered significant advantage over physical exercise or treatment as usual (Varambally et al. 2012). These authors concluded that Yoga holds promise as a complementary intervention in the management of schizophrenia.

5.5 Problems with the Piecemeal and Nontargeted Use of Yoga and Meditation Interventions and Need for Development of Targeted, Integrated, and Standardized Treatment Models

Yoga and meditation interventions are complex and heterogeneous and more often than not are not being used in a standardized manner. Yoga is to be used in a holistic and integrated manner rather than in *disjointed and piecemeal manner*. This fragmented use of Yoga, as often done in the Western World, restricts its scopes as well as utility and makes it more difficult for the integration of body and mind to occur. In this context, an interesting finding emerging from a review done in Vietnam veterans with PTSD is worth mentioning (Brown and Gerberg 2005). These studies find that although the physical aspects of yoga, such as physical postures (Sanskrit: *asana*), reduced some symptoms of comorbid depression in patients with PTSD, they had no impact on the hyperarousal symptoms, panic, or anger outbursts until meditative interventions including meditative breathing methods (Sanskrit: *pranayama*) and focused attention meditation were added. Thus, Yoga is more effective when its many elements are used in combined, synergistic, and targeted ways: this elaborative and integrated approach is in accordance with the ancient Indian scheme of eight-limbed Yoga (Sanskrit: *Astanga Yoga*) or the *Noble Eightfold Path* (Pali. *Atthangika Magga*) as they were proposed originally. Recent literature (Balasubramaniam et al. 2013; Pradhan and Sharma 2015) indicates that integrated use of multiple components of Yoga rather than their use in isolation or piecemeal, as individual components, is more effective in clinical trials. The piecemeal and nonstandardized use of Yoga and meditation not only limits their scope but also distorts these concepts. Also the nonstandardized and nonspecific approaches pose significant challenges in research when one tries to evaluate the comparative efficacy of the Yoga or meditation interventions across studies.

5.6 Yoga and Mindfulness-Based Cognitive Therapy (Y-MBCT©) Models and Their Adaptations for Use as Brief Therapies

Based on the insights from his *translational mindfulness* research and recognizing the strengths and limitations of traditional CBT as well as problems with piecemeal use of Yoga, Pradhan has developed seven new models of manualized psychotherapy which he calls as *Yoga and mindfulness-based cognitive therapy* (Y-MBCT). The psychosomatic adaptations for the therapeutic use of the Y-MBCT models are based on *two major themes in Yoga*: (i) *Yoga as a profound psychosomatic science* and (ii) *meditation as a science of attention*. The Y-MBCT models are holistic, translational, targeted, and standardized models of care and can be flexibly combined with other evidence-based treatments including medications and psychotherapeutic or cognitive behavioral interventions. As detailed in Pradhan (2014), the theoretical foundation of Y-MBCT models derives from the three original scriptural schools of Yoga and mindfulness, i.e., the eight-limbed Yoga (*Ashtanga*) of Patanjali (circa. fourth century BC), the mindfulness (*satipatthana*) model of Buddha (circa. sixth century BC), and the standardizations of the technique-rich style of *Tantra* (second century CE). The main meditation methods used in these models are the *samyama* (the combination of sixth, seventh, and eighth limbs of Yoga) combined with the Buddhist *satipatthana* method using the tripartite model of human experience and the five-factor model of mind. As illness-/disorder-specific models, all Y-MBCT models are extension of the wellness model (called, *Standardized Yoga and Meditation Program for Stress Reduction*: SYMPro-SR©, Pradhan 2014). Y-MBCT models combine all three main aspects of Yoga, i.e., yogic *philosophies*, *techniques*, *and practice* packaged together for their symptom-specific use in client's daily life. The results of this holistic practice are not only stress relief, symptom amelioration, or sustained calmness in daily life but also lifestyle modifications in form of creation of a balanced lifestyle and balanced life views (collectively known as the Middle Way in the Buddhist meditative traditions). This broader and integrated approach not only increases the scope of these interventions but also their efficacy and generalizability.

Conceptually and methodologically, the *Y-MBCT models*, like the dialectical behavior therapy (DBT), acceptance and commitment therapy (ACT), or mindfulness-based cognitive therapy (MBCT), could be categorized under the broader rubric of the *third wave cognitive therapy* (Kahl et al., 2012). The Y-MBCT models have been standardized for their *application* in psychiatric and psychosomatic conditions which range from depression, anxiety disorders, addictive and impulse control disorders, dyslexia and attentional disorders, psychosomatic conditions including chronic headaches, irritable bowel syndrome and dissociation/conversions disorder, and also tried lastly, in the psychotic disorders. In pragmatic and user-friendly formats, they have been standardized in developmentally informed and age-appropriate manner for their use in age group 7–70 years in multiethnic populations in evidence-based manner (for details, please see Pradhan 2014, p. 195–216; Pradhan 2015; Pradhan and Sharma 2015; Pradhan and Pinninti 2014a, b; Pradhan et al. 2014, 2015a, b). Compared to the often nonstandardized and piecemeal use of Yoga, as just a physical exercise or as a breathing technique or as an isolated meditation technique, as typically seen in the Western world, the holistic and sequential use of all eight steps of Yoga in flexible, personalized, and disorder-specific manner, as done in Y-MBCT, involves the use of Yoga *in its entirety* (i.e., *all eight steps*). These Y-MBCT interventions combine yogic lifestyle (Middle Way or lifestyle of moderation, Dalai Lama 2009; Pradhan 2014, p. 22–23,

115); the physical aspects of Yoga such as posture (Sanskrit: *asanas*, which means flexible positions *without allowing moving/fidgety*), yogic procedures (Sanskrit: *kriya*), and standardized breathing techniques; meditation techniques (both focused attention meditation and mindfulness meditation which belong to the fifth and sixth steps of Yoga) targeted toward individual symptoms and accompanying dysfunctions; and most importantly personalized counseling of the clients about the mindfulness philosophy that elucidates the workings of the human mind in normal and pathological states, as described in the scriptural traditions of Yoga (Satchidananda 1978) and mindfulness (Nyanamoli 1975). Of note, the focused attention meditation that cultivates a stable attention enhances one's executive functions including the problem-solving abilities and serves as a prerequisite for the other type of mediation, i.e., for mindfulness. The later type of meditation enhances calmness and frustration tolerance and decreases impulsivity and feelings of negative states such as anxiety, fear, depression, anger, etc. Apart from these important standardizations, in the Y-MBCT models, heavy emphasis is placed on *personalization of the meditative interventions* by using the data about each client obtained from the use of standardized instruments. These include the Assessment Scale for Mindfulness Interventions (ASMI©), the *five-factor inventory* based on the *five-factor model of human experience* (elaborated later), and *home practice log* (for detail descriptions, please see Pradhan 2014). These instruments help in enhancing adherence to the practice of the tools and generalization of the therapeutic gains to the daily life situations of the clients. In all the Y-MBCT models, the *five-factor inventory* serves as a personalized inventory for the therapist and client to elicit and quantify client's normal experiences as well as the psychopathology and pave the way to apply techniques and principles of brief CBT in targeted ways. The *five-factor inventory* is akin to the *thought record of CBT* and goes beyond the thoughts or feelings of client. As elaborated later, *it includes all five elements that form the fundamental building blocks of any human experience*, i.e., *one's thoughts, feelings, sensations/perceptions, memories, and the urges/will/impulses/energy that result in the various actionsor behaviors*.

5.7 Conceptual and Pragmatic Rationale for Y-MBCT for Psychosis (*Y-MBCTp©*) as a Brief Therapy

As described in various portions of this chapter, there are significant barriers to providing effective psychotherapy to individuals with psychosis, and these constitute the many gaps in the psychotherapeutic realms. These barriers are further exaggerated by the existing psychopathology (paranoid and hallucinatory symptoms, negative symptoms, i.e., lack of motivation, social withdrawal, etc.) These pathological symptoms also produce spurious experiences and distorted social meanings in the internal and external worlds of these individuals. This causes marked stress and dysfunctions not only in them but also can arouse negative feelings like fear, anger, frustration, etc., in the therapists, caregivers, or significant others. This can cause further alienations and may pose as significant barriers to providing empathic and effective care. Recent research shows that social isolation can, among other things, undermine our capacity to think clearly and regulate our emotions (Cacioppo and Patrick 2008). Also sociocultural barriers like stigma, therapist's own misconceptions that psychotic individuals are very prone to be violent on the therapist, etc., can come in the way of delivering care. On top of these ground realities, therapeutic resources for these individuals are quite limited. It is unfortunate that it is actually a luxury for these individuals to have a psychiatrist every month and to have a therapist frequently for their care. Even rarer is availability of a partial hospitalization program or an intensive case manager (ICM). Hence, development of better models of care including effective self-help models is necessary in which the clients and their families can be active and effective collaborators for their own healing. Also family members experience enormous caregiver burden that is not addressed adequately by the mental health system. Good news is that for many of these individuals, their families are involved in care and are their main support system. Yoga and mindfulness interventions are resilience promoting and effective self-help tools, both for clients and their families. Also they are inexpensive, accessible, and when culturally acceptable, can be combined with the pragmatic principles and tools of CBT. These can be standardized for their targeted use to ameliorate the impacts of stress, psychopathology, and attending dysfunctions. Thus, they are ideally suited to potentially circumvent some of the abovementioned important hurdles in care of these individuals and their families.

As an evidence-based and translational mindfulness therapy, Yoga and mindfulness-based cognitive therapy for psychosis (*Y-MBCTp©*) is designed to target some of the major clusters of psychopathology and attending dysfunctions. This therapy integrates, in a client-centered way, the concepts and tools of CBT with those of Yoga and mindfulness. In this translational psychotherapy, the *five-factor inventory* (Pradhan 2014; elaborated later) serves as a personalized inventory to elicit client's psychopathology. This rich and *experiential database obtained firsthand* from the client enables the therapist and client *to apply techniques of brief CBT in a targeted way* for amelioration of symptoms and attending dysfunctions. All the Y-MBCT models (*illness models*) including the Y-MBCTp© are adaptations and modifications of the *wellness model* (*Standardized Yoga and Meditation Program for Stress Reduction*, SYMPro-SR©; for more description, please see Pradhan 2014, p. 193–195). The two components in Y-MBCTp© are (a) the wellness component which is directed toward stress reduction in clients and their caregivers and (b) the symptom-specific component which is targeted toward amelioration of symptoms and associated dysfunctions. Taking into account the important role of stress in altering the individual's perceptions and its seminal role in perpetuating the dysfunctions, the SYMPro-SR model, as the name suggests, focuses on stress reduction. The *SYMPro-SR model* combines the integrated insights from the mindfulness philosophies with those from the stress-vulnerability hypothesis (Goh and Agius 2010; Zubin and Spring 1977) and makes the practice of the scriptural models of Yoga and meditation feasible to a common man. Thus, the interventions in the Y-MBCTp© model fit well not only with the symptom cluster model of psychosis but also with the stress-vulnerability model as well. The philosophies involved in the *SYMPro-SR* and

Y-MBCTp© models are based on a common fact that all human experiences lie in a continuum from normal to anomalous experiences. As elaborated in Chap. 2 of this book, the study of psychotic experiences (PE) in normal populations reveals that PE are seen in up to 15 % of the normal population at some point in their lives (Balaratnasingam and Janca 2015). Interestingly, many of these individuals do function normally although they are not in treatment. Research findings also support the notion that psychotic symptoms are best considered as "trans-diagnostic" entities on a continuum from normal to pathological and also that psychotic symptoms can be conceptualized with reference to normal psychological processes, whereby the content of symptoms is understandable and amenable to CBT (Harvey et al. 2005; Haddock and Slade 1996). These anomalous experiences are conceptualized as exaggerations of the normal experiences which become pathological based on the context of their origins and the dysfunctions they may cause to the individuals harboring them. The various cognitive models of psychopathology are in line with this fact. According to these models, hallucinations and delusions become transformed to severe pathological symptoms when these anomalous experiences that are commonly seen in the normal population are *misattributed in a way that has extreme, very personalized, and threatening personal meanings* (Garety et al. 2001; Morrison 2001). The concepts in these models elaborate upon the role played by the client's faulty beliefs, increased attention to threat-related stimuli, biased information processing of confirmatory evidence, and exaggerated safety behaviors (i.e., avoidance of specific situations) while the client is experiencing the psychotic symptoms. The emphasis in these is on the distress resulting not only from these difficult experiences but also and *more importantly from the meaning placed on those very experiences and the attending emotions and behaviors that influence these meanings in a personalized way*. SYMPro-SR not only introduces the client to the essential skills needed to subsequently master the *Y-MBCTp*© tools, but also its experiential style requires the therapist to actually practice this wellness model with the client during the initial training sessions. This wellness model for stress reduction serves as a foundational building block for both the client and the therapist that not only serves to reduce the stress in the individual with psychosis but also primes the client to successfully use the disorder-specific *Y-MBCTp*© model. *In addition it serves an important purpose of establishing the therapist's empathic attunement to the client's sufferings.*

These aspects greatly foster the adoption by the client of the subsequent home practice which is no longer just a *home work* but becomes a self-exploratory therapy in which the clients use meditative contemplation to practically link the five components of the human experience (behavior, thoughts, feelings included) and thus is able to access the insights and *become their own therapist*. In this *simultaneously* therapist-assisted (in-session) as well as self-help (at home or in the community) form of therapy, the therapist guides the client during a session, while the client uses the *Y-MBCTp*© tools as self-help during the period between two sessions. These unique aspects of *Y-MBCTp*© and its emphasis on the *continuum* from normalcy to anomaly (i.e., the illness models being extension of the wellness model) help in establishing a better therapeutic relationship and more effective delivery of and better adherence to these interventions. *In this experiential format, therapy is no longer just a verbal exchange of jargons* ("parroting") between patient and therapist but becomes more experiential and bring about a change in the individual that is carried on into the real world.

So far we have used *Y-MBCTp*© in combination with pharmacological or somatic treatments for individuals with psychosis.

5.8   *Y-MBCTp*© Is a Self-Exploratory Therapy That Uses Pragmatism of CBT and Amalgamates the Scriptural Mindfulness Philosophies with the Neurobiological Insights on Learning and Memory

In *Y-MBCTp*© the main method is the self-exploration of the client's inner world using the Yoga and meditation tools as well as the five-factor inventory (described later) in a detached and nonreactive manner which provides rich and real-world information about psychopathology, dysfunctions, as well as client strengths. This personalized and client specific information is used to decide on the appropriate interventions for the clients. The body of research on the nature of psychosis and its determinants indicates that many factors are relevant to the development of the symptoms in psychosis, ranging from neurodevelopment parameters and altered connectivity of brain regions to impaired cognitive functioning and social factors. There is increasingly emerging consensus to conceptualize *psychosis as a learning and memory disorder* (Tamminga et al. 2010; Liu et al. 2012; Ivleva et al. 2012). The hippocampus is altered in schizophrenic psychosis, with structural, functional, and molecular pathology. Psychosis is associated with increases in basal hippocampal activity and *reductions in associational and contextual memory processing* (Tamminga et al. 2010). These authors propose that psychosis is dependent on a pathologically increased level of neuronal function in CA3 (a crucial region of hippocampus that regulates memories), which exceeds the associational capacity of this subfield and results in mistaken and false associations, some with psychotic content. These mistaken associations are subsequently consolidated as normal memory, albeit with extreme personal and threatening meanings that are attached to relatively innocuous information. This learning process eventually makes these become the contents of the psychotic features, i.e., transform them to the *psychotic memories*. These pathological memories utilize normal neural pathways involved in the declarative memory that include the limbic and prefrontal cortical regions, even though they have psychotic content. One can also note that when an individual's mind feels threatened, as happens in the psychosis experience, the mind tries to collect all the information or evidences (factual, circumstantial, conjectural, contextual, perceived, and imagined) to substantiate that threat. Other body of evidence from cognitive neuroscience validates this fact. For example, Beck et al. (2009, p. 122) point out that in voice hearers, Wernicke's area which is responsible for the comprehension and processing (i.e., the *input aspects* of the speech) and Broca's area which is responsible for expression and fluency (i.e., the *output aspects* of the speech) are excessively coupled. In these brains, unlike in the normal brains, these two areas of the brain excessively feed each other and become less reliant on other areas of the brain, i.e., *they function in semiautomatic manner*. Also in this process, the language production area (Broca's area) "dumps" the language representations into the auditory language reception area (Wernicke's area), thereby creating hallucinatory percepts of the spoken speech in these individuals. Similarly, in the delusional experiences, abnormalities in functioning of the frontal lobe of the brain that includes but not limited to deficits in executive functions have been noted. As mind becomes preoccupied with *these misattributed information and their personalized meanings*, over time, *stress-vulnerability diathesis ensues, and* mind constructs and reconstructs the psychosis experience, layers over layers, using all these information obtained from all the five components of human experience, i.e., thoughts, feelings, sensations/perceptions, impulses/actions/behavior, and memories (described earlier). This is a new learning, and thus, *it is imperative that any in-depth therapy for the psychosis experience is essentially to reverse this process by another form of new learning* (or unlearning), i.e., to initiate a process of *deconstruction* of this multilayered experience. This *deconstruction* of the psychosis experience will require *novel approaches* that may include convergent and integrated insights from many disciplines, i.e., psychotherapeutic realms; experiential disciplines such as spirituality, cognitive neuroscience, multimodal brain imaging, and human tissue chemistry; and of course, behavioral testing. *Y-MBCTp©* attempts to incorporate some of these concepts and may promote new learning in these individuals.

As outlined in various literatures on the therapeutic utility of mindfulness techniques (Kabat-Zinn 1990; Lang et al. 2012; Pradhan 2014), the essential elements in mindfulness are cultivation of stable and focused attention and ability to flexibly shift it, self-introspection or self-exploration using the detached self-observation and reflection that provides insight into the fundamental building blocks of one's experience (the five factors, i.e., the thoughts, feelings, sensations/perceptions, will/urges/impulses that result in actions or behaviors, and the memories that accompany one's experience; described in more detail later). The result is development of compassion and non judgmental attitude towards self and others. These core elements are therapeutic in clients suffering from psychiatric disorders including the individuals with psychosis. It is well known from literature on psychodynamic psychotherapy that many of the dysfunctional thoughts and behaviors (delusions, hallucinations, etc.) of individuals with psychosis can be explained by *projection*, a core defense mechanism. *Meditation (concentration and mindfulness: the sixth and seventh limbs of Yoga) is an introspective self-analysis in which one uses one's own mind, body, and breathing as the tools to analyze one's own self and thus is conceptually anti-projective* (Pradhan 2014). Fact remains that because mind is the locus of all experiences, to effect a change of experience, one needs to work on one's mind and that work is nothing but meditation, a contemplative self-analysis in a detached way. However, because of the projective mechanisms (Sans. *vikshepa*), the mind, in a centrifugal manner, is constantly running away from this inner locus of experience, and the five components mentioned above are constantly assisting the mind in this process: mind with these five factors are co-creating and coloring these experiences at each moment. Because of this constant change and the centrifugal tendency of the mind to run away from the inner locus of all experiences, the person who is experiencing (the *experiencer*), the things being experienced, and the medium/interface one uses to experience these things (the mind with its associated thoughts, feelings, sensations, perceptions, will/urge/impulses that result in actions/ behaviors, and memories) are not able to work in a harmonious manner. This internal disharmony leads to the *distortion of our experience* (or illusion, Sanskrit: *maya*), leading to a state of cognitive-emotive-perceptual dissonance. Modern science calls it *stress*; yogic and meditative philosophies variously call it *dvanda* [Sans.] or *klesha* [Pali]. Projective mechanisms become markedly exaggerated in the psychotic or agitated or anxious (unmindful) states. Mindful or meditative states reverse the projective mechanisms in the mind by turning the mind inward (introversion) so that an introjective state ensues that is conducive for development of cognitive insight. Taking into account many of these factors mentioned above, we strategically conceptualized the *Y-MBCTp*© model with the aim to promote new learning in these individuals with severe mental disorders. The meditation component in the *Y-MBCTp*© is essentially cultivation of many important brain functions in the client that includes but not limited to cultivation of stable attention, enhancement of client's power of observation, and ability to reevaluate and reappraise the stressful situations/psychopathological symptoms in a detached manner so that extreme personal and threatening meanings are prevented from being consolidated. These are essentially important executive, evaluative, and regulatory functions governed by the frontoparietal and temporal areas of the brain which lower the impulsivity and enhance executive functions so that calmness ensues and *thought-driven* (rather than impulse driven) actions result. The wellness model (Standardized Yoga and Meditation Program for Stress Reduction:SYMPro-SR) which embraces the physical parts of the Yoga (posture, meditative breathing) and the lifestyle and life views of moderation (as done using the Middle Way philosophy which negates the extremes of lifestyle or life views) improves client's physical and social activity and the physical functioning (which mitigates the negative symptoms), promotes feelings of connectedness, and thus instills more hopes, optimism, and feelings of wellbeing. The added brief CBT interventions enhance these abilities further.

The self-help format of the *Y-MBCTp*© incorporates interested and available family members as co-practitioners and co-therapists. This serves three different purposes: (i) it could go some way mitigating the limited mental health resources available in treatment of these individuals and utilizing the family members as therapy extenders; (ii) *Y-MBCTp*© model has the wellness (SYMPro-SR) component that can help the family members to address their stress through practice; and (iii) a conjoint practice takes away the stigma associated with the client having to do something for their illness and changes the paradigm from *client-only* to one of *shared responsibility* for maintenance of health. Fortunately, now the social and healthcare system is involving peers in the delivery of mental health services, and training the peers in *Y-MBCTp*© can complement their lived experience of illness with skills that they could bring to the table. Below we describe some of foundational cornerstones of this model.

5.9   The Conceptual Foundations of the *Y-MBCTp*© Model

The following concepts about human mind and human experiences form the heart of the *Y-MBCTp*© interventions. These are succinctly described in the scriptures on yogic/mindfulness philosophies, i.e., the *Yoga Sutras*, the primary source textbook of Yoga (Satchidananda 1978), and the *Visuddhimagga*, the primary source Buddhist encyclopedia of meditation (Nyanamoli 1975). The *five-factor inventory*, the balanced views on life experiences (Buddha's *Middle Way*), and induction of detached observation, monitoring, and reappraisal of the psychosis experience using the *staged meditation protocols* (SMPs) form the foundational cornerstones of the *Y-MBCTp*© model. Below we describe some of these concepts:

(i) *Mind, the creator of all human experiences, is a bundle of five things*: One's mind, in mindfulness philosophies, is just another sense organ and is known as the *inner apparatus* (Sanskrit: *antah karana*, Pradhan 2014, p. 46). Mind is the creator and locus of all human experiences which are co-created by the five components, otherwise called as *aggregates* (Sanskrit, *skandhas*; Pali, *khandas*), i.e., one's thoughts, feelings, sensations/ perceptions, memories, and urge/ will/impulses which result in actions or behaviors (Fig. 5.1).

These components are *cemented together in a composite form* by the attending memories which provide a *personalized* context to the other four components which engage in a dynamic interplay and build up the total experience in a composite manner. Thus, these five components, by their dynamic interplay,

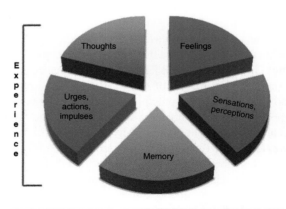

Fig. 5.1 Five factors model: any experience is co-creation of the five aggregates of the mind (Buddha, 6th cent. BC; Pradhan 2014)

co-create all the experiences including the experience of stress, happiness, sadness, the psychotic experience, etc. Importantly, *by changing these individual components of the experience, the composite experience as a whole can change.* Of note, memory (Sanskrit: *smriti, pratyaya*) is a crucial factor in this five-factor model because it tends to color the other four components, provides a contextual and temporal matrix for their expressions in an ongoing manner, and thus heavily influences one's learning processes.

The *five-factor inventory* (Fig. 5.2), developed by Pradhan (2014) based on the five-factor model, is another main tool in *Y-MBCTp*©. This is used to generate data on the content as well as the sequence of the five components as they come up during expression of the psychotic features in client's daily life or in therapist's office during trial of breathing meditation (elaborated later). Also this inventory helps to delineate the cognitive distortions and to identify maladaptive feelings, memories, or life experiences including the client's maladaptive urges/impulses, safety behaviors, and avoidance behavior that maintained the symptoms and dysfunctions in a vicious cycle. This inventory provides rich and personalized information on the psychosis experience of the client and helps the therapist to target the individual components of this experience using the brief cognitive behavioral therapy interventions in an individualized yet symptom-specific and structured way. This is akin to the *thought record* of traditional CBT but is more inclusive. The triadic model used in traditional CBT focuses primarily on one's *cognition, conation (behavior), and affect,* whereas the *five-factor model of human experience touches upon all five and thus is more inclusive.*

(ii) *All experiences are* representations *which can be changed by promoting new learning*: Mindfulness philosophies assert that all of the information derived by the mind based on the five components of human experience are just *represen-*

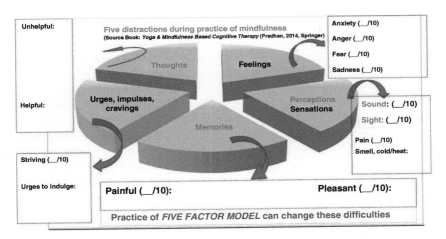

Fig. 5.2 The five-factor inventory: provides a rich data base to change one's difficult experiences

tations in the mind (Pradhan 2014). These representations, as the name suggests, are symbolic (akin to map rather than territory) and dependent on the quality/ state of the mind and brain during their acquisition and subsequent expressions. Also they change with change of the conditions that invoked these representations and thus are amenable to new learnings that result in new memories. This is true for the psychosis experience as well, which is amenable to new learning that provides new meanings or new associations to the existing information (i.e., the psychotic memories as described before). Recent research from cognitive neuroscience upholds this view and asserts that memory is *state dependent and changeable* (Pally 1997, 2005), and thus experience is prone to change as well. Meditative wisdom informs us that a*melioration of stress and healthy reappraisal of situations is possible by modification of the internal representations*: *this is done by achieving the meditative insight about the nature of these representations so that premature actions or cognitions* (*judgments, conclusions or biases,* etc.) *are prevented. Y-MBCTp©* model utilizes these principles for treatment of psychosis. Thus, breaking down the individual psychotic experiences (hallucinations, delusions, acting outs, etc.) which are a composite of the five basic components as mentioned above and eliciting the details of their sequence, form, and contents by using the quantitative *five-factor inventory* paves the way for modifying them further with mindfulness tool and the brief CBT interventions. The targeted and specific *Y-MBCTp©* tools help in de-escalation of arousal or fear symptoms in response to the psychotic experiences and also help to deconstruct the psychotic experience by inducing the detached observation and reappraisal of the five components of the psychotic experience. This detached observation helps the individual to move from the reactive state to a responsive state and also prevents the client from acting on the psychotic experience. This provides the *insight* (Pali. *nanna*) into the psychotic experience and thus provides new learnings and new meanings to the psychosis experience which eventually becomes no longer distressing or dysfunctional.

5.10   *Y-MBCTp©* as Brief Therapy and How It Attempts to Bridge Some of the Existing Gaps

Pradhan and Pinninti (2014a, b) recognized that CBTp could be used with *Y-MBCT* and after making some key adjustments, these could be applied in a brief format to individuals with psychosis. *Y-MBCTp©* is a brief therapy because it could be delivered in the brief format, i.e., using six to ten sessions conducted within a 4-month period. On average, sessions are about 30 min long. However, we also realize that sometimes sessions have to be shorter based on the mental state and preference of the client or when they are incorporated into medication management visits. Most of the data presented below if from therapy added to medication management visits. *Y-MBCTp©* as a brief therapy consisted of six to ten individual therapy sessions taken over less than a 4-month period (two initial training sessions taken weekly followed by next four to eight sessions taken at twice a month frequency) that includes one (or more) session(s) for the family member(s) who acted as co-therapist(s). Wherever possible, the involvement of family member should be in the first or second session to get their involvement from the beginning and also for added support that could enhance motivation and therapeutic engagement of clients. After stabilization of symptoms and dysfunctions using the six to ten sessions of *Y-MBCTp©*, the clients can be stepped down to less intense model of care for maintaining the therapeutic gains. In some instances the six to ten sessions may open up avenue for conducting more extensive trauma work, more so in clients with *traumatic psychosis* (for details, please see Kingdon and Turkington 2005). Hence, further sessions may be necessary to use the TIMBER© (trauma interventions using mindfulness-based extinction and reconsolidation of trauma memories, Pradhan 2014; Pradhan et al. 2015a, b) therapy, a model designed to specifically address the significant trauma symptoms in clients. For example, in author (Pinninti)'s case load, one client is currently in the 20th session and engaged in dealing with extensive childhood trauma that triggered psychotic symptoms whenever she tried to deal with it in the past. With the use of TIMBER©, she has currently developed the resilience to process her trauma experience without relapsing into psychosis.

Although *Y-MBCTp©* sessions are conducted flexibly and in personalized manner, the sessions typically focus on the following: (i) case formulation and psychoeducation; (ii) normalization and introduction to stress-vulnerability model and how human mind has been conceptualized in the mindfulness philosophy, as described before; (iii) establishment of a personalized, client-centered schedule for practice of standardized meditation protocol (SMP) in a culturally competent manner; (iv) working with hallucinations by STOPP module (an acronym) and by mindfulness-based graded exposure therapy (MB-GET, Pradhan et al. 2014); (v) working with delusions by STOPP module (an acronym, Figs. 5.3 and 5.4) and by behavioral experiments; (vi) working with negative symptoms by activity scheduling and by utilizing physical aspects of Yoga (postures, energizing breathing methods); and finally, (vii) termination of work and relapse prevention.

In the *Y-MBCTp©* model, stigma is addressed in three ways: (a) *normalizing* the human experience, i.e., by providing information that some of these experiences are actually fairly common in the general population; (b) that all experiences are derived from the same five factors of mind that are universal; and (c) that human experiences are changeable by changing each of the five components and thus can be controlled or modified in therapeutic ways. Also clients are provided with reading and audio-visual materials on the Yoga and meditation tools, the Middle Way philosophy, the five-factor model, the stress-vulnerability model, and brief CBT techniques including the mindfulness-based graded exposure therapy (MB-GET) and coping mechanisms. Client's negative beliefs and assumptions about the diagnosis and prognosis of psychosis are identified, and they are counseled about the role of stress and how that can be handled by the mindfulness tools as used in the SYMPro-SR model of wellness. Compared with CBT sessions for other disorders, these sessions are often shorter in length and much more flexible. Also in these sessions, homework is simplified, and the therapist practices meditation with the client. This makes it easier for client to model into and reduces the perceived power

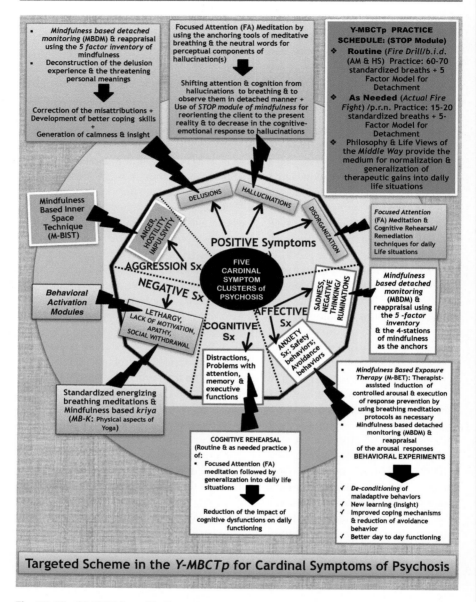

Fig. 5.3 The *Y-MBCTp*© graphic. Targeted scheme in the *Y-MBCTp* for cardinal symptoms of psychosis. Details on concepts, techniques & practice of mindfulness intervention can be found in the book: *Yoga & Mindfulness Based Cognitive Therapy: a Clinical Guide* (Pradhan 2014, Springer Publishers)

differential between the client and the therapist. The five-factor inventory is used to generate data on the content as well as the sequence of the five components present in the expression of the psychotic features, to delineate the cognitive distortions, and to identify maladaptive feelings, maladaptive urges/impulses, safety behaviors, the avoidance behaviors, as well as other coping skills. Cognitive biases are directly

STOPP Module for Mindfulness Practice©

AS NEEDED PRACTICE (FIRE FIGHT): to be practiced in the stressful situations

➤S-Stress!!   STOP for a moment !

➤T-Three mindfulness breaths THROUGH NOSE; NO MOVEMENT except breathing.

➤O-Observe (*the 5 components of the stress experience: thought/feeling/sensation/urge-action/memory; just acknowledge them by using neutral words; gently redirect attention to the breath*). This is the profound MIDDLE WAY philosophy of the mindfulness traditions.

➤P-Practice (establish *breathing home base* + induce further *detached observation of the 5 things & how sequentially they created the stress experience*).
Usually **20 slow breaths are enough** to bring back the calmness: **takes < 5 minutes !**

➤P-Proceed with planning the next course of action after calmness is attained.

ROUTINE PRACTICE (FIRE DRILL)
(routine practice enhances the as needed practice in daily life situations & vice versa)
❏ **70 breaths: ONCE daily minimum (no fidgety: just breathe slowly from belly through nose)**
❏ **After 70 breaths: Take 2 minutes to plan the next set of actions you want for the day**

❏ **SELF-MONITORING of meditation routine-By PRACTICE LOG**

Fig. 5.4 STOPP module for symptom-specific mindfulness practice

addressed by CBT predominantly through focusing on the content of thoughts and styles of thinking and inducing the detached reappraisal and reattributions to correct this in a *compassionate manner*. The individual's personal meaning, understanding, and coping with symptoms are actively encouraged, and safety/avoidance behavior is handed by mindfulness-based graded exposure therapy (MB-GET, Pradhan 2014, p. 197; Pradhan et al. 2014). Thus, rooted in the ancient Eastern wisdom in form of the *five-factor model* of human experience and the balanced view and lifestyle of the Middle Way philosophy and embracing the Western pragmatisms involved in the concepts and therapeutic tools of the CBT, the *Y Y-MBCTp©* model is a translational, tiered, and targeted (3Ts) therapy and serves as a bridge builder that attempt to meet some of the complex treatment needs of the individuals with psychotic disorders in their real-life situations. In this stepped care approach, depending upon the clinical needs, cultural background, and the level of readiness of the client, the *Y-MBCTp©* interventions can be upgraded in a tiered, client-centered, and disorder-specific manner to handle other comorbid psychiatric conditions. Some of these are TIMBER© for PTSD symptoms; Depression-Specific Y-MBCT (*DepS Y-MBCT©*, Pradhan 2015) for depression and non-OCD and non-PTSD type of anxiety symptoms; Mindfulness-Based Graded Exposure Therapy (*MB-GET*) for OCD symptoms; Mindfulness-Based Rehabilitation of Reading, Attention, and Memory (*MBR-RAM©*) for cognitive disorders; and Mindfulness-Based Inner Space Technique (*M-BIST©*) for addictive disorders and Mindfulness-Based *Kriya* (*MB-K©*) for psychosomatic symptoms (described in Pradhan 2014). The *Y-MBCTp©* graphic below (Fig. 5.3) demonstrates the symptom-specific applications of the various *Y-MBCTp©* interventions in this regard.

5.11   How the *Y-MBCTp*© Interventions Are Conducted?

In *Y-MBCTp*©, after the initial two to three therapist-assisted training sessions of the clients, the self-help format using the home practice module can be quickly introduced to the clients. Identification of a caregiver as a co-therapist definitely expedites this process. The main are in-depth assessment, gathering personalized data from client by using the *five-factor inventory* (Fig. 5.2) and engaging him/her in a *trial of breathing meditation*. The five-factor inventory, in addition to providing very important data about clients' inner world including the cognitive distortions, tendency to act out, inner feelings, and the important (traumatic) memories, also helps them to discover the obstacles that present naturally during practice of meditation at therapist's office or at home. The data obtained from the five-factor inventory are used to formulate a treatment plan in order to implement the *Y-MBCTp*© interventions through therapist-assisted sessions as well as by home practice sessions after the initial training process is over. These sessions have specific goals. For example, the session goals for delusion and hallucinations are (i) engaging and sharing of information about the paranoid beliefs and the voices; (ii) exploring client's level of understanding about the stress-vulnerability model of psychosis and how SYMPro-SR model of wellness training can help with stress reduction and better coping; (iii) exploring client's beliefs about hallucinations and the delusions; (iv) elicitation of a controlled arousal response (stress response) in the clients due to these voices and the paranoid beliefs by the use of the tools of mindfulness-based graded exposure therapy and training them on *STOPP module of mindfulness* (an acronym, Fig. 5.4) to quickly desensitize them and to de-escalate this controlled arousal and to prevent their outbursts; and (v) developing effective coping strategies including personalizing an overall model of coping with the voices. Throughout the whole course of Y-MBCTp, provision of optimism, hope, and positive reinforcement is maintained to improve adherence to practice of *Y-MBCTp*© and to improve self-esteem.

Toward the end of each session, the discussion is typically focused on establishing a personalized and targeted home practice schedule using the *standardized practice log*, how to handle obstacles to practice, and setting the agenda for the next follow-up session.

The *trial of breathing meditation* consists of asking the client to stay focused on 10–15 standardized breaths as demonstrated by therapist (usually done over less than 5 min period) and to note the distractions that take client's focus away from the breath. The distractions are neutralized by categorizing them under any of the five components mentioned before, and thus instead of letting the mind run behind any of these five things at any time (the elaborative mode of mind), client can mentally say "just a thought and come back to the breath"; "just a feeling, come back to the breath"; and try to shift the focus to the meditative breath. These phrases are not content laden: they are "neutral" rather than "extreme" and thus follow the philosophy of Middle Way (i.e., behaviors and life style of moderation rather than extremes). This attentional practice using the meditative breathing and the neutral phrases shifts the focus from the psychopathology to one's breathing and helps them to start developing the detached/nonreactive monitoring style. During this trial, client's psychotic symptoms can be a source of distraction from the breath and are handled in the abovementioned detached/nonreactive way. Once the *focused attention* (FA) is established, then the client can further proceed in the *detached monitoring mode* by maintaining the same meditative breathing established earlier and using neutral words for each of the five components as they ensue in the awareness. Once this second stage, i.e., *mindfulness-based detached monitoring* (MBDM), is established, client can mentally note the sequence in which the five components arise in the awareness during this practice without reacting to them using the FA and MBDM methods. Once client is calm enough, he/she can use the five-factor inventory to elicit detailed information on the contents of the psychosis experience present at that time. This is a *guided self-exploratory way* and may include getting the details of the sequence of one's thoughts, feelings, impulses, memories, and bodily sensations/hallucinations (sounds, visions) in the imaginative exposure situation in presence of the therapist. This method encourages the client to *just monitor and reappraise these components without reacting*. This detached reappraisal not only prevents acting on the psychotic symptoms (which in uncontrolled states usually results in outbursts or on some occasions dangerous behavior including violence) but also provides better coping mechanisms, prepares client for doing more in-depth work using five-factor inventory and brief CBT, and, if practiced consistently over a period of time, will result in new learning in which the meanings and associations are much less threatening or anxiety provoking. It is important to understand that although the focused breathing meditation that forms one of the cornerstones of the *Y-MBCTp©* is a simple method, we have observed that if not explained properly and the therapist is not careful enough to notice, clients may get caught into a *striving mode* in which *rather than meditating on the breathing, they will be striving to do the perfect breath*. In our experience, this *striving* becomes the biggest obstacle to the practice of meditation. Thus, it is important, particularly during the training sessions, to *let the model fit the client and not to try to fit the client into the model*, which we believe is a cardinal principle in any client-centered therapy. Also, for a successful application of the *Y-MBCTp©* model, the therapist has to have training and should be practicing the wellness model himself/herself.

5.12 The Structure and Flow of the *Y-MBCTp©* Therapy Sessions

Below is a brief description of the structure and flow of the *Y-MBCTp©* sessions:

(A) *Assessment Phase* (therapist assisted two sessions, once a week frequency):
   Session 1 (*mindful* assessment and psycho-education): The initial history taking involves having the client's spontaneous narrative account of the psy-

chosis experience in first person, while the therapist maintains a mindful state by practicing the SYMPro-SR model. Of note, establishment of a mindful and nonreactive state in therapist engages the mirror neuron system that modulates empathy and compassion circuits in the brain and helps the client to move toward a mindful state (Pradhan 2014). Individuals with psychosis show deficits in mirror neuron system (Pridmore and Dale 2009), and therapist being in a mindful state can help bring this state in clients. As part of this assessment, the Assessment Scale for Mindfulness Interventions (ASMI, 2014, 1015a) is done, while client is in waiting room. This scale provides rich information on client's level mindfulness, his/her deficits in the seven dimensions of mindfulness, and how to personalize the interventions to address these deficits. In this session, administration of psychopathology-specific rating scale(s), e.g., Psychotic Symptom Rating Scales (PSYRATS, Haddock et al. 1999), can be done as well. However, we do recognize that busy clinicians in routine clinical may not use these scales and would rely on clinical evaluations. Psycho-education of client and family on the *SYMPro-SR* model and *Y-MBCTp*© tools is done at this session.

Session 2 (trial breathing meditation and introduction of the five-factor inventory):

This session involves practice of 15–20 standardized mindful breaths. This is followed by psycho-education on mindfulness philosophy and techniques. Also client is trained on how to establish a home practice of SYMPro-SR (wellness) model. In SYMPro-SR, the client is trained on the staged meditation protocol (SMP) by which he/she converts the breathing (which is a physical action) into a *breathing meditation* by sequential use of the third to seventh limbs of the eight-limbed Yoga. In *breathing meditation*, both focused attention (FA) and detached monitoring of the breathing are established gradually. This module takes about 10 min initially, but with practice, even 5 min is enough. Once this basic action, i.e., the breathing, is transformed to a breathing meditation, then generalization is ensured by encouraging the client to transform other actions in daily life (e.g., walking, eating, etc.) to a meditation. This involves cultivating the focused attention state as well as establishing awareness and detached monitoring or non-activity (detachment) in one's daily life situations. If there is more time available in the first session, the interventions of the first and second sessions can be done in one session.

(B) *Symptom-Specific Intervention Phase* (therapist assisted four to eight sessions, once every 2 weeks):

This phase is geared toward the symptom-specific application of *Y-MBCTp*© which is broadly in two types: (i) the in-session, therapist-assisted training to gain mastery over the symptom-specific application and (ii) the home-based training of the client for application of these tools at home or in the community for quick control of symptom exacerbation or dysfunctions. The brief CBT interventions incorporated in this phase help client to use the meditation interventions in more individualized, client-centered, systematic, targeted, and measurable ways. The goals at this phase are to train the client on the imaginative exposure (to controlled situations that triggers outbursts) and mindfulness-based graded exposure therapy (MB-GET, Pradhan 2014, p. 197; Pradhan et al. 2014) and symptom-specific STOPP module and to establish more regularities and quality in the home practice. This is done in the following ways:

(i) To establish in the client his/her awareness of body, breathing, and autonomic (arousal/fear) response and the sequential involvements of the five components in the five-factor inventory in situ during a psychotic/aggressive outburst. In this step, if client is not actively experiencing symptom during the session, the techniques of imaginative exposure are employed in which during practice of meditation, client imagines a less distressing memory from his/her personal pyramid of troublesome memories about situations (graded from 10 to 100 % distress) related to the voices/delusions/anger, etc. After eliciting mild arousal response in a controlled way, STOPP module is used to quickly reorient the client to the focused attention (FA) breathing meditation and mindfulness-based detached monitoring (MBDM) method described before, to quickly de-escalate the arousal and reappraise in a calm manner. Once the client is able to do this, then he/she is asked to study the sequence of symptoms experienced in his body and mind during a psychotic/affective outburst. In this exercise, emphasis is placed upon identifying the first concrete symptom during such an outburst (which is usually a clear hallucination or a feeling of fear or anger or a bodily symptom like racing heartbeat or a-panic like symptoms or sense of discomfort, etc.) and establishing a window of opportunity to intervene before the client acts on this experience in a maladaptive way. The window of opportunity for a psychotic/affective outburst is essentially the brief time gap (usually a few seconds to a few minutes) between the first concrete symptom (the warning signal) and the client's maladaptive response. In this *window of opportunity*, the client is encouraged to practice the breathing meditation (third to seventh limbs of the eight-limbed Yoga) in sitting or lying down posture so that the client is able to de-escalate the impact of the psychotic/affective outburst including the fear/anger response or the behavioral response. The routine home practice twice daily and many times as needed ensures that the client uses this effectively.

(ii) Training on the philosophy and practice of the Middle Way (Pradhan 2014, p. 22–23, 115) to decrease extreme behavior and to generalize the therapeutic gains to daily life situations. Of note, by training clients to adopt the Middle Way lifestyle, the striving or "driven doing" mode of functioning is changed to more "doing" and "being" (experiential) modes (Pradhan 2014). The lifestyle and life views of *moderation* rather than the extremes, as advocated by the Middle Way philosophy, promote the subsequent generalization of meditation into client's daily life.

The home practice by clients involves two types of practices using the standardized practice log:

(i) The *routine* practice (*fire drill* mode of practice: longer version) involves the use of imaginative exposure technique and MB-GET. This practice involves practice of 60–70 meditative breaths over 15–20-min period, twice daily (BID: sitting posture in the morning, either sitting down or alternately lying down posture on the bed before going to bed in the night).

(ii) The *as needed* practice (*fire fight* mode of practice: shorter version) involves practice of 10–20 breaths over 5 min time, as many time needed, during the course of the day. This helps to lessen the frequency, intensity, and impact of the outbursts (due to hallucinations, delusions, affective, or anxiety symptoms) as they spontaneously arise in the client during the course of events in their daily life. This shorter version is actually intended to quickly reorient the client to the present moment and to de-escalate the arousal/fear/anger response by using the STOPP module (Fig. 5.4).

The various (nine) obstacles that may come during meditation practice are described in Pradhan (2014, p. 236–238). Throughout the course of treatment, care is taken to enhance coping, adherence to treatment, and enhancement of functioning in daily life by the use of client-centered approaches and brief CBT techniques including the use of coping cards and other behavioral modules (as shown in Fig. 5.3).

5.13   Pilot Data on Efficacy of *Y-MBCTp* as a Brief Therapy

We present the results of this pilot study which consisted of an open trial with eight sessions (30–45 min duration each) of *Y-MBCTp©* conducted over a period of 14 weeks in five female subjects (one adolescent, three adult, and one geriatric) with non-affective psychosis. The *Y-MBCTp©* sessions were feasible (with some adjustments as described later) and, contrary to our initial apprehensions, were remarkably well accepted by patients and among these five clients, there was no dropout. There was high acceptability, feasibility, and patient satisfaction in the patients (and their family members where involved) who continued the *Y-MBCTp©*. The results depicting levels of psychopathology as well as functioning pre- and post-*Y-MBCTp©* interventions are shown in Table 5.1.

Although the initial three training sessions were carried out at once a week frequency, the subsequent five sessions of *Y-MBCTp©* (includes one family therapy session which in addition to training of *Y-MBCTp©* modules also involved psychoeducation and identification of a family member as a co-therapist at home) were done at a frequency of once in 2–3 weeks. In clients 4 and 5, the sessions were once in 2–4 weeks based on therapist schedule and clients' convenience. All patients had incurred significant trauma (sexual abuse in four patients and emotional and physical abuse in one patient) early on in their lives, and all of them had significant

Table 5.1 Results of the pilot sample of *Y-MBCTp*

Clients with psychosis ($n=5$, all females)	Age (years)	PSYRATS[a] scores at baseline (hallucination, delusions, total scores)	GAF scores at baseline	PSYRATS scores after 8 sessions (hallucination, delusions, total scores)	GAF[b] scores after 8 sessions
#1	27	33/44, 17/24, 40/68	21–30	(18/44, 12/24, 30/68)	41–50
#2	36	(37/44, 19/24, 56/68)	11–20	(13/44, 8/24, 21/68)	51–60
#3	16	(41/44, 20/24, 61/68)	21–30	(15/44, 9/24, 24/68)	51–60
#4	72	(21/44, 10/24, 31/68)	51–60	10/44,4/24, 14/24	61–70
#5	29	(18/44, 19/24 37/68	35	Not completed 8 sessions	

[a]PSYRATS (The Psychotic Symptom Rating Scales, Haddock et al. 1999) has two parts: part A is for hallucinations and has 11 items (rated from 0 to 4; thus, maximum score is 44), and part B is for delusions and has 6 items (maximum score 24). Total scores on all items of PSYRATS are 68
[b]GAF (Global Assessment of Functioning scale, Luborsky 1962) is a numeric scale (1 through 100) used by mental health clinicians and physicians to rate subjectively the social, occupational, and psychological functioning of adults

anxiety and affective symptoms as well in addition to delusions, hallucinations, disorganizations, and impulsive and aggressive behaviors. One patient had prominent negative symptoms (apathy and social withdrawal) as well. Among the five clients, two patients (one adolescent and one adult) have achieved remission of psychotic symptoms, and two adults had significant reduction in symptoms. Of note, two of them could be off the antipsychotic medications after five to six sessions of *Y-MBCTp*©. By using the STOPP technique, they were able to deal with hallucinations, delusional beliefs, anxiety, and angry outbursts, and one person stopped dissociation as well. However, in the third client (adult), eight sessions of *Y-MBCTp* have resulted in marked reduction of positive symptoms, anxiety symptoms, and dissociative symptoms and the associated dysfunctions but she needed to remain on a fixed dose (600 mg/day) of Quetiapine. Her symptoms, although markedly reduced at this time, have not yet reached at the level of remission. Of note, her dissociative and aggressive symptoms including acting on her command hallucinations and delusions stopped within three sessions of *Y-MBCTp*. Of the five subjects, the geriatric subject had used a sealing over coping strategy to dealing with sexual abuse which led to intrusive sexual thoughts that were distressing (Tait et al. 2004). Using *Y-MBCTp*, she was able to unseal the experience and talk about it for the very first time leading to affective unfolding and integration of that experiences into her life. She reports significant improvement in quality of her life following the disclosure. The fifth client was showing impulsive behaviors of acting out on delusions, and hospitalization was considered. She is now able to talk about her delusional beliefs with therapist in a detached way and is not acting out on her beliefs.

5.14 Below Is a Description of Certain Modifications That Are Necessary for the *Y-MBCTp* Model Compared to the Other Y-MBCT Models

Efficacy studies on psychotherapy have informed us time and again that therapeutic alliance and adherence are the two main parameters for successful application of any treatment. As described in Pinninti et al. (2005), to develop an alliance with individuals with psychosis and to maintain their adherence to the treatment, the first task is to help them leave each session feeling understood, validated, and enjoying the therapist's company. The four cardinal principles for dealing with psychosis are normalization, universality, collaborative therapeutic alliance, and focusing on the patient's life goals and translating them into treatment goals. Because only one or two therapeutic interventions can be tried during a brief therapy session, problems need to be prioritized. One can save time by giving patients out-of-session assignments that include home practice sessions, providing simple semiquantitative questionnaires/rating scales to collect important information to review with patients during the next monitoring session and most importantly to help empower patients to manage their symptoms using self-help approach.

Apart from the abovementioned things, depending upon the individual situations, therapist may choose one or more of the following modifications:

1. In very disturbed clients, it is good to decrease verbal therapy and increase non-verbal components. Also it is better to use short sentences and neutral rather than emotional words. In general, more supportive stance is helpful.
2. Modified meditation techniques: During focused attention meditation practice, one can start with more concrete, graspable, and easy to use objects as the initial anchoring objects for cultivating focused attention. In some clients, depending upon the level of regression, transitional objects may be necessary. For example, in some of our clients with severe psychopathology, soft toys helped them relax and get inducted to focused attention state easier; this also decreased their paranoia and enhanced their level of participation. The goal is to use a firm sitting posture and hold a concrete object (like soft toy) to prevent all the movements/fidgety and then focus on body and breathing. Even lying down/leaning posture works fine.

5.15 Summary, Conclusions, Limitations, and Future Directions

Yoga and mindfulness-based cognitive therapy for psychosis (*Y-MBCTp*©) is a self-exploratory, client-centered translational therapy that combines together the pragmatism and methodology of brief CBT with the scriptural philosophies and techniques described in Patanjali's eight-limbed Yoga (Sanskrit: *Ashtanga Yoga*) and Buddha's mindfulness meditation (Pali. *satipatthana*). In this, the therapist and client practice together the wellness model first, which is followed by individualized use of the illness model. It can be done in nonverbal patients as well. *Y-MBCTp* as a standardized, client-centered, and symptom-specific treatment module not only trains the client and their caregivers for stress reduction and coping but also ensures in the client the cultivation of attention and induction of detachment from the frightening and distracting experiences of the psychotic/affective states and promotes new learning (insight) based on the client's reappraisal of the psychotic experience in a detached and calm mode. This also provides better coping and better insight and enhances the levels of functioning. These interventions are less stigmatizing and feasible in various age groups (when presented in developmentally appropriate language), have high adherence and client satisfaction rates, and have been well accepted by multiethnic populations. These interventions offer self-help and promote autonomy of patient and foster less dependence. As a psychotherapeutic modality, these can be used alone or, preferably, in combination with psychotropic medications. *Y-MBCTp as a brief therapy*, compared to the *routine Y-MBCTp* (*longer version*), uses the *expedited and stepped care approach* of brief therapy which makes goal directed in its applications but at the same time makes it more intense as well. Therefore, arguably it might not be suitable for every individual with psychosis, and some amount of planning on patient selection/suitability may be needed. As in any specialized form of therapy, there might also be differences in therapy when delivered by expert therapists compared to the non-experts. Brief CBT puts a greater burden on the patient to engage actively in treatment both during and between sessions, and thus patients with severe auditory hallucinations and delusions will need more supportive and engaging interventions during the *Y-MBCTp* sessions. Also for good reasons, there are many mysteries surrounding the evidence-based use of Yoga-meditation interventions. Thus, it is quite possible that patient's existing paranoid beliefs may interfere with adequate implementations of the *Y-MBCTp* interventions; however, our preliminary work on these five subjects and ongoing work with other patients with severe psychosis don't seem to substantiate these apprehensions. It has to be recognized that all five clients have history of significant abuse and they fit the category of traumatic psychosis (Kingdon and Turkington 2005). Whether *Y-MBCTp* works as well with other types of psychosis needs to be determined, and we are in the process of doing the same. Although preliminary, these data show that *Y-MBCTp* is feasible and acceptable to patients and is effective in inducing remission of symptoms of psychosis. Significant limitations include but not limited to its preliminary nature, open trial design, and the very small sample size. It is obvious that these findings need replication in larger trial and *Y-MBCTp* has a long way to go.

Contribution of Each Co-author to This Manuscript Development of the *Y-MBCTp* model, done by Dr. Pradhan, and conduct of *Y-MBCTp* sessions at the two sites and manuscript preparation, collaboratively done by Drs. Pradhan and Pinninti.

Acknowledgments We acknowledge and deeply appreciate the support of our clients, the clinicians, and the staff of the Psychiatry Outpatient Department at the Cooper University Hospital, Camden, New Jersey, and at the Camden County ACT Team that helped us to apply the *Y-MBCTp* model to these clients with trauma and severe psychosis.

References

American Psychiatric Association's Work group on Schizophrenia (2004) Practice guidelines for the treatment of patients with schizophrenia. Am J Psychiatry 161(29(suppl)):26–27

Balaratnasingam S, Janca A (2015) Normal personality, personality disorder and psychosis: current views and future perspectives. Curr Opin Psychiatry 28(1):30–34. doi:10.1097/YCO.0000000000000124

Balasubramaniam M, Telles S, Doraiswamy PM (2013) Yoga on our minds: a systematic review of yoga for neuropsychiatric disorders. Front Psychiatry 3:117. doi:10.3389/fpsyt.2012.00117

Beck AT, Rush AJ, Emery G (1979) Cognitive therapy of depression, 1st edn. The Guilford Press, New York

Beck A, Rector N, Stolar N, Grant P (2009) Schizophrenia: cognitive theory, research, and therapy. Guilford Press, New York

Bond FW, Dryden W (2005) Handbook of brief cognitive behaviour therapy. John Wiley & Sons.

Bridge JA, Barbe RP (2004) Reducing hospital readmission in depression and schizophrenia: current evidence. Curr Opin Psychiatry 17(6):505–511.

Brown RP, Gerbarg PL (2005) Sudarshan Kriya Yogic breathing in the treatment of stress, anxiety, and depression: clinical applications and guidelines. J Altern Complement Med 11(4):711–717

Cacioppo JT, Patrick W (2008) Loneliness: human nature and the need for social connection. W. W. Norton & Company, New York

Cehnicki A, Cichocki L, Kalisz A, Bladzinski P, Adamczyk P, Franczyk-Gilta J (2014) Duration of untreated psychosis (DUP) and the course of schizophrenia in a 20-year follow-up study. Psychiatry Res 219(3):420–425

Conley RR, Buchanan RW (1997) Evaluation of treatment-resistant schizophrenia. Schizophr Bull 23:663–674

Coursey RD, Keller AB, Farrell EW (1995) Individual psychotherapy and persons with serious mental illness: the client's perspective. Schizophr Bull 21:283–301

Dalai Lama (2009) The middle way: faith grounded in reason. (T. Jinpa, Trans.). Wisdom Publications, Boston

Demjaha A, Valmaggia L, Stahl D, Byrne M, McGuire P (2012) Disorganization/cognitive and negative symptom dimensions in the at-risk mental state predict subsequent transition to psychosis. Schizophr Bull 38:351–359

Diagnostic and statistical manual of mental disorders: fifth edition (DSM-5 2013). American Psychiatric Association

Eliade M (1969) Yoga: for immortality and freedom, 2nd edn. Princeton University Press, Princeton

Felder JN, Dimidjian S, Segal Z (2012) Collaboration in mindfulness-based cognitive therapy. J Clin Psychol 68(2):179–186

Frawley D (1999) Yoga and Ayurveda: self-healing and self-realization. Lotus Press, Wisconsin

Gangadhar BN, Varambally S (2012) Yoga therapy for schizophrenia. Int J Yoga 5(2):85–91. doi:10.4103/0973-6131.98212

Garety PA, Kuipers E, Fowler D, Freeman D, Bebbington PE (2001) A cognitive model of the positive symptoms of psychosis. Psychol Med 31(02):189–195, http://doi.org/10.1017/S0033291701003312

Goeree R, Farahati F, Burke N, Blackhouse G, O'Reilly D, Pyne J, Tarride JE (2005) The economic burden of schizophrenia in Canada in 2004. Curr Med Res Opin 21:2017–2028

Goh C, Agius M (2010) The stress-vulnerability model how does stress impact on mental illness at the level of the brain and what are the consequences? Psychiatr Danub 22(2):198–202

Habib N, Dawood S, Kingdon D, Naeem F (2014) Preliminary evaluation of Culturally Adapted CBT for Psychosis (CA-CBTp): findings from developing culturally-sensitive CBT project (DCCP). Behav Cogn Psychother FirstView 1–9. 43(2):200–208. http://doi.org/10.1017/S1352465813000829

Haddock G, Slade PD (1996) Cognitive-behavioural interventions with psychotic disorders. Psychology Press: London.

Haddock G, McCarron J, Tarrier N, Faragher EB (1999) Scales to measure dimensions of hallucinations and delusions: the Psychotic Symptom Rating Scales (PSYRATS). Psychol Med 29:879–889

Harvey PD, Green M, Keefe RS, Velligan DI (2004) Cognitive functioning in schizophrenia: a consensus statement on its role in the definition and evaluation of effective treatments for the illness. J Clin Psychiatry 65(3):361–372

Harvey A, Watkins E, Mansell W, Shafran R (2005) Cognitive behavioural processes across psychological disorders: a transdiagnostic approach to research and treatment. Oxford University Press, New York

Hayes SC, Strosahl KD, Wilson KG (1999) Acceptance and commitment therapy: an experiential approach to behavior change. The Guilford Press, New York

Insel TR (2009) Translating scientific opportunity into public health impact: a strategic plan for research on mental illness. Arch Gen Psychiatry 66(2):128–133

Ivleva EI, Shohamy D, Mihalakos P, Morris DW, Carmody T, Tamminga CA (2012) Memory generalization is selectively altered in the psychosis dimension. Schizophr Res 138:74–80

Iyengar BKS (2001) Yoga – the path to holistic health. Dorling Kindersley, London

Kabat-Zinn J (1990) Full catastrophe living. New York, NY: Delacorte Press.

Kabat-Zinn J, Massion AO, Kristeller J, Peterson LG, Fletcher KE, Pbert L, Lenderking WR (1992) Effectiveness of a meditation-based stress reduction program in the treatment of anxiety disorders. Am J Psychiatry 149:936–943

Kahl KG, Winter L, Schweiger U (2012) The of cognitive behavioral therapies. Curr Opin Psychiatry 25(6):522–528

Kane JM (2004) Long-term treatment of schizophrenia: moving from a relapse-prevention model to a recovery model. J Clin Psychiatry 64(11):1384–1385

Kimhy D et al (2013) Cognitive behavioral therapy for psychosis—training practices and dissemination in the United States. Psychosis: Psychol Soc Integr Approaches 5(3):296–305

Kingdon DG, Turkington D (2005) Explanations of schizophrenia. In: Kingdon DG, Turkington D (eds) Cognitive-behavioral therapy of schizophrenia. Guilford Press, New York

Kirkpatrick B, Fenton WS, Carpenter WT Jr, Marder SR (2006) The NIMH-MATRICS consensus statement on negative symptoms. Schizophr Bull 32:214–219

Koutsouleris N, Davatzikos C, Bottlender R et al (2012) Early recognition and disease prediction in the at-risk mental states for psychosis using neuro-cognitive pattern classification. Schizophr Bull 38:1200–1215

Kristeller J (2004) Meditation: an integrated model across six domains of function. In: Blows et al (eds) The relevance of the wisdom traditions in contemporary society: the challenge to psychology. Eburon Publishers, Delft

Lang AJ, Strauss JL, Bomyea J, Bormann JE, Hickman SD, Good RC, Essex M (2012) The theoretical and empirical basis for meditation as an intervention for PTSD. Behav Modif 36(6):759–786. doi:10.1177/0145445512441200

Linehan MM (1993) Skills training manual for treating borderline personality disorder. Guilford Press, New York

Linscott RJ, J. van Os (2013). An updated and conservative systematic review and meta-analysis of epidemiological evidence on psychotic experiences in children and adults: On the pathway from proneness to persistence to dimensional expression across mental disorders. Psychological Medicine 43(6):1133–1149.

Liu X, Ramirez S, Pang PT, Puryear CB, Govindarajan A, Deisseroth K (2012) Optogenetic stimulation of a hippocampal engram activates fear memory recall. Nature 484:381–385

Luborsky L (1962) Clinician's judgements of mental health. A proposed scale. Arch Gen Psychiatry 7:35–45

Ludwig DS, Kabat-Zinn J (2008) Mindfulness in medicine. JAMA 300:1350–1352

Morrison AP (2001) The interpretation of intrusions in psychosis: an integrative cognitive approach to hallucinations and delusions. Behav Cogn Psychother 29(03):257–276, http://doi.org/10.1017/S1352465801003010

Naeem F, Habib N, Gul M, Khalid M, Saeed S, Farooq S, Kingdon D (2014a) A qualitative study to explore patients', carers' and health professionals' views to culturally adapt CBT for psychosis (CBTp) in Pakistan. Behav Cogn Psychother 1–13, http://doi.org/10.1017/S1352465814000332

Naeem F, Farooq S, Kingdon D (2014b) Cognitive behavioral therapy (brief versus standard duration) for schizophrenia. Cochrane Database Syst Rev 4:CD010646

Nicholl D, Akhras KS, Diels J, Schadrack J (2010) Burden of schizophrenia in recently diagnosed patients: healthcare utilization and cost perspective. Curr Med Res Opin 26:943–955

Nyanamoli B (1975) The path of purification (Visuddhimagga). Buddhist Publication Society, Kandy

Nyanaponika T (1954) The heart of Buddhist meditation. Buddhist Publication Society, Kandy

Pally R (1997) How the brain actively constructs perceptions. Int J Psychoanal 78:1021–1030

Pally R (2005) Non-conscious prediction and a role for consciousness in correcting prediction errors. Cortex 41:643–662

Pinninti NR, Stolar N, Temple S (2005) 5-minute first aid for psychosis. Defuse crises; help patients solve problems with brief cognitive therapy. Curr Psychiatry 4(1):36–48

Pradhan BK (2014) Yoga and mindfulness based cognitive therapy: a clinical guide. Springer International Publishers, Switzerland

Pradhan BK, Pinninti N (2014a) Yoga & meditation: a standardized program for stress reduction in case managers for individuals with psychosis. Workshop presented in the annual conference of the National Association of Case Managers, Philadelphia

Pradhan BK, Pinninti N (2014b, ongoing work, unpublished) Workshop on Yoga and mindfulness based cognitive therapy for psychosis (Y-MBCTp) and its applicability in training the case managers of the Camden County PACT Team for delivering this therapy to individuals with psychosis

Pradhan BK, Sharma A (2015) The time has come for integrating complementary medicine into psychiatry. Adolesc Psychiatry (Spec Issue Complement Alternat Med) 5(2. Editorial (Thematic Issue)):71–72. doi:10.2174/2210676605021504301543421542

Pradhan BK, Pumariega AJ, Barnes A (2014) Successful use of mindfulness based graded exposure therapy (MB-GET) in adolescents with PTSD: a case series. Presented in the 21st world congress of the International Association for Child and Adolescent Psychiatry and Allied Professions (IACAPAP), Durban

Pradhan BK, Gray RM, Parikh T, Akkireddi P, Pumariega A (2015a) Trauma interventions using mindfulness based extinction and reconsolidation (TIMBER©) as monotherapy for chronic PTSD in adolescents: a pilot study. Adolesc Psychiatry 5(2. special issue on Complementary and Alternative Medicine):125–131. doi:10.2174/2210676605021504301550381

Pradhan BK, D'Amico JK, Makani R, Parikh T (2015b) Nonconventional interventions for chronic post-traumatic stress disorder (PTSD): ketamine, repetitive trans-cranial magnetic stimulation (rTMS) and alternative approaches. J Trauma Dissociation. doi:10.1080/15299732.2015.1046101

Pradhan B (2015c) Chapter-24, p. 373–381: Depression specific Yoga and mindfulness based cognitive therapy (DepS Y-MBCT) model: description, data on efficacy and differences from contemporary models. In: Greenblatt J, Brogan K (eds) Integrative psychiatry for depression: redefining models for assessment, treatment, and prevention of mood disorders. Taylor & Francis Group, FL: USA

Prasad K, Wahner-Roedler DL, Cha SS, Sood A (2011) Effect of a single-session meditation training to reduce stress and improve quality of life among health care professionals: a dose-ranging feasibility study. Altern Ther Health Med 17(3):46–49

Pridmore S, Dale J (2009) Disease mongering: the overlooked legs. Internal Medicine Journal, 39(5):343–344

Ragins M (2012) Recovery: changing from a medial model to a psychosocial rehabilitation model. A program of mental health America of Los Angeles, MHA Village, http://mhavillage.squarespace.com/storage/06RecoverySevereMI.pdf. Accessed 04/2014

Rector N, Beck A (2002) CBT for schizophrenia. Can J Psychiatry 47(1):39–48

Rudd MD (2012) Brief cognitive behavioral therapy for military populations. J Mil Psychol 24:1–12

Santina PD (1997) The tree of enlightenment: An introduction to the major traditions of Buddhism. Chico, CA: Buddha Dharma Education Association Inc.

Satchidananda S (1978) The Yoga Sutras of Patanjali: translations and commentary. Integral Yoga Publications, Yogaville

Schretlen DJ, Cascella NG, Meyer SM et al (2007) Neuropsychological functioning in bipolar disorder and schizophrenia. Biol Psychiatry 62:179–186

Segal ZV, Williams JMG, Teasdale JD (2002) Mindfulness-based cognitive therapy for depression: a new approach to preventing relapse. Guilford Press, New York

Seidman LJ, Giuliano AJ, Meyer EC et al (2010) Neuropsychology of the prodrome to psychosis in the NAPLS consortium: relationship to family history and conversion to psychosis. Arch Gen Psychiatry 67:578–588

Tait L, Birchwood M, Trower P (2004) Adapting to the challenge of psychosis: personal resilience and the use of sealing-over (avoidant) coping strategies. Br J Psychiatry 185(5):410–415

Tamminga CA, Stan AD, Wagner AD (2010) The hippocampal formation in schizophrenia. Am J Psychiatry 167:1178–1193

Thirthalli J et al (2012) Prospective study of duration of untreated psychosis and outcome of never-treated patients with schizophrenia in India. Indian J Psychiatry 53(4):319–323

Vancampfort D, Vansteelandt K, Scheewe T, Probst M, Knapen J, De Herdt A, De Hert M (2012) Yoga in schizophrenia: a systematic review of randomised controlled trials. Acta Psychiatr Scand 126(1):1–9

Varambally S, Gangadhar BN, Thirthalli J, Jagannathan A, Kumar S, Venkatasubramanian G et al (2012) Therapeutic efficacy of add-on yogasana intervention in stabilized outpatient schizophrenia: randomized controlled comparison with exercise and waitlist. Indian J Psychiatry 54(3):227–232

Wang PS, Demler O, Kessler RC (2002) Adequacy of treatment for serious mental illness in the United States. Am J Public Health 92(1):92–98

World Health Organization Australia 2009 [website], Mental health strengthening our response, Fact sheet 220, viewed 1 February 2011; http://www.who.int/mediacentre/factsheets/fs220/en/

Wykes T, Steel C, Everitt B, Tarrier N (2008) Cognitive behavior therapy for schizophrenia: effect sizes, clinical models, and methodological rigor. Schizophr Bull 34(3):523–537, http://doi.org/10.1093/schbul/sbm114

Zubin J, Spring B (1977) Vulnerability; a new view of Schizophrenia. J Abnorm Psychol 86:103–126

Zylowska L, Ackerman DL, Yang MH, Futrell JL, Horton NL, Hale TS, Pataki C, Smalley SL (2008) Mindfulness meditation training in adults and adolescents with ADHD: a feasibility study. J Atten Disord 11(6):737–746

Brief Treatment of Psychosis from a Developmentally Informed Psychoanalytic Perspective

6

Theodore Fallon Jr.

6.1   Introduction

This chapter considers a developmentally informed psychoanalytic approach to brief encounters with individuals with psychosis. Such an approach in no way suggests that it is useful to employ classical psychoanalytic practice with a patient lying down on a couch and free associating. Rather, the approach put forth here is derived from psychoanalytic work with children in which patients present material in whatever way they are able, and it is the therapist's job to help them articulate the material, organize it, make meaning from it, and, from this, help them get themselves back on track developmentally (Freud 1963). This approach nurtures the process of development itself and can be used with all children, adolescents, and adults, including ones who are overwhelmed with a psychotic process, as this chapter will elucidate.

For the many readers of this book who might be expecting a prescription for how to conduct a therapy using the psychoanalytic approach that is described here, this chapter does not prescribe any such procedures. Rather, it elucidates a stance taken by the therapist. This stance is characterized by a kind of listening and being open to whatever material is presented by the patient. As such, it does not require anything from the patient other than to produce spontaneous material. For example, from this perspective, paranoia is spontaneous material to be understood and not a barrier to the work. Freud demonstrated this stance in 1905 (Freud 1905) when he discussed transference, which is a form of mistaken reality, and it has been elaborated in the psychoanalytic literature hundreds of times since then. Even catatonia is a spontaneous production that can be worked with and understood.

T. Fallon Jr., MD
Associate Professor, Department of Psychiatry; Adjunct, Department of Humanities and Community Medicine, Drexel College of Medicine, Faculty and Former Chair, Psychoanalytic Training Program for Children and Adolescents, Psychoanalytic Center of Philadelphia, Wayne, PA, USA
e-mail: TFallonJr@verizon.net

© Springer International Publishing Switzerland 2016
B. Pradhan et al. (eds.), *Brief Interventions for Psychosis: A Clinical Compendium*, DOI 10.1007/978-3-319-30521-9_6

Safety, of course, is a prerequisite to doing any work with a patient. Among other reasons, the therapist not being under threat allows the therapist to think clearly about the patient. But other than safety, there are no prerequisites and no patient attributes that would be a barrier to this approach. There are, however, two important barriers to consider in this work: those within the therapist and those in the context of the patient's environment. Both of these barriers will be discussed further below.

The chapter begins with clarification of the chapter title and continues by organizing these terms in relation to one another. Two examples subsequently will demonstrate both how to understand psychosis from this perspective and where and when one might intervene. These examples will highlight the special role of anxiety, attachment, and disorganization and bring in to bold relief the usefulness of tracking and making use of these phenomena. The challenge for the therapist using this developmentally informed psychoanalytic approach is to accept the patient however they present, use this as the starting point, and begin the therapeutic process by helping the patient organize themselves around what the patient's chaos is.

6.2   A Developmentally Informed Psychoanalytic Perspective

The term "psychoanalytic" has been used in many different ways throughout the literature. Its use here in this chapter is meant to be in the broadest sense. In that sense, "psychoanalytic" refers to the study of thoughts, ideas, feelings, and experiences (experiences in the broadest context including bodily experiences, here and now experiences, as well as experiences held in memory), with the understanding that there is much more to the thoughts, ideas, feelings, and experiences than is immediately apparent and available. That is, any thought or feeling that is presented is accompanied by a nexus of other thoughts, feelings, memories, and experiences that are not in awareness. Another way to describe this is "depth psychology."

"Development" is meant to refer to both the process and the stages of maturation. Infants are born with certain functional capacities psychologically, including cognition, emotion, self-regulation, and ability to relate to others and to organize oneself and one's thoughts. These capacities grow over time and depend on many factors including the constitutional factors and the encounters that the infant has with the world. With these forces at play, the personality takes on its own unique patterns and evolves. So, "development" as used in this chapter refers to the expected maturation of the functional capacities and also refers to the unique evolution of the individual personality.

Development is pushed forward when the person (infant or adult) encounters a challenge for which they are not presently equipped to address. This "developmental challenge" motivates the person to evolve to meet the challenge. When a person encounters a developmental challenge and develops new capacities in order to adequately address this challenge, then we recognize that there has been an evolution, a maturation, or development of the individual. If, however, a person is not prepared to meet this developmental challenge, then we begin to see a breakdown of the personality. For example, think of the development of organizational and problem solving capacities such as putting together a puzzle. The normal progression is to put together a 2-piece puzzle, then a 5-piece puzzle, and then a 15-piece puzzle. Each challenge is an incremental step and requires the capacities developed up to that point plus the additional challenge. However if a child was not given the opportunity to put puzzles together, or a puzzle demands far more than the child has developed, then the child will likely not succeed. So, for example, if a child is exposed to sexual stimulation far beyond their developmental level, this will create problems. If the child is 5 years old, that will create one possible set of problems. If the child is 15 years old and has not experienced normal developmental experimentation, that will create a different set of problems. This latter circumstance may occur due to the environment being too restrictive; it may be that the child is too anxious to experiment for constitutional reasons, or it may be that the child has been sensitized due to early overexposure/overstimulation, again leaving the child too anxious to proceed.

6.3   Psychoanalytically Informed Developmental Conceptualization of Psychosis

Using the terms mentioned above, consider a conceptual model of mental and behavioral phenomena that is different than thinking about disease or illness. Consider the possibility that symptoms are a manifestation of unmet developmental challenges. For example, a developmental challenge for adolescents is to operate within an adult body. Adolescence is considered here because psychosis more often than not presents in the context of adolescence. The adult body presents challenges for boys to tolerate and manage the increased feelings of aggression and sexual drive created by increased levels of testosterone. Likewise, girls face challenges with increased estrogen and progesterone, with increased drive to relate to others and be comfortable with their own boundaries. Another challenge for adolescents of both genders is to manage their new adult sexual body itself.

Yet another overlapping developmental challenge for adolescents to manage is the increased independence that comes with adult capacities. There are many implications here, one of which is that a child's mind must take on organizational capacities that the newly minted adult's body now demands. These organizational capacities must take on new social and interpersonal demands, as well as make meanings of internal experiences, feelings, thoughts, fantasies, impulses, etc.

In addition, these demands must be taken on with much less support and oversight from parents (Erikson 1956). This is likely why psychosis most commonly presents at this stage of life – parents are not there to stop the free fall of degrading ego functions that can occur under the pressure of development (this is described more below) (Browning 2011). These are tall demands, and if the child's mind has not been equipped and prepared for these challenges, but solutions to these challenges are demanded, as one cannot escape one's body, then there are unmet developmental challenges of epic proportion. The child is between the devil and the deep blue sea.

There are many possible solutions to this epic challenge, depending on the various conditions including those of the preadolescent development. But if no adequate solutions are reached, anxiety will escalate to the point of overwhelming the individual's psyche including the ego apparatus, and thus disorganization of thought processes ensue. It is not uncommon to see short episodes of disorganized thoughts in adolescents, which resolve when solutions are found. However, if the challenge continues to go unanswered, disordered thought takes over the various functions of the mind more and more. At that point, in an effort for the person to preserve their psychological integrity, they will reach for models of reality that do not match reality itself, such as those seen with delusions and hallucinations. This is a psychoanalytically informed developmental conceptualization of psychosis (Fallon 2014). It also fits in with the stress-vulnerability model of schizophrenia proposed by Zubin and Spring (1997) in which the challenging event is the developmental challenge from within.

Let us approach this concept again anew, this time from another direction. Let us consider that the mind develops and holds a map or model of the reality that the person has experienced. The mind uses this model to navigate and make decisions as to how to proceed, considering what it knows of the outcomes and consequences according to that model. Some of this model may be articulated, but much of it will be contained in bodily experiences and will be detected only by the actions and inactions taken or not by the individual. Psychoanalytic work aims at helping to articulate and give meaning to the model and the actions/inactions.

Development can be conceptualized as a progressive evolution of this model of reality. The first model of reality for the infant is "I feel bad; I cry; I feel better." This model is soon displaced by another that includes "someone out there who does something that makes me feel better." These preliminary models are simple and in the beginning lean heavily on built-in responses such as crying in response to over-stimulation. Through successive evolutions of this model of reality that are more and more complex, the child is able to take into account more and more properties and subtleties of reality and themselves, becoming acquainted with more and more parts of themselves and the world outside themselves. The evolution of these models of reality aims to create a model that more closely predicts real outcomes. There are moments when the individual encounters information or events which can't be accounted for by these models. The distress of the unmet needs in addition to a sense of not knowing what is going on (something is happening for which the model of realty is not reflecting what just happened) forces the individual to modify the model to one that better accounts for (predicts) outcomes. This is what characterizes increased maturity. With each progressive developmental challenge, the individual acknowledges that the model they have of reality is inadequate, deconstructs that model, and then formulates a new one that takes into account the new problem and a new solution.

Sometimes, however, conflicting feelings or beliefs are held and the individual has a difficult time resolving these conflicts. These conflicts then interfere with deriving a new, higher fidelity model of reality. These more difficult to resolve conflicts usually involve core or foundational aspects of the model of reality. And yet development must proceed as dictated by biology, especially, for example, in adolescence.

6.4   The Case of Jay

A clinical example will be useful to illustrate the concepts presented thus far. Jay, a 19-year-old man, presented after attempting to kill himself, knowing that he would be reborn into a new, more perfect world where men were women and women were men. The idea of a more perfect world was a manic defense to an underlying despair in which he felt he could not go on in his world. One of the first statements that he made as he began his therapy was that it would be a lot easier if he was homosexual. His next thought was a question – was he homosexual? From there, the details of the material he presented for the next 6 months were a confusing chaos of words, even as his movements were stiff and uncoordinated and his speech was halting and fragmented.

After 3 years of four to five times per week listening and trying to sort out this chaos, during which a minimal amount of medication was used, he came to an understanding of his unresolvable adolescent developmental challenges. During the work, when the chaos in his mind left him with anxiety that he could not bear, he requested and was given up to 1 mg per day of risperidone which he reported as turning down the volume of the anxiety, allowing him to think more clearly, albeit more slowly. He was begun on this medication in the hospital at a dose of 5 mg per day after his suicide attempt but discontinued it as soon as he was discharged because it made him feel terrible. After a month of analytic work, he complained of the chaos and anxiety and agreed to try one-quarter milligram at bedtime. After a few days, he noted that it helped a bit and wanted to try more. The dosage was increased to 0.5 mg/day, then 1 mg/day, and then 1.5 mg/day. At that point, he said he felt like his thinking was walking in thick deep mud and that evil threatened to overtake him. The risperidone was reduced to 1 mg/day and this feeling resolved. He took the risperidone intermittently under supervision, and by year 2 of therapy, he no longer needed the medication.

The psychoanalysis consisted of the therapist listening to him as he attempted to express and then organize his thoughts and ideas. Even 4 months into therapy, the therapist could not articulate much about what was being expressed. However, the act of listening and attempting to follow and make sense of Jay's productions was deeply therapeutic and even lifesaving as demonstrated by an event that occurred in the fifth month of therapy. Up to that point, the psychoanalyst listened and noticed that Jay gradually became less stiff. He completed more and more of the sentences that he would begin and there would be less vacant pauses. Later, Jay would indicate that during those vacant pauses, he was attending to his hallucinations and delusions.

His family reported that he appeared more organized and even began to participate in family activities such as meals and was sleeping regularly and attending to his hygiene. The psychoanalyst planned to be away for 3 days, working with Jay and his family for 2 weeks prior to the absence. It was arranged that Jay and his analyst would speak on the phone at an appointed time every day. On the second day of the analyst's absence, Jay again attempted suicide and was again admitted to the hospital. On the analyst's return the next day, Jay was discharged. When the analyst asked what happened, Jay indicated that when he could not sit with the analyst and work to put his thoughts together, everything again became chaos and he was left to figure it out for himself.

After some time, the therapist began to notice that when Jay talked about certain topics such as his mother, his father, or sexuality, he would become more disorganized in his thoughts, speech, and movements and have more vacant pauses. After a time, the therapist would call Jay's attention to this sequence, and after the therapist repeatedly called Jay's attention to this sequence, Jay himself began to notice it. Soon fragments of associations began to arise, for example, in association with thinking about his mother, he would mention a certain type of tree. Again, when the therapist noted this and asked about this tree, after some thought, Jay remembered that it was a tree under which he took comfort as a child. However, sometime during his childhood, his parents cut down this tree which left him feeling abandoned. If the therapist missed an opportunity to make meaning of something which Jay felt overly anxious about, Jay would begin to experience psychotic symptoms. However, if Jay became aware of his own anxiety and then could make meaning of the anxiety himself, he would experience increased clarity.

Gradually over the 3 years of psychoanalysis, Jay constructed a narrative of his life that put his psychosis and his suicide attempts into perspective. Early in his childhood, Jay was raised by his father whom he deeply admired and with whom he heavily identified. His mother was preoccupied with her own developmental challenges and unable to attend to him throughout his life. By the time Jay was 8 years old, his father had become depressed and withdrawn, leaving him without any substantial parental support. The father's depression was due to his frustrated homosexuality, as he posed as a heterosexual husband. In Jay's early adolescence, the father left the family home and resumed the gay lifestyle that he had had prior to his marriage. In his adolescence at age 17, after Jay had experienced his first intimate sexual relationship, he became psychotic. The psychosis began to resolve in the context of therapy when he began to recognize the conflict between his early identification with his homosexual father and his own newly found adolescent heterosexual desires. At one point in the therapy, he even noticed that when he found himself exhibiting his father's feminine mannerisms, he would begin hallucinating.

Prior to therapy, Jay had not been able to resolve this conflict at the bodily experience level. This unresolved developmental challenge led to a depression and psychosis. In the context of this depression and psychosis, he came to a solution that did not match reality – killing himself and being reborn into a world where men were women and women were men.

If one considers the psychoanalytic developmental model described above, it makes sense that as Jay was presenting in his psychotic state, there was much going on below the level of awareness, even as he was revealing the deep underlying conflicts in plain sight – it would be so much simpler if he were a homosexual like his father. Becoming aware, articulating, and giving meaning to these conflicts then allowed him and the analyst to intervene with reason and alternative meanings, placing the conflict in a new context. This new context changed the questions and what was previously experienced as a conflict was now experienced as simply his history.

Jay's intensive and prolonged therapy was certainly not brief, but it demonstrates that even on presentation of the psychosis, there is meaning, most of the time in plain sight, and still there is a puzzle yet to be understood.

6.5   The Case of Bernard

Let us now consider an example of a brief encounter with psychosis and how a psychoanalytic developmental model might be useful in the moment. Bernard, a 28-year-old African-American man, presented to a psychiatric emergency room very anxious, paranoid, and fearful that the devil was pursuing him. As the attending physician encountered him, sat, and talked with him for a few minutes, Bernard seemed reassured that he was now in a safe place. The resident physician then stepped in to complete a full evaluation in order to consider an appropriate disposition. As the resident approached Bernard, Bernard began screaming that the devil was among us and had come to get him. Bernard proceeded to barricade himself in a corner of the room, preparing to be attacked.

After 20 min of chaos, Bernard was placed in physical restraints. The attending physician again approached him as he had in the beginning and again Bernard gradually calmed. Agreeing that he felt safe now as he had felt safe before, the attending physician asked him what had changed and when. He said the devil had come for him and the attending physician wondered if he was referring to the resident physician that had approached him. Bernard now became more anxious. Again, the attending physician calmed him and was then able to ask him how he knew that the resident physician was the devil. "Because he's black" was the answer. The resident physician was from Africa, and indeed he was very dark skinned as was Bernard himself. The attending physician felt a momentary sense of confusion and disorientation as he heard himself say, "but you're black, too." Suddenly Bernard was saying, "That's it. That's it." With that, there was a lessening of anxiety and expression of psychotic thought. Further history revealed that Bernard had been living in a shelter that was cramped and overcrowded. He felt dependent on the shelter for food and physical protection and yet became angry and began to feel murderous rage toward the shelter staff. That was when he got the idea that the devil was after him. It is easy to imagine that he projected his murderous rage onto an imaginary devil that was in his own image and included being black. It is also likely that this murderous rage originated earlier in his life and resonated with his present situation in the shelter. By the time this history had been obtained and created into a meaningful narrative shared by both the evaluator and Bernard, Bernard appeared comfortable and happy and prior to being admitted was last seen enjoying a hospital cafeteria bagged lunch, which was not that good.

As in the case of Jay, Bernard's initial symptoms were manifestations of unconscious processes. Helping Bernard to articulate and make meaning of his present situation, as well as helping him to explore the possible origins of his symptoms in the context of his present life, was useful. Useful longer term work would be to explore the origins of his symptoms in the context of his development. As was suggested in the case of Jay, longer term work with Bernard would be slow and would likely need to be intensive and very supportive. Nonetheless, even in brief encounters, keeping in mind this psychoanalytic developmental perspective can help guide the initial evaluation. It will then be important to pass on information gathered during this initial evaluation, even as the disordered thoughts are unintelligible loose pieces to a yet-to-be-put-together puzzle. Also such psychoanalytically informed developmental models provide an in-depth understanding of the client's symptoms and dysfunctions, and this deeper understanding on the part of the therapist may serve to make better decisions with regard to the patient's reality and can pave the way to deliver better therapeutic care to individuals with psychosis.

6.6   Brief Therapy

Since this book is focused on brief interventions with psychotic individuals, it is pertinent to comment on how brief is brief. The model used for the psychiatric emergency service in which Bernard was seen, operated in the context of a public mental health community system of care. In that context, patients were not triaged and disposed of, but rather were held continuously in a nexus of services and agencies. If a patient was being served in one agency such as the psychiatric emergency room, as long as the patient needed that service, there was no rush to move that person to another setting. The service that was provided in the psychiatric emergency room was a place where acute behavioral and mental health crisis were contained, and data gathered, making contact with as many entities as could be garnered to create the most robust picture of the person who presents in crisis. This meshed well with the developmentally informed psychoanalytic model in which insight came in a moment of understanding. A psychoanalytic moment might be just a moment in time as in an acute traumatic moment or the aha moment of insight or a moment that could last a lifetime as in the traumatic moment that is relived again and again or a relived moment that sustains a person through a holocaust. In Bernard's case, the attending physician spent perhaps 25 min with him in total during this evaluation. Bernard's moment was in the terror that he experienced. Exploring that moment led to the understanding that his moment of terror was also his moment of rage at those around him, who were supposed to be caring for him. The aha moment for the attending physician and then for Bernard came when the lived experience was also lived/shared with the attending physician, and together they made meaning of his fear and rage. The process of an evaluation, just as the process of a meditation, cannot be hurried, if one is really going to move the process forward. As daunting as it may seem, to evaluate crises, especially psychotic crises, a big advantage in the setting of psychiatric crises such as one sees in psychiatric emergency rooms is that it is quite common to see a blatant revealing of underlying unconscious conflicts. The difficulty is in making meaning of these psychotic symptoms. In psychoanalytic jargon, it is id material without any ego to help us understand or interpret.

Habib Davanloo (1995) articulated a model of short-term (1 year) psychoanalytic psychotherapy called the intensive short-term dynamic psychotherapy (ISTDP). In his model, Davanloo does an initial interview in which he methodically strips away ego defenses, allowing him to "stroll through the unconscious." In the case of psychosis, those ego defenses are already stripped away, allowing a stroll through the unconscious without any of the preliminary work.

It is not recommended that one induce psychotic states in order to examine unconscious processes. It is also not recommended to attempt to externally contain the feelings and expressions of the psychosis, although it is also important to be sure that physical safety is maintained at all times. Efforts to contain the feelings will be experienced by the patient as people not wanting to hear how they are feeling or what they have to say, or feel rejected, or that their feelings are dangerous and must be suppressed. These efforts to contain the feelings may be made by therapists and staff to avoid making contact with the patient's chaos. This phenomenon will be addressed below.

On the other hand, as in the case of Jay, when the therapist comes to know the patient, attending to what stimuli leads the patient to become more disorganized provides clues as to the underlying conflicts. In that case, focused interventions to provide the patient with a modicum of structure and organization will result in a lessening of psychosis. In the acute setting, as in the case of Bernard, maintaining physical safety and then a review of the events and a cooperative exploration by patient and therapist of what is going on in the patient's mind frequently leads to a lessening of anxiety, intrapsychic chaos, and psychosis.

A note here is that none of this work can be done unless the therapist is mindful of his environment and a sense of safety. If the therapist is not in that state, then this work cannot be done. Trainees should be instructed from the beginning and repeatedly that if they have any sense of insecurity, especially in working with psychotic patients, they should not be in that place, should immediately get up without explanation, and leave the room for a place in which they feel safe.

6.7 The Role of Anxiety, Attachment, and Disorganization in Psychosis

In thinking about developmental challenges and the evolution (maturation) of a person's model of reality, anxiety, attachment, and disorganization have key roles. These processes become particularly important when thinking about psychosis as a maturation process gone awry and especially if considering assisting with getting this developmental process back on track.

Anxiety, from a psychoanalytic perspective, is an internal signal for danger (Freud 1923; Gray 2005). When this signal is at a tolerable level, it motivates the person to address the danger. However, when it moves beyond tolerable limits, the signal is distorted, like an overpowered loudspeaker. Beyond this level, the signal becomes psychically painful and interferes with cognitive and ego capacities, creating disordered thought as evidenced by disorganization. In the context of a developmental challenge and the disorganization that precedes the new model of reality, anxiety is very high, degrading cognitive and ego capacities. Degraded cognitive and ego capacities in the form of disordered thought then create a sense of helplessness which creates more anxiety, which leads to more disordered thought. And so it goes round and round, spiraling down. In this feedback cycle continues, eventually there will be complete collapse of the ego. This is when thought disorder becomes psychosis.

When there is an attachment and a trust with another, that other, in this case the therapist, if effective, will dampen the destructive feedback of anxiety and disordered thought. The attachment or bond being talked about here is not specifically the attachment that occurs between mother and child (although that kind of attachment would be included in the definition). What is meant is something broader – the sense that another person, the therapist in this case, is there, aware of the patient's state, and the patient is trusting that if need be, the therapist will lend their ego and cognitive functions just enough to create a nidus of organization, but not so much that it overwhelms the patient who will be vulnerable to being overwhelmed. What fosters this attachment will be a sense of being understood.

In the face of psychosis, it is difficult to know how to be supportive and allow the patient to feel understood in the midst of such chaos if one just listens to the content, which many times does not make sense or is contrary to what we know of how reality works. This is where monitoring anxiety and disorganization is key, as they will rise and fall with internal disordered thought. Most therapists are attuned to monitoring anxiety. However, with psychotic individuals, it is difficult to monitor anxiety since the anxiety is overwhelming and not tolerated. Here anxiety is usually hidden among the myriad of defenses and the chaos of psychosis.

Although most clinicians are not attuned to disorganization, in a psychotic individual, disorganization appears everywhere and can be monitored in every facet of the patient's functioning including qualities of speech, movement, generated thoughts or sudden disruptions in continuity of thought, verbal productions, and actions. Attending to and monitoring this disorganization can be cultivated. The most difficult part of training this attunement is tolerating the internal experience of chaos. This is discussed more below.

Allowing the patient to express themselves, even as the material is disorganized, and thinking with the patient about that material as much as the patient can tolerate will foster a lessening of disorganization, and hence there will be a lessening of disordered thought. This will then allow more underlying disorganized and conflictual material to surface. When this underlying conflictual material begins to surface, disorganization will again increase. This was seen, for example, in the case of Jay when he noticed his feminine mannerisms and began to have hallucinations. This observation is done using what Paul Gray refers to as close process monitoring (Gray 2005). When there is an increase in disorganization, and especially when this begins to degrade the ego capacities and move toward that downward spiral described above, this is the point at which the therapist needs to lend organizing ego capacities to the patient.

The aim here is to provide some small interpretation that brings a new meaning that the patient can accept regarding the conflict. For example, in the case of Jay, he became more disorganized in the session and began to hallucinate after he noticed that his movements mimicked his father's mannerisms. When the therapist saw this increased disorganization, he said, "You notice that you are hearing voices now and a moment ago you were noticing your mannerisms that remind you of your father. I wonder what the connection might be." If there is a lessening of disorganization, then you have got it close enough. However, if the disorganization worsens, the intervention was either too much, too little (not very likely), or wrong. In any case, if the disorganization worsens after your intervention, you call the patient's attention to your intervention, noting that what you said does not seem to be correct and empathizing with the patient that it is painful when one is not understood. Then see if you can clarify with the patient what was not correct.

The result of persistent close process monitoring is a sense the patient has of being understood. Here a quick clinical vignette will illustrate.

6.8   The Case of Terry

Terry, a 14-year-old child in the autistic spectrum, had been admitted to a psychiatric inpatient unit in a psychotic state. For his entire 3-month stay, the therapist met with him almost daily, listening, providing close process monitoring, and organizing support when needed. For example, Terry began a session talking about school, saying it was going well for him and he was ready to go home. When asked what was going well, he pulled out a textbook, opened to page 279, and pointed to the page number. After 15 minutes of wondering about what Terry was trying to convey, the therapist noted the sequence as just stated above and wondered if Terry was uncomfortable with the specific question of what was going well. Terry nodded yes. The therapist suggested that maybe Terry felt some pressure about school. Terry again nodded yes. The therapist then followed up with the question: What was in Terry's mind when he decided to reach for the textbook? Terry responded that he really wanted to play a game of catch rather than do schoolwork. Terry and the therapist then proceeded to have a lively game of catch which, as Terry said, made him feel like he was communing with the therapist. As they played catch, Terry began to talk about his inner experiences.

As the work continued over the next few months, Terry's overt psychotic state subsided, although there were still many aspects of his state that had not been addressed and much of the source of the psychotic material was still not understood by his therapist or anyone else. Despite the remaining questions, as discharge drew near, Terry asked his therapist if the therapist would talk with his parents.

What is it that you would like me to talk to them about?
Tell them about me. You know about me. Just like when we played catch, tell them so they can understand too and they can help me like you have. This example illustrates the importance of feeling understood and allowed Terry to explore his chaos even in the face of not knowing.

6.9   Barriers to a Psychoanalytic Developmental Approach

6.9.1   Barriers Related to the Therapist

As simple as this approach would seem, there has been little written about it over the past 50 years. Prior to that, there were a number of authors who wrote about psycho-analytic work with psychotic individuals (Arieti 1966; Gottschalk et al. 1988; Searles 1961, 1976). Recently, there has been a resurgence of interest (Garrett 2012; Knafo 2012; Kocan 2012; Lotterman 2011; Marcus 2012; Slevin and Marcus 2011). One might wish that with the advent of newer medications, a psychoanalytic approach might be antiquated. However, recent data continues to show poor out-come for psychosis. So why would a simple and useful psychoanalytic development approach to psychosis be ignored? The difficulty may be found in the therapist's experience when doing this work. Using the close process monitoring as described above, one must use empathic capacities and in this way comes into intimate contact with the psychotic state of the patient.

Development is occurring in all of us and is the progressive evolution of our model of reality that we carry with us. That evolution requires that we have decon-structed and reconstructed this model repeatedly throughout our lives. However, to be in that moment after we have deconstructed our old model but before we have reconstructed our new model is a moment of chaos. This experience of chaos that each of us has had over and over is a dysphoric experience and one that all of us want to move away from as quickly as possible. That wanting to move away from this experience quickly gives us motivation to work hard at and quickly reconstruct our model of reality that serves us well evolutionarily as it would not be adaptive for us to be wandering around the world lost and defenseless. However, if we are to help others with this chaos, we must be able to tolerate it. With that intimate contact with a psychotic patient, the chaos that reigns in the patient resonates in the therapist. That is, the therapist can feel like they themselves are psychotic.

The experience of that moment is extremely dysphoric, has been referred to as annihilation anxiety (Benveniste et al. 1998), and is a state that few, if any of us, wish to tolerate for long (Fallon 2014). Therefore it is a reflex that we avoid this state in ourselves and also in our patients, since to be empathic with this state in another means that we allow it to resonate in ourselves. As therapists, we reflexively distance ourselves to avoid the extreme dysphoria that the chaos of psychosis brings.

Being aware of the dysphoria that empathic contact with the psychotic state engenders in us and developing the tolerance for this level of uncertainty and chaos are important qualities of a therapist who endeavors to use this approach. Open awareness (mindfulness) meditation is one way to practice and develop tolerance for this uncertainty in ourselves as therapists as a prerequisite for tolerating it in those who we might want to help. Be warned, however, that asking a patient to do medita-tion and tolerate this state when they are already suffering from an overload of uncer-tainty and chaos will likely lead to increased disordered thought in the patient. Therefore, we see that there is resistance within us as therapists to being empathic to the psychotic state in another. However, without this empathy, it is impossible to monitor the disorganization, anxiety, and disordered thought in another.

6.9.2 Barriers Related to the Family

The powerful deep conflicts in development which are the primordial nidus for most psychoses arise most if not all of the time in the context of developmentally important relationships that always contain strong ambivalences, particularly with parents, siblings, or even offspring as in the cases of postpartum psychosis. One can hypothesize that these conflicts occur because the attachment role needed in the development of new models of reality was not adequately fulfilled during the person's early development. This failure may have been due to attachment figures not functioning or to the maturing individual not being able to accept the support that was offered, or a combination of the two.

Nonetheless, we see the critical role of the failure of these relationships in the development of psychosis. This understanding is well established, and in fact one of the most effective interventions is to educate the family of the psychotic individual in providing support (Gottschalk et al. 1988). This education has been labeled as training the family in techniques of low expressed emotion. Its effectiveness is in providing support to the psychotic patient and avoiding increasing anxiety.

In addition, because development has gone awry, parents in particular continue to be critical elements in the patient getting back on developmental track. This is true even for adults who are psychotic. In fact it is quite common that adults who are chronically psychotic continue to be strongly tied to their parents, many times in a relationship that has a strong negative valence. This is why it is critical that family and, in particular, parents be involved in the work if they are available.

With the family involved, information about the core conflicts frequently comes to light, although it is important to be careful in engaging these core conflicts with the family, as manifestations of these conflicts, still unresolved, may be continuing within the family and the parents. Many times, resistance will develop within the family when the identified psychotic patient begins to get to the core conflicts. Occasionally, there will be opportunities to help the family and parents work through some of these core conflicts. Even in brief encounters, efforts should be made to include the family. It is important to respect this ecology. Chapter 8 addresses this topic further.

Conclusion

A developmentally informed psychoanalytic approach to individuals who are psychotic can be very useful, even in brief encounters. In order to do this work, to begin with, the therapist must tolerate considerable feelings of discomfort and internal chaos with empathic contact with the psychotic state. Therapists can be trained to develop tolerance to these feelings. A variety of methods such as regular supervision and mindfulness meditation are helpful in this regard. This empathic contact is necessary in order to track anxiety and disordered thought. This tracking is done by monitoring disorganization. Disorganization can be monitored through observing posture, physical moment, and speech production including porosity, cadence, and content. This monitoring then guides the therapist to provide minimal organizing support when increased disorganization is detected with the aim of preventing a downward spiral of degrading ego function. The effectiveness of this support is dependent on the patient's trust in the therapist's persistent ability to be empathic to the patient's internal experiences.

References

Arieti S (1966) The psychoanalytic approach to the psychoses. Am J Psychoanal 26:63–66

Benveniste PS, Papouchis N, Allen R, Hurvich M (1998) Rorschach assessment of annihilation anxiety and ego functioning. Psychoanal Psychol 15(4):536–566

Browning DL (2011) Testing reality during adolescence: the contribution of Erikson's concepts of fidelity and developmental actuality. Psychoanal Q 80:555–593

Davanloo H (1995) Intensive short-term psychotherapy with highly resistant patients. I. Handling resistance. In: Selected papers of Habib Davanloo. Wiley, New York, pp 1–27

Erikson EH (1956) The problem of ego identity. J Am Psychoanal Assoc 4:56–121

Fallon T (2014) Disordered thought and development: chaos to organization in the moment. Jason Aronson, New York

Freud S (1905) Fragment of an analysis of a case of hysteria (1905 [1901]). The standard edition of the complete psychological works of Sigmund Freud Volume VII (1901–1905): a case of hysteria, three essays on sexuality and other works

Freud S (1923) Freud S (1923) The ego and the Id., Volume XIX (1923–1925): the Ego and the Id and other works, 1–66., XIX (1923–1925), 1–66

Freud A (1963) The concept of developmental lines. Psychoanal Study Child 18:245–265

Garrett M (2012) Psychoanalysis and the severely mentally ill. Am Psychoanal 46(1):20 & 22

Gottschalk LA, Falloon IRH, Marder SR, Lebell MB, Gift TE, Wynne LC (1988) The prediction of relapse of schizophrenic patients using emotional data obtained from their relatives. Psychiatry Res 25(3):261–276, http://doi.org/10.1016/0165-1781(88)90097-2

Gray P (2005) The ego and analysis of defense, 2nd edn. Jason Aronson, Lanham

Knafo D (2012) Working at the limits of human experience. Am Psychoanal 46(2):17–18, 20

Kocan M (2012) Treating patients vulnerable to psychotic regression. Am Psychoanal 46(1): 21–22

Lotterman M (2011) Psychotherapy can benefit schizophrenic patients. Am Psychoanal 45(4): 12–15–16

Marcus E (2012) Creativity in psychosis. Am Psychoanal 46(2):19

Searles HF (1961) Anxiety concerning change, as seen in the psychotherapy of schizophrenic patients—with particular reference to the sense of personal identity. Int J Psycho-Anal 42:74–85

Searles HF (1976) Psychoanalytic therapy with schizophrenic patients in a private-practice context. Contemp Psychoanal 12:387–406

Slevin M, Marcus E (2011) Introduction. Am Psychoanal 45(4):1

Zubin J, Spring B (1977) Vulnerability: a new view of schizophrenia. J Abnorm Psychol 86(2):103–126

Application of Motivational Interviewing in Working with Psychotic Disorders

David Rubenstein

7.1 Introduction and Historical Context

Motivational Interviewing (MI) was developed by William R. Miller, and his work in this area was first published in 1983 following experiences in working with alcohol use patients and the difficulties they experienced. This treatment approach was later explained more fully, with Stephen Rollnick, in their publication, Motivational Interviewing: Preparing People for Change (1991), as a combination of strategies aimed at resolving ambivalence in facilitating behavior change across different potential problem areas. This treatment was a patient-centered approach which highlighted the elicitation of a patient's own intrinsic motivation and ability to change. Prochaska and DiClimente's Stages of Change model (1983) was also incorporated into Motivational Interviewing (Miller and Rollnick 1991) and this model is commonly referred to as the trans-theoretical model, secondary to its incorporation of different theories of how and why behavior change occurs. Over time, this treatment approach which started with application to alcohol use has grown into application for use with smoking cessation, substance abuse, HIV risk reduction, treatment of sex offenders, eating disorders, self-injury, medication adherence, and a whole host of other health-related issues in which behavior change is a primary aspect of treatment. Miller and Rollnick went on to publish 2nd and 3rd editions of their book, with each discussion of Motivational Interviewing growing in terms of conceptualization and richness of treatment strategies and approaches.

This chapter focuses on the application of Motivational Interviewing (Miller and Rollnick 2013) strategies in working with individuals with psychotic disorders.

D. Rubenstein
Associate Vice President for Student Wellness Rowan University, Adjunct Clinical Professor, Philadelphia College of Osteopathic Medicine, Adjunct Clinical Associate Professor of Psychiatry, Drexel University College of Medicine, Camden, NJ, USA
e-mail: Rubenstein@rowan.edu

© Springer International Publishing Switzerland 2016
B. Pradhan et al. (eds.), *Brief Interventions for Psychosis: A Clinical Compendium*, DOI 10.1007/978-3-319-30521-9_7

103

Mental health clinicians across disciplines – psychiatrists, psychologists, social workers, psychiatric nurse practitioners, nurses, case managers, counselors, etc. – should all find the strategies discussed in this chapter helpful in their work with client/service users' suffering from these disorders. While there have been studies evaluating the efficacy of Motivational Interviewing on health-related behaviors (Britt, Blampied, and Hudson, 2003) and some studies evaluating the application of Motivational Interviewing to psychotic disorders, clearly there is the need for further evaluation in assessing the empirical evidence for the use of Motivational Interviewing with psychosis. Although research is limited in this area (Romano and Peters 2015), the need to study the use of Motivational Interviewing with individuals with psychotic disorders is particularly important given the enormous potential that different elements of Motivational Interviewing can have on enhancing different provider interventions and facilitating readiness on the client/service users' part toward making gains and progress on the various aspects of life impacted by psychosis.

Many individuals with psychotic disorders have a history of disconnectedness, experiencing social isolation and stigma that lowers their self-esteem, and can suppress motivation for embracing all facets of life and of living to their potential level of functioning. Motivational Interviewing's collaborative approach which focuses on absolute worth, autonomy, affirmation, and accurate empathy as being central aspects of acceptance of the client/service user (Miller and Rollnick 2013) along with emphasis and respect for facilitating and bringing to the surface and then working with their own intrinsic strengths makes it a treatment approach well worth applying and integrating in work with individuals with psychotic disorders.

7.2   Psychosis

The DSM-V (American Psychiatric Association 2013) has classified psychotic disorders within the Schizophrenia Spectrum and Other Psychotic Disorders section (see Chap. 1 for further discussion). Specifically, these include delusional disorder, brief psychotic disorder, schizophreniform disorder, schizophrenia, schizoaffective disorder, substance/medication-induced psychotic disorder, psychotic disorder due to another medical condition, catatonias, other specified and unspecified schizophrenia spectrum and other psychotic disorders, and schizotypal personality disorder (as this personality disorder is part of the schizophrenia spectrum). The DSM-V (2013) notes that these psychotic disorders all have "key features" which include delusions, hallucinations, disorganized thinking (speech), grossly disorganized or abnormal motor behavior, and negative symptoms. Secondary to these symptoms, individuals with psychotic disorders have historically been a difficult population to treat given the severity and chronicity of symptoms, impact on the family and potential supportive, waxing and waning of symptoms over the lifecycle, potential problems with medication adherence, vulnerability to isolation from society, and vulnerability for exacerbation of symptoms due to alcohol and substance use.

From a treatment standpoint, medication management has been most helpful in the management of problematic symptoms (see Chaps. 1 and 2 for further discussion). Medication coupled with supportive psychotherapy and/or milieu therapy has added the benefit of closer monitoring of mental status and stability, reducing social isolation, allowance of social support, and work toward the development of life skills coping strategies given the vulnerabilities that these disorders generate.

7.3 Rationale for Use of MI for Individuals with Psychosis

While there has not been a clear indication of one type of psychotherapy as working "best" for individuals suffering from psychotic disorders, rather a combination of elements of supportive, cognitive, behavioral, family education and support, life skills coping, etc. is common. The application of Motivational Interviewing strategies can be quite applicable, helpful, and effective in addressing many different features commonly associated with individuals with psychotic disorders. These strategies can be well integrated into existing treatment modalities as we will discuss. Many of these strategies have universal applications, so family members are also encouraged to learn and use these strategies. Westra et al. (2011) recommend ongoing study of the efficacy of Motivational Interviewing as applied to the treatment of various major mental health disorders secondary to the "promising preliminary findings" that have been established in various studies that have been done. This chapter will explore different principles, strategies, approaches, and techniques in working with individuals experiencing varying challenges common with psychotic disorders. Motivational Interviewing from this author's opinion may be perhaps one of the best matches in working with patients suffering from psychotic disorders. Patients experiencing the severity of these mental health issues, as noted earlier, are often profoundly stigmatized by society with significant amounts of shame, humiliation, embarrassment, and even secrecy coloring a patient's (and their family) efforts at coping with severe mental illness. Client/service users with psychotic disorders frequently display problematic behaviors related to medication nonadherence and substance abuse which can affect the course of the disorder (Barkof et al. 2006. Motivational Interviewing, capable of addressing all of the issues noted above, is guided by a spirit of *acceptance* which is defined from an MI standpoint as (1) *conveying a sense of "absolute worth" or unconditional positive regard (Rogers) for the patient in accepting them fully, with complete respect and without judgment*, (2) *conveying "accurate empathy" (which we'll discuss in more detail later) of communicating an understanding and appreciation of your patient's experiences as they are experienced by the patient*, (3) *conveying "autonomy support" for the patient's own right for self-direction*, and (4) *full "affirmation" of the patient's strengths, efforts, and resources in their living of life, rather than from a strength rather than deficits standpoint.* The spirit of Motivational Interviewing expresses "compassion" in patient care described as, "… a deliberate commitment to pursue the welfare and best interest of the other" (Miller and Rollnick 2013, pg. 20). Miller and Rollnick (2013) discuss fundamentally, the belief that individuals have a "deep well of wisdom" (pg. 21) that can be unearthed and drawn upon in efforts to address areas being focused on in treatment. For client/service users who have had many experiences in which their sense of independence, autonomy, and efficacy have been squelched, ignored, or not trusted, this can be a welcome treatment approach.

Perhaps of primary importance is the development of a strong working therapeutic alliance. For individuals suffering from this disorder where periods of reality testing are challenged, episodes where judgment is compromised, and the ability to make decisions and choices that prioritize health and are difficult to make, the importance of the therapist developing a therapeutic alliance marked of trust is critical. Most therapies place a strong emphasis on the development of a therapeutic alliance; Motivational Interviewing places a very strong emphasis on the development of treatment relationship where maintenance of the therapeutic alliance is central to the work being done in treatment.

7.4   OARS: Acronym Describing the "How" of MI for Individuals with Psychosis

Within Motivational Interviewing, specifically, the acronym of *OARS* describes facets of the work that place a premium on the maintenance of the therapeutic alliance. OARS refers to open-ended questions, affirmations, reflection, and summarizing. Asking open-ended questions is particularly important in working with psychotic disorder client/service user, as it reveals for the clinician information, both content and process, related to thought processes, mood congruence, reality testing, and general ego functioning. It of course also puts centrality on the clinician's efforts to understand as fully as possible the patient's inner experience and their efforts of coping with external environmental demands that are part of everyday life. The process of the clinician putting their understanding of the patient's experience as front and center has the benefit of allowing for a stronger treatment relationship to develop which will facilitate a process in which the patient begins to trust the clinician to consider that they are trying to fully understand and appreciate who they are and their experiences, concerns, needs, and hopes.

Asking open-ended questions "fills the sails" so to speak, with information and opportunities for "affirmations." Affirmations from a Motivational Interviewing standpoint refer to efforts by the clinician to recognize and support areas of strengths and effort in the patient. Sometimes, finding these pockets of strength and effort can be challenging in working with client/service user whose judgment is compromised and reality testing is impaired or when they have impulsivity. However, this challenge can be addressed with wonderful therapeutic opportunity with a clinician emanating a nonjudgmental stance coupled with a trained eye and proper perspective. With this approach, the strengths of the individual can be identified as the example below illustrates.

7.5   Clinical Example

A 45-year-old client came to see her psychiatrist of 10 years with increase in delusions that the sensations in her back are from implants placed there by doctors several years ago. She also believed that there is a conspiracy to kill her and her psychiatrist was part of it. When asked specifically, she told her psychiatrist that she could not trust him and he was "in with others." Here the psychiatrist instead of focusing on the delusions of persecution against him focused on the help-seeking behavior that prompted this individual to ignore her delusions and come to see him. He said "J, I appreciate your honesty in expressing how you feel about me. It takes courage to do so and what to me is even more important is you putting aside these questions about me and coming to speak with me. Looks like there is this trusting part of you who does not believe that I am part of the conspiracy." This is a good example of the psychiatrist affirming the part of the patient that was able to reach out and seek help. Within Motivational Interviewing, affirmations allow for focus to be placed on explicitly recognizing any areas of strength and effort. This process as it plays out in treatment and the positive experience a patient can have when this is recognized, when so many other areas of their life may be challenged or difficult, is extremely helpful in the facilitation of the working alliance. As the process of asking open-ended questions and making affirmations unfold, the emergence of more clinical material and information about the patient's life will also, hopefully, emerge. In working with client/service users with psychotic disorders, the process of uncovering history, past experiences, current experiences, past and current relationships, and understanding the symptom picture can be complicated. This process can sometimes proceed slowly, move quickly, or sometimes be challenging in terms of understanding the content of the information and its relationship to their experiences. Nevertheless, clinical information emerges related to content and process, and this allows for clinician reflections to occur. Reflections allow for the clinician to be "accurately empathic" toward the patient, that is, clarifying and amplifying what a patient is attempting to communicate, without interference of the clinician's interpretation and judgment. Reflection is done purely for the purpose of the clinician attempting to more fully understand and appreciate the patient's experience and then convey that understanding to them. For example, the client/service user states, "I am hearing all of these voices that are telling me to do things and I am just not sure if they are real or not." The clinician, in giving a simple reflection, would state, "There are so many voices that you are hearing in your head and it is just so hard to tell what are real and what is not. I can see how you are really trying to figure this out." This simple response communicates to the individual that they understand the experience that he/she is trying to communicate and does so without further intervention. This can have a powerful impact on deepening the therapeutic alliance and the patient's experience of a clinician attempting to understand their inner world and efforts to cope with this in combination with environmental experiences. This also allows the patient the ongoing opportunity to "correct" the clinician helping to ensure that the clinician does, at least for the moment, have an accurate understanding and appreciation of their experience. The patient being in a position to correct the therapist is an empowering experience and reduces the power differential for a brief period of time. The therapist can facilitate this by explicitly stating that he would like to get the client's experience accurately and hence would appreciate the client correcting his understanding. Finally, "Summarizing," from a Motivational Interviewing perspective, allows for the process of collecting information that is shared, linking information that is shared, and using information to transition to other important areas. Summarizing, MI can be both extremely effective and challenging in working with client/service user with psychotic disorders as getting a handle on the content of the information can be challenging, particularly with reliably gathering historical information. However, the process of the clinician continuing to attempt to understand the information presented, linking this information contextually, and bridging to other important related areas of treatment communicates to the patient an ongoing attempt by the clinician to understand them and their experiences and their efforts to work with them, which is meaningful and therapeutic, even when this is not obvious. For example, following a client/service user's expression of ambivalence of taking their medication and their ambivalence about this, a clinician using a summarizing intervention might state, "In this case you found yourself wondering if you should take your medication. You remembered in the past that sometimes when you did not feel well physically, not taking your medication made you feel a little better and on the other hand, you also remembered the risk you were taking of hearing voices again in not taking your medication. You thought of our conversations weighing the pros and cons of taking your medicine and you felt really stuck on what to do. What should we talk about that can help you make a decision that will both keep you healthy and have you feeling better?" Here the clinician demonstrates a summarizing intervention by reflecting back to the patient their summary of what they understood the patient to be struggling with presently while tying in previously discussed historical information in such a way to set the stage for the patient and the clinician to discuss next steps, therapeutically moving forward. The clinician who is demonstrating OARS in clinical practice is also demonstrating the four central processes of Motivational Interviewing. These processes are engaging, focusing, evoking, and planning. Miller and Rollnick (2013) describe examples of each (pg. 32). Engagement addresses attempts by the clinician to strengthen a working relationship with the patient. This is particularly important in working with client/service users with psychotic disorder, many who have had multiple treatment providers over time and a revolving door of care providers. The clinician who spends significant time on engagement with the patient allows for a stronger and more trusting working relationship. Focusing illustrates the clinician and patient working to choose a direction and specific path to walk down in deciding what areas to focus on in treatment. After choosing the specific direction and areas to work, evoking refers to the clinician's attempt to elicit the patient's own motivation to change specific problematic behavior. Here again, this experience may feel new, potentially empowering, and maybe even a little scary to a patient with severe mental illness who may have had a long history of decisions being taken out of their hands. Planning reflects both a commitment to change as well as the identification of specific steps one needs to take in this course of action.

7.6   Clinical Examples

This author has selected examples of some of these questions within each process (Miller and Rollnick 2013, pg. 32) and believes that these are helpful for working with client/service users with a psychotic disorder. They include engagement ("How comfortable is this person talking to me?" and "do I understand this person's perspective and concerns?" and "does this feel like a collaborative partnership?"), focusing ("What goals for change does this person really have?" and "are we working together with a common purpose?" and "do I have a clear sense of what we are doing?"), evoking ("What are this person's own reasons for change?" and "is the reluctance more about confidence or importance of change?" and "am I steering too far or too fast in a particular direction?"), and planning ("What would be a reasonable next step toward change?" and "what would help this person move forward?" and "am I retaining a sense of quiet curiosity about what will work best for this person?"). These specific questions reflect the sometimes challenging experience with the client/service user with psychotic disorders and the difficulty in developing working relationships, trust, specific areas to focus treatment, motivation to work on these areas, and actual efforts and developing treatment plans toward this end. These four central processes of engaging, focusing, evoking, and planning, though, highlight what is needed in working with client/service users with psychotic disorder; they emphasize respect for the patient; they highlight the importance of developing an accurately empathic connection; they emphasize strong collaboration with the patient that facilitates the allowance of a patient-led uncovering of areas to address in treatment and they acknowledge the patient's own well of potential resources to address these areas of concern.

In this treatment approach, clarifying values and goals is another element of Motivational Interviewing and is a process that should be ongoing throughout the clinical work. This is another area in working with client/service users with psychotic disorders which can be challenging, but quite therapeutically rewarding, in the process. Attempting to ascertain what the patient you are working with "values" in their life is extremely important and an area vital for exploration. Sometimes, working with individuals with psychotic disorders, it can be difficult as a clinician to understand what these areas are and this might not always be clear, depending on the current nature and state of their disorder and how impaired reality testing and judgment are. However, even when reality testing and judgment are compromised, the clinician is encouraged to listen closely to the content that the patient is sharing, which may reveal both subtle and not so subtle elements in their life of what they feel are important to them. Understanding what your patient values also helps to get a clearer picture of the goals that they have established in their life. From a Motivational Interviewing standpoint, it is not about the clinician establishing their goals for treatment, but more about helping the patient to unearth their goals in their life and where their behavior might be discrepant from what they value and what their goals are. This process, once again, puts the patient's experiences, hopes, values, and goals – whatever they are – front and center. Goal setting can be challenging in working with psychotic disorder and the trap that clinician's from this perspective can fall in is making assumptions about patient values and becoming overly directive in the goal setting process. It can be challenging to work with patients with compromised reality testing and not become overly directive. Of course, sometimes this is necessary as it relates to direct needs to ensure safety of self and others, but that aside, the clinician should work alongside the patient, collaboratively, in establishing goals for treatment that emanate from what the patient values. A clinical example here to identify values of the client and addressing them to change a behavior that is discrepant with goals will be helpful.

A 38-year-old Caucasian male with schizoaffective disorder lives with his parents and takes clozapine medication. He always verbalizes desire to move out and live independently. However he would frequently drink alcohol and take medication only partially and would end up in hospital. When the discussion was about preventing hospitalization, he would blame his parents or neighbors for calling cops on him. Therapist used MI to address the stated value of client for independence and some barriers in reaching that independence. In this discussion, hospitalization was discussed as a barrier and then the discussion was about client working with therapist to address and remove all barriers to his independence. That led to discussion of going out with friends to drink, missing some doses of medication, and changes in behavior that are construed by others as risky or dangerous leading to hospitalization. Now client was able to see what he could control to give expression to behaviors that are consistent with his values and preventing hospitalization became not an end in itself but a means to the end of trying to live his value of independence.

As values and goals have been further clarified, "agenda mapping" is another process within Motivational Interviewing and refers to the process of the clinician and patient working together to decide on areas in treatment to choose to work on. Agenda mapping is greatly enriched by preceding processes in which a strong therapeutic alliance has developed, reflected by openness and trust of the patient feeling able to share their experiences, concerns, anxieties, what is important to them (e.g., values), and what they value, wish, and hope for (e.g., goals). In psychotic disorder client/service users, these goals can range from coming to appointments, self-care routine, hygiene, adherence to medication, to finding and sustaining employment and to developing and maintaining relationships. Similarly, depending on the current stability of the patient, identification and decision of which goals to work on may fluctuate, sometimes, rapidly during treatment. The process of agenda mapping with the patient conveys respect for the patient in being the primary author of the "map" so to speak. This is important particularly for client/service users suffering from psychotic disorders to experience. Frequently, these client/service users are underestimated and have had the experience of being told too often what "they need to do." While this may be true in some areas of their life (e.g., support for adherence to medication), it is not necessarily true in many other areas of their life. Through agenda mapping with client/service users, the clinician respects the client/service user's areas of independence and autonomy in making decisions and choices regarding what areas to work on in treatment. This process allows client/service user to establish several "destinations" of areas they would like to address in treatment. This can have the relieving impact of unburdening the patient who might experience treatment historically as over-focusing on one area. It also allows an opportunity for the patient and the clinician to discuss and establish several different areas in which to work and prioritize.

Typically, the development of the "agenda map" and the development of "goals" in treatment also uncover obstacles or "problem areas" which need to be addressed to enable work on a particular goal. If, for example, clear thinking and mood stability happen to be a goal in treatment, medication nonadherence might be considered a potential problem area which gets in the way of achieving the goals of intact reality testing and mood stability. In working with client/service user with psychotic disorders, identifying "problem areas" may be obvious and clear to the clinician, but not necessarily the patient. This is why the use of OARS is so fundamental in accurately establishing the agenda map, values and goals, and problem areas to address in treatment.

7.7 Rationale for Motivational Interviewing Working with Psychosis

In working with client/service users with psychotic disorders, from a Motivational Interviewing perspective, the application of Prochaska and DiClimente's Transtheoretical Stages of Change model is applicable and integrated within the Motivational Interviewing process. In treatment, following the establishment of an understanding of patient unique values, their goals, and "problem areas," assessing what stage of change the patient is fundamental for and how to proceed from a matching intervention standpoint in treatment. Typically, there are many problems that unfold over the course of treatment and it is critical for the clinician to assess, separately, what stage of change client/service users are at with each specific problem, as this answer will dictate the type of interventions that are most appropriate. The Stages of Change include pre-contemplation, contemplation, preparation, action, and maintenance. The following are characteristics that illustrate each stage of change. Pre-contemplation is marked by denial or an unwillingness to see or accept a certain problem area. Contemplation is characterized by an acknowledgment of the problem area and ambivalence around change. Preparation is illustrated by a patient acceptance of a problem area with beginning efforts to developing a plan for change. Action is characterized by the patient's engagement in actual, observable behavioral changes in relation to the problem area. Maintenance is marked by longer term investment in having made changes to address the problem area and continuing to maintain those changes. This Stages of Change model is based on various biopsychosocial theories of change and is stepwise in nature. An individual can enter at any point and move through these stages or fall back. The clinician's role is to facilitate movement from one stage of change to the next.

7.8 Obstacles in Conducting MI in Individuals with Psychosis and Some Ways to Navigate Those

With psychotic disorder client/service users, common problems might be medication adherence, keeping appointments, substance abuse, etc. So it is critical to address specifically the nature of the problem and what stage of change the patient is in. If, for example, substance abuse and medication adherence are identified as problem areas, the clinician would assess what stage of change the patient was in for each of these areas. Each stage of change requires different types of interventions. For example, if the patient was in pre-contemplation regarding their substance use, the intervention would be to increase the perception of risk in the patient's mind of continuing the problematic behavior. If they were in contemplation regarding medication management, the clinician's task would be to unearth the ambivalence around change and tip the scale, by weighing the pros and cons on both sides of the behavior (e.g., taking medication vs. not taking medication), both short term and long term. For a patient who reported that they are ready to stop drinking alcohol, in preparation, the clinician's task would be to help the patient come up with the best plan of action and help tweak that plan of action as necessary. For a patient who was now taking their antipsychotic medication as prescribed, the clinician's task would be to reinforce and support the behavior. And for a patient who had made a commitment to not using cocaine and had been abstinent for longer than 6 months, the interventions appropriate for the maintenance stage of change would be to identify alongside the patient strategies they could employ to sustain recovery and non-drug use behaviors while identifying potential high-risk situation coping strategies. It is important that in employing the Stages of Change model with client/service users with psychotic disorders, taking into account their overall level of psychosocial functioning and reality testing, mood stability is critical in making assessments regarding what specific stage of change they are at as well as decisions around matching interventions.

Once areas for focus of treatment have been collaboratively agreed upon and specific problem areas identified and the specific stage of change carefully assessed the clinician from an MI standpoint, works to facilitate "change talk" on the part of the patient, both from a "preparatory and mobilizing" standpoint. Preparatory change talk can be characterized by four different elements, desire, ability, reason, and need. Evoking change talk (Miller and Rollnick 2013, p. 171–173), in the process of preparation for change as the patient moves closer to addressing and changing problematic behavior, involves uncovering and evoking desire (e.g., "How would you like for things to change?"), ability ("What do you think you might be able to change?"), reasons ("What might be the three best reasons to change?"), and need ("What needs to happen, how important is this, and where do we start?"). Miller and Rollnick (2013) suggest the mnemonic, DARN, that can be used to remember these elements. As treatment progresses and the patient moves toward change, concretization of this process occurs, and within motivational interviewing, this involves increased "commitment," "activation," and "taking steps" or better remembered by the mnemonic CAT. Commitment is seen through the verbally expressed intention of change, whereas activation reveals more specifically what a patient is willing, ready or prepared to address, and taking steps, finally, involves specific activities the patient has done toward behavior change. Facilitating the verbalization of "mobilizing change talk" involves evoking activation talk ("Are you willing to give that a try?"), asking for commitment ("Are you going to do it?"), getting more specific ("How would you get ready?"), setting a date ("When could you do this?"), and preparing ("What would be a first step?") (Miller and Rollnick 2013, p. 272). Application of DARN CAT (Miller and Rollnick 2013) and the process of mobilizing change talk, as applied to client/service users with psychotic disorder, can be extremely helpful in helping them to identify areas of concern, their own beliefs about efficacy for changing behavior, why change in a particular area might be important, and identification what needs to happen next, a commitment toward attempting to make a change, increased specificity regarding next steps, and when, specifically, they can put the plan for change into action. The clarity and specificity of this process alongside keeping patient values, goals, and intentions front and center, in working collaboratively with a clinician who supports this process, are conducive to good and effective clinical work.

7.9 Application of the "How" in Motivational Interviewing with Psychosis

Eliciting motivation for change from a Motivational Interviewing standpoint can be done through several strategies. Querying extremes ("If everything stays the same and nothing changes, what is the worst that can happen?" and "If you were to make a change, what is the best thing that could happen?"), "looking back" ("Do you remember a time when things were going well? What changed?"), and "looking forward" ("If you were to make a change, what would things look like for you five years from now?") (Miller and Rollnick 2013, p. 176–177). This process keeps the patient's thoughts, feelings, and needs about problem areas and behavior change central. For psychotic disorder client/service users, it can also strengthen the ability for client/service users to increase their awareness of their current situation, experiences, values, problems areas, and goals for better functioning.

Sometimes, client/service users are deeply connected to behaviors that are problematic and there is "resistance" in considering change. In the area of psychotic disorders, these can include medication adherence, problematic beliefs, social isolation, unusually routinized/ritualistic behaviors, etc. Motivational Interviewing puts forth a number of strategies to manage resistance (Miller and Rollnick 2013). Some of these include simple reflection (simply conveying back to the patient what you understand them to be saying and expressing, without evaluation) which can be used at any stage of change; amplified reflection (amplifying one side of the ambivalence to draw out the behavior on the other side of the ambivalence) best used in contemplation; double-sided reflection (in which the clinician reflects back to the patient what they have heard them say, both sides of the ambivalence) used during contemplation and for later stages; and emphasizing personal choice and control (expressing the clear truth that a patient's decision regarding their behavior they have complete freedom, responsibility, and accountability for) which is good intervention for client/service users in pre-contemplation and reframing (giving the patient an alternative way to consider their experiences that may allow for potential change) applicable for any of the stages of change. As noted above, these techniques for managing resistance to changing problematic behavior should be matched with the appropriate stage of change, for example, a patient with a psychotic disorder who reports using substances and while it "improves how I am feeling in the short run… seems to make my auditory hallucinations worse later." A simple reflection would be, "using substances seems to make you feel better in the short term, but seems to result in increasing distress and auditory hallucinations in the long run." In simple reflection, you are just trying to convey that you understand how they think and feel. This has the effect of strengthening the therapeutic alliance, or at the very least maintaining it, in the face of resistance to change. An example of an amplified reflection would be, "It seems like your drinking really does make you feel better, maybe you should actually drink more," and for a patient who is in the contemplation stage of change, this will actually elicit the other side of the ambivalence (e.g., patient response: "No, I can't do that... the drinking actually makes the voices I am hearing worse... I have to figure out a different way feel better rather than drink!"). Giving a double-sided reflection, the clinicians might say, "On the one hand, there is a part of you that really would like to continue to drink because it makes you feel better and on the other hand, the drinking that you are doing, over the longer term, seems to make you more distressed"). This technique is used for client/service users in contemplation or higher and used to convey to the patient that you as a clinician understand their ambivalence, dilemma, and conflict regarding change. Emphasizing personal choice and control is a strategy that highlights the patient's own responsibility for the decisions they make and is particularly good for client/service users in pre-contemplation, who are already struggling with the difference between what they would like to continue to do in their life and the pressure they are getting from others to change and then becoming further entrenched in their behavior. In this example, the clinician might say, "Tom, it is entirely up to you whether you decide to continue using substances. What impact, one way or the other, do you think your drinking has on your mental health? At the end of the day, you have to decide how important your overall health and stability is to you."

7.10   Broader Applications of MI in the Context of Psychosis

Elements of Motivational Interviewing can be readily applied by professionals across different treatment professions and over the course of treatment within most sessions, the physician who is trying to have their patient with psychotic symptoms adhere to their medication, the psychologist who is trying to have the patient share more information with them about their experiences, the counselor who is trying to have their patient attend their sessions with more frequency, the nurse who is encouraging the patient to "open up" more in group, the substance abuse counselor who is attempting to engage the patient in relapse prevention strategies, the family member who is attempting to have their son (patient) attend the appointment with the psychiatrist, etc. Motivational Interviewing can be used across professional disciplines and modalities. Developing the therapeutic alliance has been shown to improve outcome and medication adherence in client/service users with schizophrenia (Julius et al. 2009), and one of the strongest elements of Motivational Interviewing, as has been discussed, is working to develop and sustain the therapeutic alliance. Targeted use of MI can potentially be beneficial in improving medication adherence with certain groups of patients (Barkhof et al. 2013).

7.11 Integrating MI with Other Evidence-Based Interventions

Motivational Interviewing can also be integrated across treatment approaches, e.g., cognitive-behavioral therapy, dialectical behavior therapy, family systems, psychodynamic therapy, etc. For example, each of these theoretical treatment approaches noted above places an emphasis on developing the therapeutic alliance where the development of accurate empathy is important. Each of these theoretical approaches involves varying degrees of collaboration as well as patient or family centeredness in which the patient's involvement and participation is vital. Each of these orientations involves "agenda mapping" and some decision making process involving what to work on in treatment and some efforts at planning how to proceed. Of course within each theoretical orientation, the contribution to these processes is different, but most treatment orientations can involve elements of motivational interviewing. Why? It is because the characteristics that define and describe the "spirit" of motivational interviewing are universal to the human experience and, in many regards, draw on fundamental universal needs as human beings, e.g., understanding, acceptance, collaboration, compassion, affirmation, worth, value, commitment, etc. Motivational Interviewing in its spirit addresses these areas. The therapist, who defines themselves as psychodynamic, or cognitive-behavioral, or family systems, or eclectic, is recommended to become thoroughly versed on Motivational Interviewing as it can be readily integrated into most contemporary treatment approaches. These treatment approaches share elements of engaging the patient, to some degree focusing treatment, addressing areas where needs for change are identified and the ability and readiness to do so, as well as treatment planning. Motivational Interviewing can also enhance the efficacy of other treatment approaches, for example, the cognitive-behavioral therapist that is attempting to teach the patient cognitive-behavioral relapse prevention strategies to reduce or prevent substance use secondary to efforts to cope with auditory hallucinations. Haddock et al. (2003) report significant improvement in patient functioning with combined cognitive-behavioral therapy and motivational interviewing. Instruments used to assess adherence to integrated Motivational Interviewing and cognitive-behavioral approaches for psychosis and substance abuse have also been developed (Haddock et al. 2012). Another example is the primary care physician who is attempting to improved attendance, medication adherence, and substance abuse. Westra et al. (2011) found that Motivational Interviewing can increase engagement, reduce substance use, and increase medication compliance and, that in this area, the evidence for the clinical support of Motivational Interviewing is the strongest. Possidente et al. (2005) also note that Motivational Interviewing can be used to increase medication adherence. For the psychodynamic therapist working with the psychotic disorder patient, attempting to increase greater awareness of the impact their behavior has on their own level of functioning, Rusch and Corrigan (2002) also suggest that there is some empirical evidence that Motivational Interviewing can increase insight and treatment adherence in schizophrenia. For the dialectical behavior therapist that is attempting to help the patient employ distress tolerance skills to reduce cutting secondary to mood dysregulation, the Motivational Interviewing strategy of developing discrepancy in the patient's mind between current self-injurious coping behaviors and the achievement of patient-identified moderate term goals might be helpful. Similarly, applying the stage of change model in assessing readiness to employ identified alternative healthy strategies of coping with distress and intervening with matching intervention to facilitate change. Also the family therapist who is attempting to improve a family member's communication strategies to increase their patient's attendance at psychiatrist appointments can be taught to be accurately empathic in strengthening their support and engagement with the patient to improve overall adherence and reduction in relapse.

In each of these scenarios described above, the clinician can apply the Stages of Change model in assessing readiness for changing problematic behavior and this will allow the clinician, regardless of the treatment model they are working from, to employ Motivational Interviewing strategies, as a precursor to facilitate readiness to respond to treatment interventions. These strategies are applicable for anyone who is working with clients to facilitate a behavior change, whether one is a primary care physician, psychiatrist, psychologist, social worker, nurse practitioner, nurse, counselor, or family member.

In a similar fashion, the learning and application of Motivational Interviewing strategies of family members can only improve the quality of relationships, communication, and efforts to promote healthy behavioral change. Improved medication adherence and decrease in relapse result in family members who have received some level of intervention and are actively engaged and supportive of client/service users (Julius et al. 2009). Many of the fundamental elements of motivational interviewing, for example, the importance of conveying acceptance, absolute worth, affirmation, compassion, exploring values and goals, and autonomy, are all vital in healthy and growing relationships. Efforts of one family member attempting to be accurately empathic toward the patient in their efforts to understand and appreciate their experience of living with a psychotic disorder and communicate this understanding are vital to the establishment of trust in the relationship and the enhancement of further communication and sharing of experiences. Demonstration of OARS by family members with the patient is a healthy communication style which enhances the family relationship. For example, a family member who practices asking open-ended questions (rather than close-ended) to learn more about the patient's experiences, then being affirmative of their experiences and accurately empathic toward what they are experiencing, will only deepen the trust in the relationship. Summarizing has the effect of both conveying to the patient that the family member has understood what has been said and also allows for correction and further learning. This is particularly important as client/service users with psychotic disorders can have difficulty describing and explaining their experiences, often distrustful, choosing to limit what is communicated. The four processes of Motivational Interviewing – engaging, focusing, evoking, and planning – can all be expressed by family members in their efforts to improve and enhance communication with the patient through efforts to communicate and interact with them, helping to work with them in allowing them to make appropriate decisions regarding behavior and change, emphasizing personal choice and control, eliciting their commitment, and "agenda mapping" and planning alongside them for preparation for specific steps to take toward change. Similarly, specific techniques to manage resistance such as simple reflections and double-sided reflections, emphasizing personal choice and control can be helpful in demonstrating both understanding and respect of the patient's experiences and can be easily learned.

7.12 Training of Staff in Motivational Interviewing Can Occur in Any Number of Different Ways

Healthcare providers across disciplines can be easily trained to integrate and deliver Motivational Interviewing strategies to assess and increase client/service user readiness and response to respective treatment. Psychiatrists, nurse practitioners, psychologist, social workers, and other healthcare professionals can all implement Motivational Interviewing techniques – whether addressing medication adherence, attendance to appointments, follow-up with discharge planning, therapeutic homework, and other psychosocial needs that are common in working with individuals with psychotic disorders. Motivational Interviewing techniques can be easily learned and adopted. Certainly reading any number of different books or articles on Motivational Interviewing is necessary. Miller and Rollnick's most recent edition (3rd) of Motivational Interviewing: Helping People to Change (2013) is highly recommended as a good starting place. Reading the first two editions of this book as each builds upon the last is also encouraged. Reading each of these books gives breadth and depth in understanding the principles, assumptions, strategies, and application of Motivational Interviewing. Attending workshops on Motivational Interviewing, attending formal training, reviewing online training resources, and receiving supervision by professionals skilled in Motivational Interviewing are all good practices in learning Motivational Interviewing. The healthcare provider working with client/service user with psychotic disorders who is also actively working with family members is encouraged to communicate and teach Motivational Interviewing strategies to enhance communication, quality of relationships, and health behavior change as the research suggests that improved family relationships marked by support and engagement improves outcomes.

It is worth noting that incorporating technology into the application of Motivational Interviewing can enhance accessibility and application of specific strategies, for example, the client/service user who has already written in information related to their own specific goals and values and healthy lifestyle behaviors that are consistent with these goals and values and, similarly, the client/service user who has written in benefits and risks or short- and long-term medication adherence or the client/service user who has documented their plan of action toward sustaining behavior change of consistent attendance at healthcare appointments. These are just a few examples of where technology and the use of mobile devices can be used as part of strategies within treatment by the provider and client/service user as a vehicle for accessing motivational enhancement information toward sustaining health.

7.13   Summary and Conclusion

Motivational Interviewing is a treatment approach which is quite compatible with the treatment needs of individuals with psychotic disorders. Its emphasis on a patient's own intrinsic value, worth, and individual "well" of resources, in and of itself, allows for growth and development in the patient. The processes of accurate empathy, acceptance, agenda mapping, assessing stage of change, eliciting motivation for change, and strategies for managing resistance and the strategies within can all be readily used by professionals across healthcare professions and well integrated into existing major mental health psychotherapies. For these reasons, Motivational Interviewing could be considered as an important modality of treatment in working with client/service user with psychotic disorders.

References

American Psychiatric Association (2013) Diagnostic statistical manual of the mental disorders, 5th edn. American Psychiatric Association, Arlington

Barkhof E, Haan L, Lieuwe M, Meijer CJ, Fouwels AJ, Keet IPM, Hulstijn KP, Schipper GM, Linszen DH (2006) Motivational interviewing in psychotic disorders. Curr Psychiatry Rev 2(2):207–213

Barkhof E, Meijer CJ, de Sonneville LMJ, Linszen DH, deHaan L (2013) The effects of motivational interviewing in medication adherence and hospitalization rates in non-adherent patients with multi-episode schizophrenia. Schizophrenia Bull 39(6):1242–1251

Britt D, Blampied NM, Hudson SM (2003) Motivational interviewing: a review. Aust Psychol 38(3):193–201

Haddock G, Barrowclough C, Tarrier N, Moring J, O'Brien R, Schofield N, Quinn J, Palmer S, Davies L, Lowens I, McGovern J, Lewis S (2003) Cognitive-behavioural therapy and motivational interviewing for schizophrenia and substance misuse. Br J Psychiatry 183(5):418–426

Haddock G, Beardmore R, Earnshaw P, Fitzsimmons M, Nothard S, Butler R, Eisner E, Barrowclough C (2012) Assessing fidelity to integrated motivational interviewing and CBT therapy for psychosis and substance use: the MI-CBT fidelity scale (MI-CTS). J Ment Health 21(1):38–48

Julius RJ, Novitsky MA, Dubin WR (2009) Medication adherence: a review of the literature and implications for clinical practice. J Psychiatr Pract 15(1):34–44

Miller WR, Rollnick S (1991) Motivational interviewing: preparing people to change addictive behavior. Guilford Press, New York

Miller WR, Rollnick S (2013) Motivational interviewing: helping people to change, 3rd edn. Guilford Press, New York

Possidente CJ, Bucci KK, McClain WJ (2005) Motivational interviewing: a tool to improve mediation adherence? Am J Health Syst Pharm 62:1311–1314

Prochaska JO, DiClimente CC (1983) Stages and processes of self-change of smoking: Toward an integrative model of change. J Consult Clin Psychol 51(3):390–395

Romano M, Peters L (2015) Evaluating the mechanisms of change in motivational interviewing in the treatment of mental health problems: a review and meta-analysis. Clin Psychol Rev 38:1–12

Rusch N, Corrigan PW (2002) Motivational interviewing to improve insight and treatment adherence in schizophrenia. Psychiatr Rehabil J 26(1):23–32

Westra HA, Aviram AM, Doell FK (2011) Extending motivational interviewing to the treatment of major mental health problems: current directions and evidence. Can J Psychiatry 56(11): 643–650

Brief Family Interventions in Psychosis: A Collaborative, Resource-Oriented Approach to Working with Families and Wider Support Networks

8

Frank R. Burbach

8.1 Family Intervention

Family intervention (FI) is a generic term for a range of therapeutic approaches to working with someone with psychosis and their family. Working with the significant others as well as the patient – in other words focusing on the relationships within which the patient's problem behaviors/symptoms are manifested – is known as a systemic intervention or therapy. All systemic practitioners work with as many as possible of the key people involved with the patient (and affected by the behaviors). In some cases, this is the partner/spouse and in others the immediate family, wider family, or support network. The field therefore includes couple, family, and network approaches, and in this chapter, the author refers to both "systemic" and "family/network" approaches to denote this range of approaches which all focus on relationships.[1] Even in a brief systemic intervention, the family/network members attending therapeutic sessions will often vary from one session to the next. Ideally this will be decided by the family and therapist on a session-by-session basis to enable particular topics to be addressed, but sometimes the attendance at a family meeting is determined by practical issues such as availability.

---

[1] It is also possible to work systemically with an individual if the focus of the conversation is on relationships; an empty chair technique is often used in such cases: "If x were here, what would he say…?"

F.R. Burbach
Somerset Partnership NHS Foundation Trust & University of Exeter, UK
e-mail: Frank.Burbach@sompar.nhs.uk

© Springer International Publishing Switzerland 2016
B. Pradhan et al. (eds.), *Brief Interventions for Psychosis: A Clinical Compendium*, DOI 10.1007/978-3-319-30521-9_8

8.2   Rationale for Working with Families

In light of the disabling effects of psychosis on an individual's functioning (see Chaps. 1 and 2), it is not surprising that there is considerable evidence that concerned family members and other individuals within the support network are adversely affected. This has been most extensively demonstrated with people experiencing long-term disability (see research literature on "objective" and "subjective burden," e.g., Fadden et al. 1987; Schene et al. 1994), but there is also considerable evidence of the adverse effect on families in the early stages. The first episode of psychosis often develops when the person is in close contact with their family of origin, and concerned family members are often pivotal in their initial engagement with mental health services. Families are often extremely worried about their relative and feel let down and unsupported by services, resulting in particularly high levels of distress and a range of mental health symptoms such as anxiety and depression (Addington et al. 2003; Onwumere et al. 2011b; Patterson et al. 2005). Numerous clinical guidelines (Bertolote and McGorry 2005; Dixon et al. 2010; IRIS 2012; NICE 2014; Worthington et al. 2013) therefore explicitly recommend actively supporting families and involving them as partners throughout the care pathway, with a particular emphasis on active engagement with relatives from their first contacts with services (creating a "Triangle of Care").

Personal reports of recovery in memoirs (e.g., Saks 2007) or in journals such as the Schizophrenia Bulletin also attest to the importance of having the support of family members and friends. Family supporters often play a crucial role as navigators and advocates, helping their loved one through a maze of often fragmented health care services. It may be useful to briefly summarize the extensive evidence base for family interventions (FI) at this point. Systematic reviews of clinical trials indicate that FIs are clinically effective and cost-effective (Pharoah et al. 2010; NICE 2014; Mihalapoulos et al. 2004). Adding FI to standard care (medication and supportive follow-up) more than halves the relapse rates, and the cost of this additional intervention is more than covered by the savings made, particularly because of reduced hospital admissions. Most of these studies have been conducted with long-term service users, and the evidence is less well developed for first-episode psychosis (FEP), but a systematic review and meta-analysis by Bird and colleagues (2010) demonstrated that FI also significantly reduces relapse and readmission rates for this group of patients.

Evidence supporting the involvement of significant others in mental health treatment can also be found in the systemic therapy and couple therapy literatures (von Sydow et al. 2010; Stratton 2011; Baucom et al. 2012). A radically different mental health service which has been developed in Western Lapland in Finland arguably provides even stronger evidence for a family-/network-based approach (Seikkula 2003; Seikkula et al. 2001). This service, which provides a family/network crisis intervention and minimizes use of psychotropic medication, has achieved remarkable clinical and functional outcomes e.g., around 75 % of those experiencing psychosis returned to work or study within 2 years and only around 20 % were still taking antipsychotic medication at 2-year follow-up (Seikkula et al. 2006).

8.3   A Note About the Historical Context of FI

A casual reader of FI literature might be confused about the plethora of models described, and it is useful to be aware of the phases of development in the field. Psychoeducational family management approaches developed from the "expressed emotion" (EE) studies contrast their approach with the earlier systemic family therapy approaches (Burbach 1996). Systemic family therapy, however, has been developed through a number of phases, and contemporary practice is socio-constructionist in nature (see Dallos and Draper 2010). Psychoeducational approaches have also developed over time – they are now more cognitive than behavioral in orientation. This has led to a fifth phase of family intervention in psychosis (Bertrando 2006) – the integration of systemic and psychoeducational approaches. In Somerset, UK, our group has developed a range of services based on an integrated approach since the mid-1990s (Burbach 2013b). This chapter presents a pragmatic brief intervention suitable for use in routine clinical practice, based on this integrated approach.

A historical understanding is helpful because it explains fundamental shifts in values underlying the approaches. Early approaches were "modernist" – believing that therapists, as "experts," should reeducate family members or restructure family relationships. In contrast, contemporary "postmodern" approaches acknowledge the subjective nature of reality, the need to work within people's belief systems in a collaborative and respectful way, and the importance of self-reflexivity. This shift to a constructivist/social constructionist approach predominates in the field of family therapy, but it can also be seen in the CBT field with the development of concepts such as "radical collaboration and acceptance" and a focus on strengths and solutions (e.g., Chadwick 2006; Padesky and Mooney 2012; Rhodes and Jakes 2009). Recently a number of these therapeutic approaches have been categorized as "resource-oriented therapeutic models" (Priebe et al. 2014).

Historical differences in the FI field have also narrowed because there is now greater understanding of the processes underlying empirical measures of distress and family tension (Burbach 2013a; Kuipers et al. 2010). Different interventions are required to address the specific maintenance factors involved in the three common care giving relationships in psychosis – "positive," "over-involved," and "critical/hostile" – in order to optimize therapeutic outcomes. It is worth noting that while both over-involved and critical/hostile styles of interaction are clearly associated with poor clinical outcomes and that the former style has a poorer outcome with psychoeducational family management approaches, it is now recognized that these EE styles reflect normal coping strategies and develop over time (McFarlane and Cook 2007; Patterson et al. 2005; see Burbach 2013a for a detailed review).

These interaction patterns can be addressed in a number of ways, but the typology developed by Baucom and colleagues (2012) in their work with couples provides a useful framework[2]:

---

[2] Baucom differentiates "partner-assisted," "disorder-specific," and "couple" therapies.

1. Some interventions simply enlist the support of significant others (e.g., relatives) as "assistant therapists"; for example, the clinician may model how to gently help the patient to test out whether his/her thinking is supported by the evidence or a family member could support the patient to carry out a planned "homework" task.

2. Other interventions may be focused on particular family interactions which are maintaining problems – for example, a withdrawn inactive patient may not have any incentive to go out to the shops if their partner has taken over this role (encouraging both parties to change this pattern is much more likely to result in rapid change than to focus solely on the patient's motivation in individual therapy sessions).

3. In other cases, the intervention would focus on more pervasive relationship problems (especially couple issues) because the ongoing high stress levels would not be conducive to recovery. Only the first two types of interventions ("significant other-assisted" and "disorder-specific" family work) would generally apply to brief FI. Longer term couple or family therapy would usually be required to address long-standing and severe relationship distress.

The literature on solution-focused brief therapy (SFBT) is also pertinent. This is a well-developed systemic therapy approach which explicitly focuses on the patterns of interaction which are most directly relevant to the symptoms (cf. Baucom's type 2 FI), but it pays particular attention to the solutions ("noticing what already works") and uses techniques such as miracle questions, scaling, and focusing on exceptions (de Shazer 1985; Trepper et al. 2012). A systematic review of 43 studies concluded that they provided "strong evidence that SFBT is an effective treatment for a wide variety of behavioral and psychological outcomes and, in addition, it may be briefer and therefore less costly than alternative approaches" (Gingerich and Peterson 2013: 266). The reader will see that the integrated brief family intervention described in this chapter contains many aspects of SFBT.

Despite its origins in working in a more manualized way (using a standard package) with people with long-standing disability resulting from psychosis and its treatment, it is also worth noting that the new consensus in the field is that FI should be tailored to the individual family's needs (the problems they are concerned about). This is especially the case when working with families coping with early psychosis when it is important to focus on the emotional distress and to discuss psychotic symptoms rather than diagnosis (Burbach et al. 2010; Gleeson et al. 1999; Onwumere et al. 2011a).

Research into the real-world implementation of evidence-based FI is also noteworthy. It has proved a challenge to develop routine FI services in comprehensive mental health services such as in the UK even following staff training (Fadden 1997). The challenge is even greater in more fragmented health systems such as in the USA where "family services are rarely utilized as part of routine care, and the majority of families are not having regular contact with the treatment team" (Cohen et al. 2010: 32). The literature indicates that there are a range of barriers to successful implementation of FI – systemic (especially organizational) issues are often paramount, but there are also individual factors such as the service user not wanting to involve family members (often because they do not want to "burden" their relative) or being estranged from their families, family members not responding to invitations to undertake FI (this is usually not the case if this is offered from the family's first contact with a service), and staff attitudes (e.g., "families are dysfunctional or toxic") and perceived lack of skill to deal with the complexities of family work (fear of "opening up a can of worms"). Training can overcome many of these barriers, but systemic issues such as lack of time, little or no supervision, services not being reimbursed by medical insurance companies, or legal barriers such as the HIPAA[3] rule have to be addressed if formal FIs are to be successfully offered.

These are the wider historical, theoretical, and service contexts within which the integrated brief family intervention presented below can be situated. The author would argue that clinicians need to feel empowered to take any opportunities that present themselves to work with families, however brief. Where possible this can then be boosted by more formal FI. The next section will attempt to provide a "nuts-and-bolts" description of a flexible, integrated approach.

8.4   The Clinical Approach

A *brief, focused, resource-oriented approach* to working with families and wider support networks which would be widely applicable is now described. At the heart of this approach is the collaborative therapeutic relationship where everyone's views are valued and respected. If the therapist creates a sufficiently safe space, the patient and family/network members will be able to share their thoughts and feelings and find more effective solutions to their current concerns. During such conversations, it often becomes clear that significant others have inadvertently reinforced the problem behaviors and the whole system can be enabled to change unhelpful interactional patterns through shifts in their beliefs, appraisals of one another's motives and actions, and by practicing new behaviors. In previous publications, our group has described this as a "cognitive interactional" approach (Burbach and Stanbridge 2006).

This brief collaborative systemic intervention can be described in terms of seven overlapping phases:

1. The provision of information and emotional and practical support
2. Identification of patient, family, and wider network resources
3. Encouraging mutual understanding

---

[3] The US Health Insurance Portability and Accountability Act (HIPAA) Privacy Rule and the UK Information Governance laws (Caldicott Guidelines) require health professionals to protect the privacy of health information. These legal frameworks attempt to strike an appropriate balance between the protection of the patient's information and the use and sharing of such information to improve care, but their emphasis on confidentiality often results in defensive practice with family/carers being excluded from care.

4. Identification and alteration of unhelpful patterns of interaction
5. Improving stress management, communication, and problem-solving skills
6. Relapse prevention planning
7. Ending

8.4.1   Phase 1: The Provision of Information and Emotional and Practical Support

At times of crisis, such as when a family member develops psychotic symptoms, takes a turn for the worse, or exhibits an extreme behavior, family members are often in a state of "shock" and feeling confused, overwhelmed, upset, despairing, or angry. Their attempts to get help have often been frustrating, and they may have had traumatic experiences due to their loved one's reactions and contacts with police, compulsory admissions, etc. Other experiences of the mental health services such as seeing chronically disabled psychiatric patients when visiting their relative, as well as possibly seeing their loved one's adverse reactions to their treatment, commonly leave relatives feeling afraid and despondent about the future. The reactions of the wider community due to the stigma still surrounding mental illness in many societies often compound both the patient and the family members' sense of hopelessness.

The most important first step in any family intervention is therefore to provide family members with tailored support and information. Providing families with emotional support primarily involves listening to the family members' experiences and validating them. This often involves undefensively accepting that the family feels that they have been let down due to gaps or inadequacies in mental health services. Normalizing their reactions to these traumatic events is the next essential step before exploring their understandings and offering information in order to help the family to feel more empowered to cope. This approach is sometimes called psycho-education (Xia et al. 2011) to contrast it with other forms of therapy, but there is a danger that clinicians might see their roles as "teachers" and that the family will feel "talked down to" and disempowered (Szapocznik and Williams 2000). Good clinical outcomes should not be evaluated in terms of family members' increased understanding of the medical model. What is required is much more than the provision of information leaflets; and if these are used, they should simply be adjuncts to the process. What needs to occur is a conversation where the clinician finds out how the different family members make sense of the psychotic experience and help them to build on this foundation so that they develop a more coherent, helpful understanding. For example, in a family session, we had a useful discussion about psychosis by exploring the client's description of it as "an ugly monster" and the family members' view that this behavior was her adopting a childlike persona and playing a role. This led to them making a connection with their regular game of playing different characters and speaking in different accents during family meals. A subsequent exploration of the way in which her father and oldest brother were very expressive with their anger while her mother and her second oldest brother denied and avoided such feelings led to a helpful understanding of the psychosis as a way of expressing unbearable feelings. In essence this is a therapeutic process rather than an educational one, and the clinicians should resist the temptation to impose their framework of understanding.

> In particular professionals should not insist that people agree with the view that experiences are symptoms of an underlying illness. Some people will find this a useful way of thinking about their difficulties and others will not. (Cooke 2014: 105)

Many people make sense of their experiences as a response to life's stressors and trauma, or in terms of a spiritual experience, and will find such personalized understandings more helpful for regaining optimum functioning following an episode of psychosis than an "illness model." The clinician's role is to tentatively and respectfully provide information which helps to develop these personalized understandings of the psychosis. There is also a great deal of general information that can helpfully be shared – information about services, what to do in a crisis, additional sources of support, etc.

8.4.2   Phase 2: Identification of Patient, Family, and Wider Network Resources

Besides listening and acknowledging problems that are facing the family, it is also important to take any opportunity to identify individual's strengths and competencies. Solution-focused therapy, narrative therapy, and other competency-based therapeutic techniques are useful in this regard (Bertolino and O'Hanlon 2002). For example, a clinician might comment "you are coping really well with…" or "what did you draw on to find the strength to go on at that point?" In the initial meeting(s), it is useful to explore the potential contributions of members of the family/wider network and the things that they have tried to do to help ("attempted solutions"). During times of crisis, when the patient may be acting irrationally and may even present as a danger to himself/herself or others, the wider network can be an invaluable resource. It is often important to keep an eye on the patient and help him/her to occupy his/her time, but this can become unhelpful if the patient feels overly scrutinized or pressured. Some members of the network may have less complex relationships with the patient and may be better suited to take on this task, or they may be able to help share this role.

Besides harnessing the network to solve particular problems and taking any opportunities for reinforcing competencies, it is also important to notice exceptions to problems and when they have found solutions to their problems (e.g., "It is good to hear that there are times when x is able to ignore the intrusions of the voices"). People often report partial solutions to their problems but discuss them as failures. By gently exploring these, the clinician can help family members to recognize that they *are* able to deal with their difficulties and thereby encourage them to renew their efforts. Often a potentially useful strategy is only partially implemented because people expect it to fail. Any discussions which increase the patient and significant others' sense of agency and hope for the future will be a therapeutically useful conversation, and this should be the overarching aim of the clinician.

8.4.3   Phase 3: Encouraging Mutual Understanding

Relationships often become fraught when a family member develops the confused thinking, perceptual abnormalities, and fears, becomes withdrawn or displays odd behaviors, or develops a lack of interest in everyday activities which are commonly associated with psychosis. A brief intervention is most likely to be effective if available as early as possible, before these problems have become entrenched. Systemic therapists refer to the way families/networks change and adapt to the new stressful situation as "trauma-organized systems" (Bentovim 1996). Trauma-organized systems are often unhealthy for all concerned: family members commonly become angry, critical, or hostile, and the patient becomes angry and fights back or, more often, withdraws (and in both cases is more likely to relapse). In other cases, family members may be overly fearful, watchful, and over intrusive, and the patient feels "smothered" and may become stuck in a "chronically disabled role." Again, in this scenario, the patient is more likely to have a further episode of psychosis, and the family members are more at risk of developing common mental health problems such as anxiety and depression.

Besides creating a safe space for all family/network members to express their fears, frustrations, and other feelings and responding with active listening, validation, and other general (nondirective) counseling skills, family/network sessions offer the opportunity to increase mutual understanding. Clinicians should try to get each person present to his/her their thoughts and feelings as a first step. This will require facilitation skills, with the clinician "bringing in" the different contributors and making sure no one feels silenced and no one dominates the conversation. This role can be likened to that of a Conductor of an Orchestra – most of the time only a light touch is required, for example, using humor, asking a question, or reflecting on a process in the room (Burbach 2016; Stanbridge and Burbach 2007). On some occasions, a firmer, more active approach may be needed to steer the conversation. Clinicians should stop discussions which are excessively blaming or otherwise harmful if the family members don't appear to be able to do this themselves.

A safe conversation in which everyone feels heard and validated is often a powerful emotional experience and in itself can be enough to help people to develop more positive, mutually supportive relationships. Commenting on the positive aspects of family/network relationships can benefit the emotional atmosphere in the session and help to move the session forward to a point where the family can successfully resolve their problems. It is therefore useful to make observations such as "you are a close, supportive family," "that really shows how much you care for x," or even "the fact that you are here today shows that you care and want to help." However, sometimes the clinician will need to explore issues in more detail and to more explicitly address unhelpful interactional patterns (see Phase 4 (Sect. 8.4.5)).

8.4.4   Commentary

We find that as little as one session, encompassing the first three phases, can be an effective brief intervention. This can be conceptualized as helping the family "back on track" and is most likely to suffice if the family members have previously had reasonably positive relationships and if the family's unhelpful coping strategies have not yet become "set in concrete." However, even in cases where we are able to intervene early, it is often necessary to provide further sessions as part of a brief intervention. This would often involve addressing unhelpful family patterns and developing coping skills.

8.4.5 Phase 4: Identification and Alteration of Unhelpful Patterns of Interaction

Families often report their problems in a generalized (and blaming) way, and it is useful to explore specific situations and help family members to recognize that they are often part of a repeated pattern to which they all contribute. An exploration of sequences of behaviors (or "circularities") regarding specific incidents (e.g., "Let's look at what happened yesterday evening") allows a detailed exploration of the feelings, beliefs, and actions of the participants. A "cognitive interactional cycle" can be drawn out on paper with the family by clarifying a (problem) behavior and then asking about the circumstances leading up to it and the appraisals, emotional reactions, and response to the behavior. An example of a cognitive interactional cycle is provided below (and other common examples are detailed in Burbach 2013a) (Fig. 8.1):

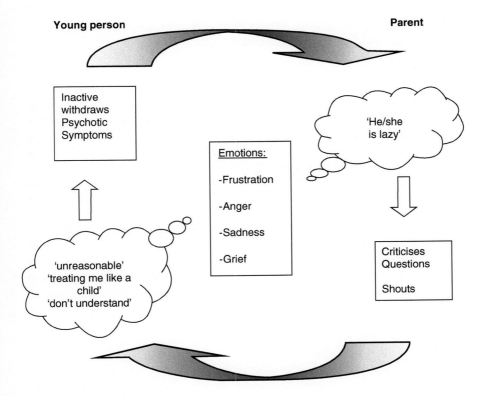

Fig. 8.1 Cognitive interactional cycle

As mentioned previously, the exploration of such cognitive interactional cycles can be a powerful therapeutic experience as the different family members all realize that they have been misinterpreting each other's motives and have inadvertently been reinforcing the problem behavior. This technique not only results in increases in mutual understanding and a consequent improvement in the emotional climate in the family but can also help identify specific targets for intervention. In the example above, working with either party could result in a new, more positive interactional cycle developing. Behavioral techniques with the patient such as goal setting and positive reinforcement of approximations of the desired behavior and communication training with the parent could result in the patient becoming more active and less withdrawn and the parent becoming less critical. Focusing on their appraisals of each other (exploring alternative understandings) is another avenue to engender helpful change. For the patient, more helpful alternative cognitions that may develop could be "They are getting upset with me because they are concerned/care about me and want to help" and for the patient might be "She is struggling with (difficult symptoms) and doing the best she can. I'll try to support her without pressurizing her."

If the exploration of interactional cycles is not sufficient, and the "spontaneous" alteration of feelings, beliefs, and feelings does not occur, then more structured cognitive-behavioral skills training may be required (see Phase 5 below (Sect. 8.4.6)).

8.4.6   Phase 5: Improving Stress Management, Communication, and Problem-Solving Skills

It is often not enough to provide information regarding the stress-vulnerability model (phase 1) in order to reduce the emotional tension in the family (and reduce the likelihood of relapse and the family members developing their own mental health symptoms); helping them to develop specific stress management skills is often required. A range of techniques can be adopted, and, again, if this is decided in collaboration with the family and fits with their values and beliefs, the techniques are more likely to be used and to be of benefit. Yoga (see Chap. 5), meditation, relaxation, exercise, or simple breathing exercises such as 7–11 breathing (breathe in for a count of 7 and out for a count of 11) can be very useful. Different family members may be more or less receptive to these ideas, but even a reduction in one person's stress levels can benefit the overall family atmosphere and is therefore worthwhile. These activities can also help to strengthen couple or family relationships, so finding one that everyone is prepared to join in with is the ideal.

Communication difficulties are at the heart of many stressful family interactions (whether the family has someone struggling with psychosis or not!). Some families with psychosis have specific communication difficulties (Doane et al. 1981), but many people in the "normal population" have poorly developed communication skills. Specific guidelines for clear, direct, and positive communication have been developed (Falloon et al. 2004), and many families benefit from practicing and following these. For example, rather than criticizing, family members can practice calmly asking a person to carry out the desired behavior: "It really makes me feel

Table 8.1 Communication skills training (based on Falloon et al. 2004)

Active listening
Look at the speaker and attend to what is said
Nod head, say "Yes, Uh-Huh"
Ask clarifying questions (e.g., "What happened next?")
Check out what you heard (e.g., "So what you are telling me is …")
Expressing positive feelings
Look at the person
Say exactly what she or he did that pleased you
Tell the person how it made you feel
Making a positive request
Look at the person
Say exactly what you would like that person to do
Tell how it would make you feel
In making positive requests, use phrases like:
"I would like you to …"
"I would really appreciate it if you would …"
"It is very important to me that you help me with the …"
Expressing negative feelings
Look at the person: speak firmly
Say exactly what the person did that upset you
Tell the person how it made you feel
Suggest how the person might prevent this from happening in the future

cross when you… please do…" Similar communication skills guidelines have been developed for active listening, expressing positive feelings, and expressing negative feelings (see Table 8.1).

Some families also find it helpful to improve their problem-solving skills. Providing families with information about the 6 problem-solving stages (Falloon et al. 2004; see Table 8.2) and helping them to practice these can provide a useful family ritual which can reduce stress and help prevent problems from becoming entrenched. Many families will set a regular time each week for a family meeting in which problems are worked through, with family members rotating the roles of chairperson and scribe/ secretary. This structured format enables difficult issues to be addressed in a safe way.

8.4.7 Phase 6: Relapse Prevention Planning

Most people with psychosis and their friends/relatives are concerned about the possibility of relapse, and thus, this often becomes the agreed focus for family sessions. Exploring the factors which led up to the psychotic episode – predisposing ("background issues") and precipitating factors ("triggers") as well as the sequence of prodromal and psychotic symptoms – is very useful as a therapeutic technique.

Table 8.2 Six-step problem-solving approach (based on Falloon et al. 2004)

Step 1: *What is the problem or goal?*
Talk about the problem/goal – get everybody's opinion; ask questions to clarify. Then write down the agreed problem/goal
Step 2: *List all possible solutions*
What has worked in the past? What would a friend say? Get everybody to come up with at least one possible solution. Put down all ideas, even if you think they won't work. List the solutions *without discussion*
(1) _____
(2) _____
(3) _____
(4) _____
(5) _____
Step 3: *Consider pros and cons of each solution*
Quickly discuss the main advantages and disadvantages (pros and cons) of each possible solution
Step 4: *Choose the solution that seems best*
Choose the solution that can be carried out most easily to solve the problem
Step 5: *Plan how to carry out the best solution*
Be specific: Who? What? When? Where? How?
What could cause problems and how could you get around this? What resources are needed? Practice difficult steps. Plan time for review
(1) _____
(2) _____
(3) _____
(4) _____
Step 6: *Do it*! *try out the solution and review results*
Did it work? Which aspects worked? Focus first on *what worked well. Praise all efforts. Revise as necessary/try out another solution (return to Step 3 and 4)*

"Storying" or "integrating" the psychotic experience results in better outcomes than "sealing over" or "burying it" but also enables the patient, family, and professionals to identify specific "warning signs" of relapse and to agree an intervention plan should this "relapse signature" occur again. In some services, it is also possible to agree "advance statements" or "directives" where the patient specifies his/her preferred options for treatment should he/she becomes ill again. For example, he/she may express a preference for a particular medication or specify that a particular relative should be contacted even if, when acutely unwell, he/she is likely to express the wish that no one be told that he/she is in the hospital.

8.4.8   Phase 7: Ending

Whatever the components of the intervention, it is good practice to review progress and reflect on the key "learning points" at the end of each session and at the end of the course of therapy: "How did you find today's session? Can you think of one thing that you can take away from our meeting today?" It is also useful to encourage the family to make some notes/provide them with a bullet point summary of "key points." If the family then decides not to continue with the meetings, each session will feel like a completed "mini intervention," and this will help consolidate the work.

It is also useful to discuss how new strategies can be kept in place/practiced and to consider how to prevent or respond to "lapses" at the end of certain sessions and at the end of therapy. This should be done in detail in the last planned session: "What will you notice if your voices/fears/worry start to invade your life again? What triggers should you need to look out for? What will you do if you notice your unhelpful habits/problems creeping up again? What strategies will you use to 'nip this in the bud'? What qualities will you draw on to overcome this? Who else can support you to beat (the problem)? How can they best support you?"

8.4.9 What Would This Brief Intervention Look Like?

With some families, the sessions can touch on all seven phases even if the family intervention is only two or three sessions. However, in most cases, the meetings will not be able to include the development of specific skills without an agreement to devote sessions to this work (and thus a longer series of sessions – *typically up to ten* would need to be agreed). If a typical brief family intervention of three to five sessions is offered, this often proves sufficient to improve the emotional climate, help the family to (at least begin to) change some unhelpful patterns, solve some immediate problems, and feel prepared and supported should they need to access services again.

Brief family interventions can also be incorporated into routine practice such as monitoring visits by psychiatrists or care coordinators/case managers where a 5- or 10-min addition to the visit could focus on FI. This can be done by arrangement but can also take place "spontaneously" by involving a family member who happens to be present at a routine home visit. The family member does not even need to be physically present, as illustrated by the case vignette provided by Dr. Narsimha Pinninti, one of the book editors, below.

Case vignette

JH, a 37 year old male living with his elderly divorced mother of 66 was being treated in a partial hospitalization program and carried a diagnosis of schizo-affective disorder and OCD. One of the chronic sources of stress for both the mother and son was their frequent negative interactions triggered by him expressing delusional thoughts. He believed that sounds on the road were from his neighbors, the leaves that blew into their house were them trying to send a message and bully him. He would express them several times a day, that would frustrate his mom and she would retort by saying that everything was in his mind and that he is bothering her. He would feel guilty about it and would be withdrawn and then she would get upset that he was sad. Their perception of each other was "we get on each other's nerves".

In a medical monitoring visit, the psychiatrist specifically enquired if he had positive interactions with his mom lately and he was able to describe that on one occasion she did not get angry when he talked about neighbors and instead explained that he should not let others' actions bother him. The clinician explored his feelings following this positive interaction and he was able to describe both relief and appreciation of what his mom said and how she said it. With his permission, the psychiatrist called his mom and had her on the speaker phone and asked the client to express his positive feelings and appreciation towards his mom. She was pleasantly surprised to hear this from him and after thanking him explained that she does not know how to stop his delusional thoughts as they are not true. The Psychiatrist explained that she should not feel responsible to stop his thoughts. The Psychiatrist also explained what he found helpful in working on these thoughts with the client. One was to try to gently explore with the client if there was any evidence for the belief. This was framed to mother as 'tapping into his logical thinking part' and working with it to examine his belief. The client then said that he would be happy if his mom listened to him and did not ask him to stop thinking those thoughts. His mom said that she would not be so burdened if all she had to do was just listen and not having to think that she has to do something to make his thoughts go away. Next the psychiatrist asked mom to describe something positive JH did in the last week and she was able to say that he expressed concern about her physical health and helped her with cooking. JH was pleased to hear positive comments from mother. Then the psychiatrist asked them both how often they express positive feelings and both agreed that they usually do not. It was suggested that they try to express positive feelings to each other. This intervention did not take more than 6 or 7 minutes and led to both of them feeling good about each other and that they had a way of moving forward.

8.5   Cultural Considerations

It may be reasonable to assume that "collectivist" and "individualist" cultures hold differing views on the role of the family and that this may affect family participation and involvement in mental health services. Despite needing to be sensitive to such issues, however, most family members are likely to be highly concerned about their loved one and can be successfully engaged in services, especially if this is done early on.

It has been shown that family interventions can be successfully adapted to a range of cultural contexts (NICE 2014), but there is also some evidence that with particular cultural groups, a manualized approach can result in increased stress levels and worse outcomes (Telles et al. 1995). In contrast, the flexible approach described in this chapter is based on a collaborative therapeutic relationship, with the clinician adopting a position of *respectful curiosity*. Whether one is working with people who appear to be from a different cultural background or not, adopting a respectful, cautious, curious position (guarding against making assumptions about how people should live their lives) is essential. This does not mean ignoring one's ethical or moral values, but being open-minded about things that are discussed, and exploring (to what extent) these is helpful to the individual and their family or not. However, if this respectful exploration reveals exploitation, abuse, or any other harmful behaviors, then this should be addressed in the sessions and appropriate safeguarding or law enforcement procedures followed.

8.6   Service Considerations

The collaborative, resource-oriented brief family/network therapy described above should not be considered in isolation. Working in this way is most likely to optimize outcomes if it is at the heart of the approach of the wider service (cf. Open Dialogue services in Finland) rather than simply added to standard care. A recent report (Knapp et al. 2014) details a range of evidence-based interventions and services which can significantly improve outcomes which would all, ideally, be available in an integrated manner. Liberman et al. (2002) review the factors related to recovery from schizophrenia and conclude that recovery is most likely with "comprehensive, evidence-based, continuous, coordinated, and consumer-oriented services" (p. 267).

Although the above may sound like a call for a "revolution" in the delivery of mental health care, perhaps the most radical and also achievable change would be to develop more family-oriented services. The author has argued (Burbach 2012, 2015) that this can be done by slowly increasing the "menu" of services for families and that, especially if we intervene early, the "sufficiency principle" (Cohen et al. 2008) can be utilized – providing a range of family-based services so that the needs of clients and family members can be met with the least intensive intervention. Employing a few family specialists can lead to the development of a cost-effective "stepped care" service if part of their remit is the wide-scale training of frontline mental health staff in family inclusive practice and family interventions (Stanbridge and Burbach 2014). Although good listening and basic counseling skills go a long way, these fundamental skills would ideally be augmented by training in at least foundation-level systemic (and solution-focused) therapy as well as behavioral family therapy (BFT). The relevant courses vary in length: the BFT skills used in phase 5 usually require 4–5-day training, numerous workshops and courses in systemic therapy are available, and Open Dialogue is taught on courses lasting a minimum of 1 year.

While the barriers to family interventions can best be overcome by people who have some influence on the delivery of mental health care, all clinicians can choose to begin to practice in a more family-oriented manner. This is possible even when someone has more long-standing mental health problems and family members are estranged or geographically distant. In such cases, family interventions may be more appropriately delivered to relatives without the patient present. Such programs can be successfully delivered by peers (Lucksted et al. 2013) or professionals (Lucksted et al. 2012). Technological solutions such as Internet-based FI programs and the use of smartphones and computer tablets also show great promise in this regard (Ben-Zeev et al. 2015).

Conclusion

The approach described in this chapter has been simplified into seven phases, but the reader will have recognized that many of the therapeutic skills have been drawn from different therapy models, all of which may be of use to a clinicians wishing to develop their therapeutic practice. What this work has in common, however, is a focus on reinforcing strengths and enabling people to feel able to solve their own problems. While many will find it helpful to use the seven phases as a guide to providing brief family interventions, it should be recognized that these are fluid and that clinicians should not try to impose a structure on the family but should rather construct a therapeutically useful conversation with families based on their main concerns. These may vary from session to session, and it is therefore helpful to start each session by asking how they would like to use the time today.

Although the seven phases can helpfully structure therapeutic work, perhaps *the greatest benefit of any therapeutic model is that it makes the clinician feel more secure and hopeful*, and it is then possible for them to enable the regeneration of these feelings in the people they are trying to help. In Somerset we find these phases helpful, but we are also intrigued by the Open Dialogue approach, and while we have many aspects in common, we are moving toward this less structured and even more collaborative way of working (Seikkula and Arnkil 2014; Burbach et al. 2015). Hopefully this chapter will encourage all clinicians, whatever their level of training, to engage with and collaborate with families in their struggles with psychosis and that, in itself, will be greatly valued and is likely to lead to better outcomes.

References

Addington J, Coldham EL, Jones B, Ko T, Addington D (2003) The first episode of psychosis: the experience of relatives. Acta Psychiatr Scand 108(4):285–289

Baucom DH, Whisman MA, Paprocki C (2012) Couple-based interventions for psychopathology. J Fam Ther 34(3):250–270

Bentovim A (1996) Trauma-organized systems in practice: implications for work with abused and abusing children and young people. Clin Child Psych Psychiatry 1(4):513–524

Ben-Zeev D, Drake RE, Brian RM (2015) Technologies for people with serious mental illness. In: Marsch LA, Lord SE, Dallery J et al (eds) Behavioral health care and technology: using science-based innovations to transform practice. Oxford University Press, New York, pp 70–80

Bertolino B, O'Hanlon WH (2002) Collaborative, competency-based counseling and therapy. Prentice Hall, Upper Saddle River, NJ

Bertolote J, McGorry P (2005) Early psychosis declaration (EPD). International consensus statement. Br J Psychiatry 187:s116–s119

Bertrando P (2006) The evolution of family interventions for schizophrenia. A tribute to Gianfranco Cecchin. J Fam Ther 28(1):4–22

Bird V, Premkumar P, Kendall T, Whittington C, Mitchell J, Kuipers E (2010) Early intervention services, cognitive-behavioural therapy and family intervention in early psychosis: systematic review. Br J Psychiatry 197:350–356

Burbach FR (1996) Family based interventions in psychosis – an overview of, and comparison between, family therapy and family management approaches. J Ment Health 5(2):111–134

Burbach FR (2012) Family interventions: fundamental considerations when developing routine and formal family interventions services. Chapter 10. In: Anastassiou-Hadjicharalambous X (ed) Psychosis: causes, diagnosis and treatment. Nova Science Publishers, New York

Burbach FR (2013a) Towards a systemic understanding of family emotional atmosphere and outcome after psychosis. Chapter 9. In: Gumley A, Gillham A, Taylor K, Schwannauer M (eds) Psychosis and emotion: the role of emotions in understanding psychosis. Routledge, Hove, East Sussex

Burbach FR (2013b) Developing systemically-oriented secondary care mental health services. Plymouth University PhD thesis archived in PEARL: http://hdl.handle.net/10026.1/1599

Burbach FR (2015) The development of efficient family intervention services- a whole systems approach. Clin Psychol Forum 271:36–41

Burbach FR (2016) Co-work: working in pairs enables effective whole family sessions. Parental mental health and child welfare work – Volume 1. Pavilion Annuals

Burbach FR, Stanbridge RI (2006) Somerset's family interventions in psychosis service: an update. J Fam Ther 20:311–325

Burbach FR, Fadden G, Smith J (2010) Family interventions for first episode psychosis. Chapter 23. In: French P, Read M, Smith J, Rayne M, Shiers D (eds) Promoting recovery in early psychosis. Wiley-Blackwell, Chichester

Burbach F, Sheldrake C, Rapsey E (2015) Open dialogue in Somerset? Context 138:17–19

Chadwick P (2006) Person-based cognitive therapy for distressing psychosis. John Wiley & Sons, Hoboken, NJ

Cohen AN, Glynn SM, Murray-Swank AB, Barrio C, Fischer EP, McCutcheon SJ, Rotondi AJ, Sayers SL, Sherman MD, Dixon LB (2008) The family forum: directions for the implementation of family psychoeducation for severe mental illness. Psychiatr Serv 59:40–48

Cohen AN, Glynn SM, Hamilton AB, Young AS (2010) Implementation of a family intervention for individuals with schizophrenia. J Gen Intern Med 25(Suppl 1):S32–S37

Cooke A (2014) Understanding psychosis and schizophrenia: why people sometimes hear voices, believe things that others find strange, or appear out of touch with reality, and what can help. British Psychological Society. Division of Clinical Psychology, Leicester

Dallos R, Draper R (2010) An introduction to family therapy: systemic theory and practice. McGraw-Hill Education, Maidenhead

De Shazer S (1985) Keys to solution in brief therapy. Norton, New York

Dixon LB, Dickerson F, Bellack AS, Bennett M, Dickinson D, Goldberg RW, Lehman A, Tenhula WN, Calmes C, Pasillas RM, Peer J, Kreyenbuhl J (2010) The 2009 schizophrenia PORT psychosocial treatment recommendations and summary statements. Schizophr Bull 36(1):48–70

Doane JA, West KL, Goldstein MJ, Rodnick EH, Jones JE (1981) Parental communication deviance and affective style: predictors of subsequent schizophrenia spectrum disorders in vulnerable adolescents. Arch Gen Psychiatry 38(6):679–685

Fadden G (1997) Implementation of family interventions in routine clinical practice following staff training programs: a major cause for concern. J Ment Health 6(6):599–612

Fadden G, Bebbington P, Kuipers L (1987) The burden of care: the impact of functional psychiatric illness on the patient's family. Br J Psychiatry 150:285–292

Falloon I, Mueser K, Gingerich S, Rappaport S, McGill C, Graham-Hole V, Fadden G, Gair F (2004) Family work manual. The West Midlands Family Programme, Meriden

Gingerich WJ, Peterson LT (2013) Effectiveness of solution-focused brief therapy: a systematic qualitative review of controlled outcome studies. Res Soc Work Pract 23:266–283

Gleeson J, Jackson HJ, Stavely H, Burnett P (1999) Family intervention in early psychosis. In: McGorry PD, Jackson HJ (eds) The recognition and management of early psychosis: a preventive approach. Cambridge University Press, Cambridge, pp 376–406

IRIS (2012) IRIS guidelines update. IRIS Ltd. www.iris-initiative.org.uk

Knapp M, Andrew A, McDaid D, Iemmi V, McCrone P, Park A, Parsonage M, Boardman J, Shepherd G (2014) Investing in recovery: making the business case for effective interventions for people with schizophrenia and psychosis. London School of Economics and Rethink Mental Illness. http://www.rethink.org/media/1069950/Investing%20in%20Recovery%20-%20May%202014.pdf

Kuipers E, Onwumere J, Bebbington P (2010) A cognitive model of caregiving in psychosis. Br J Psychiatry 196:259–265

Liberman RP, Kopelowicz A, Ventura J, Gutkind D (2002) Operational criteria and factors related to recovery from schizophrenia. Int Rev Psychiatry 14(4):256–272

Lucksted A, McFarlane W, Downing D, Dixon L (2012) Recent developments in family psychoeducation as an evidence-based practice. J Marital Fam Ther 38(1):101–121

Lucksted A, Medoff D, Burland J, Stewart B, Fang LJ, Brown C, Jones A, Lehman A, Dixon LB (2013) Sustained outcomes of a peer-taught family education program on mental illness. Acta Psychiatr Scand 127(4):279–286

McFarlane WR, Cook WL (2007) Family expressed emotion prior to onset of psychosis. Fam Process 46:185–197

Mihalopoulos C, Magnus A, Carter R, Vos T (2004) Assessing cost-effectiveness in mental health: family interventions for schizophrenia and related conditions. Aust N Z J Psychiatry 38: 511–519

National Institute for Health and Care Excellence (2014) Psychosis and schizophrenia in adults: the NICE guideline on treatment and management in adults (update). CG 178. National Institute for Health and Care Excellence, London

Onwumere J, Bebbington P, Kuipers E (2011a) Family interventions in early psychosis: specificity and effectiveness. Epidemiol Psychiatr Sci 20(02):113–119

Onwumere J, Kuipers E, Bebbington P, Dunn G, Freeman D, Fowler D, Garety P (2011b) Coping styles in carers of people with recent and long-term psychosis. J Nerv Ment Dis 199(6): 423–424

Padesky CA, Mooney KA (2012) Strengths-based cognitive–behavioural therapy: a four-step model to build resilience. Clin Psychol Psychother 19(4):283–290

Patterson P, Birchwood M, Cochrane R (2005) Expressed emotion as an adaptation to loss: perspective study in first-episode psychosis. Br J Psychiatry 187:S59–S64

Pharoah F, Mari J, Rathbone J, Wong W (2010) Family intervention for schizophrenia. Cochrane Database Syst Rev 12

Priebe S, Omer S, Giacco D, Slade M (2014) Resource-oriented therapeutic models in psychiatry: conceptual review. Br J Psychiatry 204:256–261

Rhodes J, Jakes S (2009) Narrative CBT for psychosis. Routledge, Hove, East Sussex

Saks ER (2007) The center cannot hold: a memoire of my schizophrenia. Virago, London

Schene AH, Tessler RC, Ganache GH (1994) Instruments for measuring family or caregiver burden in severe mental illness. Soc Psychiatry Psychiatr Epidemiol 29:228–240

Seikkula J (2003) Open dialogue integrates individual and systemic approaches in serious psychiatric crises. Smith Coll Stud Soc Work 73(2):227–245

Seikkula J, Arnkil TE (2014) Open dialogues and anticipations: respecting otherness in the present moment. National Institute for Health and Welfare, Tampere

Seikkula J, Alakare B, Aaltonen J (2001) Open dialogue in psychosis 1: an introduction and case illustration. J Consultative Psychol 14:247–265

Seikkula J, Aaltonen J, Alakare B, Haarakangas K, Keranen J, Lehtinen K (2006) Five-year experience of first-episode nonaffective psychosis in open-dialogue approach: treatment principles, follow- up outcomes, and two case studies. Psychother Res 16:214–228

Stanbridge RI, Burbach FR (2007) Involving carers (part 1) chapter 5. In: Froggatt D, Fadden G, Johnson DL, Leggatt M, Shankar R (eds) Families as partners in mental health care: a guidebook for implementing family work. World Fellowship for Schizophrenia and Allied Disorders, Toronto

Stanbridge R, Burbach F (2014) Family needs, family solutions: developing family therapy in adult mental health services chapter 9. In: McNab S, Partridge K (eds) Creative positions in adult mental health: outside in – inside out. Karnac Books, London, pp 167–186

Stratton P (2011) The evidence base of systemic family and couples therapy. Association of family therapy. www.aft.org.uk

Szapocznik J, Williams RA (2000) Brief strategic family therapy: twenty-five years of interplay among theory, research and practice in adolescent behavior problems and drug abuse. Clin Child Fam Psychol Rev 3:117–134

Telles C, Karno M, Mintz J, Paz G, Arias M, Tucker D, Lopez S (1995) Immigrant families coping with schizophrenia: behavioural family intervention versus case management with a low-income Spanish-speaking population. Br J Psychiatry 167:473–479

Trepper TS, McCollum EE, De Jong P, Korman H, Gingerich WJ, Franklin C (2012) Solution-focused brief therapy treatment manual. In: Franklin C, Trepper TS, Gingerich WJ, McCollum EE (eds) Solution-focused brief therapy: a handbook of evidence-based practice. Oxford University Press, New York, pp 20–36

von Sydow K, Beher S, Schweitzer J, Retzlaff R (2010) The efficacy of systemic therapy with adult patients: a meta-content analysis of 38 randomized controlled trials. Fam Process 49:457–485

Worthington A, Rooney P, Hannan R (2013) The triangle of care – carers included: a best practice guide in acute mental health care, 2nd edn. Carers Trust, London, https://professionals.carers.org/working-mental-health-carers/triangle-care-mental-health

Xia J, Merinder LB, Belgamwar MR (2011) Psychoeducation for schizophrenia. Cochrane Database Syst Rev (6):CD002831. doi:10.1002/14651858.CD002831.pub2

Recovery-Related Brief Interventions for Psychosis

9

Geoff Shepherd

9.1 Introduction

Mental health services in most countries are facing fundamental challenges in terms of their capacity to meet ever-increasing demands with limited resources and limited powers to increase the availability of funding. Mental health conditions represent the single, largest source of disability (World Health Organization 2008), and the mismatch between demand and supply has been so great that we may have to rethink our traditional assumptions about the content and "style" of service provisions – both "what" is delivered and "who" delivers it.

This chapter will examine these themes in relation to psychosis and some of the new ideas which focus on the importance of supporting "recovery." It has long been established that for people with psychosis, their symptomatic course and their social outcomes can be heterogeneous and often not closely correlated with one another (Strauss and Carpenter 1977; Harding et al. 1987). It is also the case that while antipsychotic medications are effective in controlling symptoms in the acute phase for most people, they are not effective in a substantial minority of cases (about one in five, according to the Royal College of Psychiatrists 2014). On the other hand, effective psychosocial interventions have been relatively neglected in research and service delivery (see Chap. 1). Doubts have also been raised recently regarding the long-term use of antipsychotics since there is preliminary evidence that maintenance medication may lead to worse social outcomes in young people with remitted psychosis, despite a more benign symptomatic course (Wunderinck et al. 2013). In either case, one cannot assume that the most effective way to improve long-term outcomes for people with psychosis is simply through the administration of

G. Shepherd
Professor Geoff Shepherd, Senior Consultant,
ImROC Programme, Centre for Mental Health, 136–138 Borough High Street,
London SE1 1LB, England
e-mail: Geoff.Shepherd@centreformentalhealth.org.uk

© Springer International Publishing Switzerland 2016
B. Pradhan et al. (eds.), *Brief Interventions for Psychosis:*
A Clinical Compendium, DOI 10.1007/978-3-319-30521-9_9

symptom-oriented treatments – medical or psychological. Instead, one needs to look at how to combine traditional treatments with more social models of care in order to improve outcomes.

9.2   Supporting Recovery

One of the most well-known social models in mental health services derives from ideas about the importance of supporting "recovery" (Slade 2009). This underpins national policies across the developed world. But what does "recovery" mean in this context? What are the key practices? What is the evidence for their effectiveness – and cost-effectiveness? And what are the organizational implications of adopting such an approach?

The term "recovery" is contested, and there are different definitions used by different authors. However, most people use the term to refer to the process of building a meaningful and satisfying life, as defined by the person himself/herself, whether or not there are ongoing or recurring symptoms. This definition stems from the work of one of the intellectual founders of the recovery movement, Bill Anthony, who defined recovery as "*a deeply personal, unique process of changing one's attitudes, values, feelings, goals, skills and roles. It is a way of living a satisfying, hopeful and contributing life, even with the limitations caused by illness. Recovery involves the development of new meaning and purpose in one's life as one grows beyond the catastrophic effects of mental illness*" (Anthony 1993).

This definition emphasizes "personal recovery" (i.e., the achievement of individually chosen life goals) and may be contrasted with the more common understanding of "clinical recovery" where the emphasis is on symptom treatment and management (Slade 2009). Of course, symptom relief is desirable whenever this can be achieved, but for many people with psychosis, the key question is not simply how can we eradicate their symptoms? It is how can we help them live meaningful and inclusive lives in the presence of residual symptomatology? Repper and Perkins (2003) used their study of the narrative accounts of people with mental health problems to suggest that the process of recovery contains three essential components: "hope," "control," and "opportunity." "Hope" consists of maintaining a belief that it *is* possible to pursue one's personal goals despite the difficulties of intractable symptoms and negative social reactions (stigma). Achieving some sense of control over symptoms and life choices is then a prerequisite for maintaining hope and taking "opportunities" to build a life "beyond illness" and participating in the community in the same ways that everybody else does. This formulation of recovery has been supported by a systematic literature review conducted by Slade and his colleagues (Leamy et al. 2011) which confirmed the importance of hope, control, and opportunity and added two additional themes – "connectedness" and "meaning."

In this chapter, an argument will be presented that one of the central tasks of staff is to support personal recovery in the sense defined above. This means supporting the development of key interventions, based on sharing knowledge, power, and responsibility with service users and their families. It does not involve an increase in workload, rather the opposite. It also does not mean that we shouldn't offer evidence-based treatments like medication and CBT. However, it may mean sometimes we have to carry hope for the person when he/she has lost it himself/herself. It certainly means a change in attitudes, with staff looking all the time to help people function in key social roles – e.g., in safe and secure housing of their choice, in meaningful occupation, in supportive relationships, and in feeling a part of the community in which they live. This is what the therapeutic "work" does. Staff thus have to prioritize supporting the person in pursuit of these goals. This does not take extra time. Staff may also have to be prepared to work together with service users and carers to "coproduce" new services.

9.3   Coproduction

The term "coproduction" was originally introduced by a political economist (and later Nobel Prize winner), Elinor Ostrom, in the 1970s. She had been asked by the Chicago Police Department to investigate why crime rates had apparently increased when the city's police officers changed their operations from being mainly on the "beat" to being mainly in cars. Ostrom (1973) concluded that the key reason for this was that by moving into cars, the police became detached from the communities they were supposed to be serving. As a result they lost access to the wide range of knowledge, experience, assets, and skills of members of the community – including some of the criminals themselves – who also had an interest in controlling crime. Edgar Cahn, a human rights lawyer, then took this idea and coined the notion of the "core economy" to describe the networks of formal and informal relationships that make up local communities (Cahn 2001). The core economy – as distinct from the market economy – is the platform upon which "specialist programs" in society (e.g., public services) are actually built. This gives us a new way of defining "capacity" in public services which takes us beyond the services themselves.

In England, the New Economics Foundation and NESTA, two radical, independent "think tanks," have applied these ideas to thinking about the organization and delivery of public services in a time of austerity (Boyle and Harris 2009). They identified coproduction as an alternative model of engagement to the dominant model where "professionals design and deliver services for needy users" and brought together a number of examples from across the health and social care field (see Nesta/Innovation Unit/*nef* 2012). These included projects from across the age range (children, teenagers, adults, and older people) and with various special populations (offenders, homeless, people with acquired brain damage, learning disabilities, HIV). These programs demonstrated the value of a range of coproduced interventions including information and advice services, mutual support and self-help, personalization, pooled budgets, Time Banks, and life coaching.

Boyle and Harris were careful to clarify that coproduction was not the same as what is sometimes called "task shifting" where staff with lower levels of education and training take on the delivery of interventions previously the province of more highly paid professionals, i.e., attempting to solve the capacity problem by simply having the same services delivered more cheaply. By contrast, coproduction calls for new partnerships between professionals and service users (and carers) to deliver different kinds of services to local communities which better meet their needs as defined by the people on the receiving end of services.

At the heart of this new perspective is the recognition that people who are receiving services are not simply passive recipients of care – problems for services to "fix." They are also part of the solution of what to do and how to do it. But to release this capacity, they must be made equal partners in the process: equal but different. If this perspective is adopted then it opens up a vast pool of talent and resources which are more than adequate to meet the capacity problem. However, this is not easy. There is often a fear of what may be lost, as well as what may be gained, by rebalancing the power relationships in mental health services. This fear is perhaps most acutely felt by those who currently have the greatest power and status in the system.

With these ideas in mind, the reader can now turn to the questions of how to make supporting recovery a reality in mental health services (Shepherd et al. 2008). This will begin by considering what this means in practice by looking at supporting recovery under two headings: (a) at the level of individual care practices and (b) in relation to the organizational context.

9.4 Supporting Recovery at an "Individual" Level

At an individual level, Slade and his colleagues have made a helpful distinction between "recovery-promoting relationships" and "pro-recovery working practices" (Bird et al. 2011). The former relates to the general quality of the therapeutic relationship and applies to all relationship-based interventions; the latter refers to specific, pro-recovery working practices relating to the support of recovery. In addition, a number of approaches can be added which, although not necessarily derived directly from recovery ideas, are nevertheless highly consistent with supporting recovery for individuals. These three sets of individual-level practices are summarized in Box 9.1.

Box 9.1: Effective Individual-Level Recovery Practices (From Shepherd et al. 2014)
Staff should aim to:

Facilitate recovery-promoting relationships
- Establish shared values
- Demonstrate good, basic relationships skills (empathy, warmth, respect)
- Support personal hopes and aspirations
- Promote a sense of control ("agency")

Use "pro-recovery working" *practices*
- Narrative accounts (recovery stories)
- A "strengths" approach
- "Coaching" methods
- Personal recovery plans (WRAP, STAR)
- Self-management
- Illness Management and Recovery (IMR)
- Shared decision-making
- Person-centered "safety planning"

Use specific approaches which support the achievement of common recovery goals
- Joint Crisis Plans (JCP)
- "Housing First"
- Individual Placement and Support (IPS)
- Use of "personal budgets" (social and health)

9.4.1 Recovery-Promoting Relationships

Relationships are at the heart of recovery. The creation of supportive relationships depends upon establishing shared values and demonstrating empathy, warmth, respect, and a willingness to go the "extra mile" (Borg and Kristiansen 2004). These qualities form the bedrock for all forms of care (National Institute for Health and Care Excellence 2014). Some would argue that they have been undermined in recent years with the increasing fragmentation of service structures and disruptions to continuity of care. There has also been an increasing emphasis on "treatment as technology," associated with the "marketization" of healthcare and service models based on "transactions," rather than the relationships within which these transactions take place. It has been argued that models of care which neglect the importance of these basic human qualities are at much greater risk of neglecting the needs of individuals and even of abuse. Recent examples in England of the neglect of older people in hospitals underline these dangers and highlight the responsibility of managers and policy makers, as well as frontline staff, to ensure that these conditions do not arise (Francis 2013).

9.4.2 Pro-recovery Working Practices

In terms of recovery-oriented practices, the best starting point for most people is to encourage them to tell their story. Narrative accounts are the oldest, and probably the most powerful, ways in which we make sense of the world and build relationships. Everyone has a story to tell, and the process of storytelling is almost always experienced as positive and validating. Narratives are inherently meaningful and are expressed in a form and language that is accessible and relevant (Greenhalgh and Hurwitz 1999). They also provide a source of information and explanation which is complementary to a conventional "evidence-based medicine" approach (Roberts 2000). Narratives should therefore be the beginning of any supportive relationship, and most practitioners will naturally start by inviting the person to *"Tell me a bit about yourself..."* These stories can then be shaped over time until there is a version that both the person and their key worker can agree upon as a basis for moving forward (similar to CAT formulations in brief analytic therapy, Ryle and Kerr 2002). Such documents can sit alongside more formal assessments and are particularly useful in terms of helping people formulate personally relevant goals and in monitoring outcomes (see below). The use of narratives is therefore a quick and easy way of ensuring that a therapeutic contract is couched in a way that is meaningful and engaging for the person. Because of their direct relevance, they are often more suitable for routine outcome measurement than standardized questionnaires (see below) and can be enhanced with some form of quantification (e.g., Goal Attainment Scaling, Kirusek and Sherman 1968).

A second important practice is the consistent use of a "strengths" approach (Rapp 1998). This is a way of recording information that seeks to identify the person's competencies and their environmental resources (friends, neighbors, local opportunities) which might be used to further their personal life goals. They provide a useful alternative to simply listing their problems. A strengths assessment often develops from encouraging the person to tell his/her story as this can provide important clues to activities and interests that were pursued in the past and might be used again in the future.

Another recovery-supporting practice which has been developed in the last few years is known as the "coaching" model (Bora et al. 2010). This uses many of the same techniques as the strengths approach, e.g., an emphasis on the service user taking the lead, the importance of identifying personally relevant goals, and a focus on strengths and natural supports. However, there is greater emphasis on the importance of staff behavior as a "coach," or learning partner, and on the service user's responsibilities to make a commitment to action. Although there is good evidence for the effectiveness of coaching in relation to the management of long-term health conditions (O'Connor et al. 2008), there is little evidence as yet regarding its specific effectiveness in relation to supporting recovery in mental health services.

The use of narratives, building on strengths, and a coaching approach can then form the basis for developing a personal "recovery plan." This may use formal tools such as the "Wellness Recovery Action Plan" (WRAP), (Copeland 2015) or the Recovery STAR (McKeith and Burns 2010), or simply be developed through informal discussions (e.g., narratives). WRAP is a framework which is aimed at helping the person develop a plan to cope with distressing symptoms, prevent relapse, manage crises, and stay "well." It was designed by a service user for service users and has been used widely in many countries. The Recovery STAR has also been developed to provide a structure for personal recovery planning. It contains ten recovery "domains" and the service user and staff member work together to rate each domain area on a 10-point scale. The results are then presented visually on a star diagram. It is an attractive, easy-to-understand format and most service users seem to find the ten domains helpful for identifying personal goals, although some report that it needs to be more personalized.

Both WRAP and the STAR are useful methods for engaging people, assisting with personal recovery planning, and monitoring individual progress. However, both have limitations which arise from their standardized format and therefore limited acceptability to some individuals. Neither is psychometrically very sophisticated, and they are not recommended for use as outcome measures (Killaspy et al. 2012). Whatever their derivation, personal recovery plans should contain an identification of the person's internal and external resources and a plan for how he/she can use these to take control of his/her life and achieve his/her chosen goals (Perkins and Rinaldi 2007). The person should not necessarily have to share their recovery plan with staff: they belong to the individual and are not the same as "care plans" (although it is clearly desirable that there is as much overlap as possible between the two).

As indicated earlier, an important theme in most people's recovery is the struggle to achieve a greater sense of control over their symptoms and their life in general. One needs therefore to consider attempts to improve the person's capacity for "self-management." There is strong evidence, mainly from studies in the physical healthcare field, that supporting self-management can be extremely helpful in terms of ameliorating symptoms, improving quality of life, and reducing dependency on formal healthcare interventions (Foster et al. 2007; De Silva 2011). Self-management can refer to a wide variety of methods from simply handing out leaflets to personal support through telephone monitoring, goal setting, coaching, and structured education. However, approaches which include the full and active involvement of the person, rather than the passive provision of information, are most likely to be effective.

Mueser and his colleagues (2002) have developed a comprehensive educational and self-management package designed to provide people with severe mental illness with the information and skills necessary to manage their symptoms more effectively and work toward achieving personal recovery. The "Illness Management and Recovery Program" (IMR) consists of five components: (i) "psychoeducation" regarding severe mental illness; (ii) the provision of information on medication and side effects, using a "motivational interviewing" approach; (iii) a relapse prevention program; (iv) training in coping skills and problem solving; and (v) a cognitive-behavioral approach to symptom management. The program is delivered using an educational format, but with professionals taking the lead role having determined the majority of the content. Preliminary findings have been published regarding its implementation in the USA and Australia (Mueser et al. 2006; Salyers et al. 2009) and a randomized controlled trial found that service users appeared to have increased their knowledge of illness, coping skills, personal goal identification, and attainment (Hasson-Ohayon et al. 2007). There was weaker evidence of improvements regarding hope and no significant gains regarding social support or help from others. Systematized programs like IMR provide a good summary of basic information and give general tips on self-management, but they do not really reflect "*a fundamental transformation of the patient-caregiver relationship into a collaborative partnership"* (De Silva 2011, p. vi). They therefore cannot be said to fully represent coproduction

Alongside self-management and educational approaches, there has also been increasing interest in "shared decision-making" to support recovery. This brings together two sources of expertise – the knowledge, skills, and experience of health and social care professionals and the individual's knowledge and expertise of his/her own condition. Both forms of expertise are key to making good decisions. Used together they enable the person to make choices regarding treatment and management options that are most consistent with research evidence and with his/her own preferences and priorities. "Shared decision-making" is therefore the basis of truly informed consent. Again, there are already a number of examples of the value of this approach in the physical healthcare field (e.g., Simon et al. 2009), and they are now beginning to be applied in mental health, particularly in relation to medication management (Deegan and Drake 2006; Drake et al. 2010; Torrey and Drake 2009; SAMSHA 2011). A recent article coproduced by service users, carers, and professionals places shared decision-making in relation to medication management clearly within the framework of recovery-oriented practice (Baker et al. 2013).

The assessment and management of risk are central concerns of mental health services (and the public), but in recent years, *staff preoccupation with risk has sometimes become a barrier to personal recovery.* Many services have become highly "risk averse" and are often reluctant to engage in what might have been seen previously as "positive" risk taking, i.e. working with service user to help him/her manage those risks which are necessary in order to support the person in pursuing reasonable and realistic life goals. This has happened despite clear government and professional guidance to the contrary (e.g., Department of Health 2007). To compensate for this, recovery-oriented professionals have developed new approaches to managing risk which are based on involving service users fully in the development of a plan to support the pursuit of their life goals in ways that are safe for them and for those around them. This is known as person-centered "safety planning" (Boardman and Roberts 2014). Again, at its heart is an assumption that *the best – and most effective – methods for risk assessment and management will be those that fully involve the person in the process.* Managing risk is an inherent part of all our lives and surely those whose risk "problems" have caused them the most difficulties have the greatest interest in managing their risk effectively. Of course, not everyone will seek to manage their own risk responsibly, but maybe it is time that we began with this as the default assumption, rather than that everyone with a mental health problem (and/or some contact with forensic services) simply wishes to pursue their own goals with no regard for the consequences to themselves or others.

All these approaches to supporting recovery at an individual level do not require much in the way of additional staff time. Indeed, if incorporated into routine practice, most involve less time because they are more efficient in focusing on what is important to the service user and they are therefore likely to save time in the long run. They do this by using a language and a sense of priority that service users can easily understand. Most also do not involve doing "new" things: they involve doing "old things" differently, with a different set of attitudes and expectations. Of course, this is not to say that they are necessarily easy for professionals who are used to being "in charge" and to determining the priorities (and the language) themselves. Nevertheless, it is a significant challenge for many professionals to be able to make a contribution which is genuinely responsive to the needs of service user, accepting their priorities, and working out exactly what skills and knowledge they have that may be useful. That doesn't require a lot of time, but is does require intelligence, sensitivity, and, perhaps, a little humility.

9.4.3 Specific Approaches Which Support the Achievement of Common Recovery Goals

It is difficult to pursue your recovery goals if you are in a hospital, and most people with psychosis would wish to avoid unnecessary admissions to hospital, particularly if these are compulsory under Mental Health legislation. The "Joint Crisis Plan" (JCP) is an intervention which has been specifically developed to achieve these aims and is based on a process of coproduction (Henderson et al. 2004). The JCP is formulated by the service user, together with peer support if available and the key mental health staff involved, including the treating psychiatrist. It is therefore similar to an "advance statement" (or the kind of crisis plan contained in WRAP) but with the explicit inclusion of the clinical staff and the treating psychiatrist in the discussion. In an initial randomized controlled trial, people who were discharged with a Joint Crisis Plan were shown to have significantly fewer compulsory admissions compared with controls over a 15-month follow-up period (Henderson et al. 2004). Qualitative data also suggested that the JCP group felt more "in control" of their mental health problems (Henderson et al. 2008). A second study produced less impressive results, but the authors acknowledge that this was mainly due to practical difficulties in ensuring that the joint planning meetings always occurred and were effectively facilitated (Thornicroft et al. 2013).

Once in the community, finding somewhere safe and practical to live which is consistent with personal preferences is at the center of most peoples' recovery (Shepherd and Macpherson 2011). There is a dearth of evidence regarding the effectiveness of sheltered housing programs, but *an exception is the "Housing First" initiative* which was developed in the USA to meet the needs of homeless people with complex mental health and substance misuse problems. It prioritizes the identification of suitable housing, based on personal preference, and then delivers other supportive services to the person once he/she is housed, without a prerequisite that their substance misuse must cease first. The use of permanent housing options and the commitment to floating support mean that the resident does not have to make continual moves between different types of accommodation as their support needs change. There is now good evidence for its effectiveness and prospective trials comparing the "Housing First" model with traditional "treatment first" approaches have found that almost twice the number of people manage to maintain stable housing after 2 years (Padgett et al. 2006). In this study, despite there being no requirement for the Housing First group to abstain from substance misuse, there was actually no significant difference between the two groups regarding their levels of drug and alcohol use. The annual per capita costs of the Housing First program were also around half of the "treatment first" program. Similar results have been reported more recently by Stergiopoulos et al. (2015), although they comment on the difficulties with implementation and remaining faithful to the fidelity of the model in different settings. This approach has been tried in England (Shelter 2008) but is not widespread.

For most people, meaningful occupation is next on the list of personal recovery goals, and here the evidence for effective intervention is much stronger. The "Individual Placement and Support" (IPS) model (Becker et al. 1994) has consistently been shown to be the most effective approach for helping people with severe mental health problems gain and retain paid employment . There is now very strong evidence, both nationally and internationally, that IPS consistently achieves employment rates two to three times better than traditional alternatives such as prevocational training and sheltered workshops (Burns et al. 2007; Bond et al. 2008; Sainsbury Centre for Mental Health 2009). Longer term follow-up studies of people placed through IPS also suggest that the higher rates of employment are maintained and have positive impact on non-vocational outcomes, e.g., improved confidence and well-being and reduced sense of stigma (for further details, see Chap. 20 in this book by Bell). IPS has a number of similarities with the Housing First approach. Thus, it is also based on placing the person in a work position of his/her choice as quickly as possible and then providing him/her with an integrated package of vocational and clinical support *in situ* rather than wasting a lot of time on preplacement assessment and training efforts which generally don't predict behavior across settings or produce generalized improvements. The one study where IPS failed to produce such impressive results was where it was not implemented with good fidelity to the research model (Howard et al. 2010; Latimer 2010).

Finally, one needs to consider the most basic form of support for recovery – financial subsistence. It almost goes without saying that adequate financial support is important in the recovery of individuals with psychosis, but the Benefits Systems in most countries are often complex and difficult to negotiate. People – especially those with mental health problems – therefore require specific advice and advocacy, and this is seldom available, even 'though there is evidence to suggest that it would be extremely cost-effective (Parsonage 2013). An approach which aims to give the person direct control over a substantial proportion of their financial support is known as "personal budgets," or "self-directed" care. This has been tried both in the USA and in England (Cook et al. 2008; Alakeson and Perkins 2012) and aims to provide the person with the resources that would otherwise be spent on services for them to spend on whatever they think will be most helpful. This sounds like it must be a good idea, but there are considerable practical problems around its implementation. These include the processes to calculate the amount of money made available, monitoring of what it is used for, ensuring that resources are effectively targeted on those in greatest need, and coping with the inevitable bureaucracy involved. It therefore remains to be seen whether a practical system to get personal budgets to work effectively can be devised and rolled out on a large scale. If it could, then this would undoubtedly be a very important development.

9.5 Supporting Recovery at an "Organizational" Level

It has been mentioned earlier that to support an individual's recovery effectively requires not just the efforts of individual practitioners but also of the organizations concerned. They need to be committed to making this a reality (Shepherd et al. 2010). Of course, for the individual, their judgment of quality of service will be mostly determined by their experiences with individual staff, but what can the organization do to ensure that this is of a high quality and remains so? Effective staff training is part of the answer, but is not sufficient in itself. This is well illustrated in a study by Whitley and his colleagues (2009) who examined the implementation of Mueser's "Illness Management and Recovery Programs" across 12 community settings. They found that while training was important, it only had a lasting effect if issues of supervision and leadership were also addressed. They also noted the importance of a "culture of innovation" within the organization which was open to changes in existing practices. If all these factors were present, then they acted synergistically, but no one element was sufficient on its own. The *ImROC program* (*Im*plementing *R*ecovery through *O*rganizational *C*hange) began with this as its starting point. It assumed that training staff on its own would not be sufficient to consistently support recovery and that it would be necessary to facilitate a range of organizational changes to support and sustain change "on the ground."

9.5.1 The ImROC Program

The ImROC program was launched by the Secretary of State for Health in England in April 2010. Its aim was to assist public mental health services (NHS Trusts), their local authority partners in Social Service departments, and local independent sector organizations, particularly user and carer groups, to improve their capacity to support the recovery of people using these services, their family, friends, and carers. The program has been delivered through a partnership between two non-government organizations (charities): the Centre for Mental Health and the Mental Health Network of the NHS Confederation (NHS Confederation/Centre for Mental Health 2012).

It began by developing a simple audit tool consisting of "10 key organizational challenges." These were drawn from workshop discussions with a number of services who had already made some progress in changing their organizations to support recovery and were prepared to share their experiences. (More than 300 health and social care staff together with 60 users and carers contributed to these discussions which were held in different parts of the country during the period 2008–2010.) The challenges were designed to assist local organizations – public and independent – to work together to review current services and then set locally agreed priorities for change (Shepherd et al. 2010). They are set out in Box 9.2.

Box 9.2: "10 Key Organizational Challenges" for Organizations Wishing to Support Recovery (From Shepherd et al. 2010)

1. Changing the nature of day-to-day interactions and the quality of experience
2. Delivering comprehensive, user-led education and training programs
3. Establishing a local "Recovery Education College" to drive the programs forward
4. Ensuring organizational commitment, creating the "culture," leadership at all levels
5. Increasing "personalization" and choice
6. Changing the way we approach risk assessment and management
7. Redefining user involvement
8. Transforming the workforce
9. Supporting staff in their recovery journey
10. Increasing opportunities for building a life 'beyond illness'

The "10 key challenge framework" was not designed as a psychometric instrument, and its test-retest or inter-rater reliability have never been systematically explored. However, it has now been widely used to support the development of more recovery-oriented services by a range of different groups – staff, service users and carers, clinicians, and managers – and has proved a useful heuristic. It also appears to have good content validity when compared with the areas identified by Le Boutillier et al. (2011) in their international review of recovery-oriented practice.

9.5.2 The ImROC Methodology: Evidence-Based Organizational Change

The ImROC methodology has been based on a set of elements which are most likely to be effective in producing organizational change. These emphasize knowledge dissemination (guidelines), the importance of choice and local ownership, clear and realistic goal setting, and continual feedback on progress. At their heart is a process of closed audit loops (goal setting, action, review) deployed in repeated "Plan-Do-Study-Act" cycles. This is recommended by leading experts as the most effective way of producing organizational change (Iles and Sutherland 2001; Berwick 2008; Health Foundation 2013). It is similar to an "Action Research" model where the results and learning from the initial intervention are used to inform future goals and future change processes.

At each stage, there is an attempt to involve staff at senior levels in the organization, particularly team leaders and managers. They are included in the training and project planning and encouraged to begin to supervise staff according to the service developments being worked on (e.g., using recovery-supporting language and behavior, spending time coproducing a course for the Recovery College with a service user, etc.). There are also usually special sessions for the most senior managers (Board) to ensure that they are familiar with what is going on and that it reflects the overall goals of the organization. They are encouraged to think how they can support the desired changes in the attitudes and behavior of the staff. The process is described in detail by Shepherd et al. (2010).

In order to sustain the service developments, sites were also offered membership of an "Action Learning Set" (Revans 1998). This consisted of groups of clinicians, managers, service users, and carers who met on a regular basis to provide opportunities for mutual learning and support. These were extremely effective in maintaining the momentum for change with staff and service users working together to solve common problems on an equal footing. The Learning Sets also sparked off inter-site visits by teams of staff and service users between the workshops, creating a learning network in which ideas and experiences could be honestly shared in a non-critical (and, largely, noncompetitive) environment.

As indicated, the program aimed to establish new coproduced services to support recovery, and it was therefore important that the process of organizational change itself demonstrated coproduction. Thus, wherever possible, the external consultants consisted of experienced mental health professionals working together with people with "lived experience" who were coached (and paid) for their contribution. Many of these service user consultants were also peer workers recruited from local services.

9.5.3   What Has ImROC Achieved?

The program has worked with more than two-thirds ($n=35$) of the NHS mental health Trusts in England and their local partners. It has supported a number of new service developments.

- The establishment of *500+ Peer Support workers* – Trained, placed, and supported to work alongside mental health professionals in a variety of positions. This has involved the development of training materials, guidance on employing Peer Support workers, and evaluation of impact.
- The opening of *30+ Recovery Colleges* – These are local facilities, modeled on educational lines, where people with lived experience, professionals, carers, and others can learn together to construct and cope better with mental health difficulties and become better integrated into their local communities.
- *New ways of thinking about the assessment and management of risk* – Staff have been helped to use recovery-focused principles to move from *a* preoccupation with "risk" and "risk management" to a process of working directly with the service user to work out strategies they can use to pursue their own life goals in ways that are safe for them and safe for the people around them.
- *A significant reduction in the use of physical restraint and forcible medication on acute wards* – This builds on previous work by Recovery Innovations in Phoenix,

Arizona, who developed an approach known as "No Force First" (Ashcraft et al. 2012) which involves coproduced training for staff and exploration of alternatives to physical methods of intervention. This initiative has been pioneered by Mersey Care NHS Trust in Liverpool (UK) and has received national recognition (King et al. 2013).

9.6   Effectiveness of Service Developments to Support Recovery

What is the evidence for the effectiveness of these service developments in supporting recovery? At this stage, no one has tried to evaluate the effects of a "whole system" change; this would be very difficult (and costly) and would pose a host of methodological and design problems. However, it is possible to look at the evidence for "specific" service developments, and there are two where there is a growing body of evidence: (a) Recovery Colleges and (b) Peer Support workers.

9.6.1   Recovery Colleges

As indicated above, the concept of the "Recovery Colleges" is based on an "educational" model and uses coproduction to develop and deliver courses to students who are a mixture of service users and staff (co-learning). "Recovery Colleges" (also known as "Recovery Education Centers") are a relatively new development in the UK, although they have been present in a similar form in the USA for several years. The first example appeared more than 20 years ago at the Centre for Psychiatric Rehabilitation in Boston (http://cpr.bu.edu/living-well/services) and the concept was then developed by "Recovery Innovations" in Phoenix, Arizona (Ashcraft and Anthony 2005). It was imported into England in 2010 and has become a central theme in the ImROC program (Perkins et al. 2012). The first UK "Recovery College" was established in South West London and St. George's Mental Health NHS Trust and officially opened in September 2011. A second was quickly established in Nottingham, and there are now almost 40 in operation, mainly in England, but also in Scotland, Ireland, Italy, Australia, and Japan.

Recovery Colleges are new, and there is little evidence for their effectiveness as yet from randomized controlled trials. Work is currently underway to identify a set of "key defining features" which might, in time, form the basis for fidelity criteria which would allow replicable interventions in a control group design; see McGregor et al. 2014. Nevertheless, there is an emerging and consistent set of findings from prospective, uncontrolled, cohort studies, mainly conducted in England, but with some support from other countries (notably Australia, Italy, and Japan) which suggests very positive findings associated with attendance at the Colleges. These are summarized by Shepherd et al. (in press). They suggest that Recovery Colleges are very popular among users, with over 90 % reporting that the course they attended was "good" or "excellent" and that they would recommend it to others (Rennison et al. 2014; Meddings et al. 2014). Students also feel that the College helps them progress toward their personal life goals and to feel more hopeful about the future (Rinaldi and Wybourn 2011). In this study of the 74 students who responded to a questionnaire (83 % of the total surveyed), almost 70 % had become mainstream students, gained employment, or started volunteering. There is also evidence in two of the prospective studies that students' quality of life and well-being were significantly improved after attending the Recovery Colleges (Meddings et al. 2015; North Essex Research Network 2014). Learning with others with similar problems and with professionals who are genuinely open to challenge also means that Recovery Colleges can often engage people who find traditional services unacceptable. Attendance rates are generally high (around 60–70 %) which is similar to mainstream adult education. Lastly, Recovery Colleges are a resource for training and developing staff skills to support recovery more effectively. As one member of staff said *"attending a recovery college course is the very best introduction to working with people with psychosis"* (Sussex Recovery College Student, quoted by Shepherd et al. in press). They therefore also have the potential to raise staff expectations and thereby change the culture of the organization in which they are located.

9.6.2 Peer Support Workers

Peer support is based on people who have direct experience themselves of mental health issues and can use this to help others in similar circumstances. It may be defined as *"offering and receiving help, based on shared understanding, respect and mutual empowerment between people in similar situations"* (Mead et al. 2001) and has a long history in mental health services, beginning with the moral treatment era in the early part of the nineteenth century (Davidson et al. 2012). The use of peer support in hospitals declined in the later part of the nineteenth century as the mental health professionals – medical, nursing, psychology, and social work – established themselves, but it made a reappearance in the 1960s and 1970s in the Therapeutic Community movement. They are now popular again, with more than half of the US states making peer support billable under Medicaid and trained peer workers being employed in many countries all over the world (Repper 2013a). Peers may be employed either in addition to traditional professional staff or instead of them in certain specific roles, e.g., as peer trainers in Recovery Colleges, support workers in community teams or on inpatient wards, as case managers, etc.

In terms of evidence for their effectiveness, like the Recovery Colleges, there have been few, well-designed, randomized controlled trials (Pitt et al. 2013; Lloyd-Evans et al. 2014). However, other reviewers have considered non-RCT evidence (Warner 2009) and taken a more inclusive approach, including "gray" as well as published literature (Repper and Carter 2011). Not surprisingly, because of the variable quality of the evidence and the use of different samples, different reviewers come to slightly different conclusions. Nevertheless, a number of consistent findings do seem to emerge.

- In no study has the employment of Peer Support workers been found to result in worse health outcomes for those receiving the service.

- Most commonly the inclusion of peers in the workforce produces the same or better results in a range of outcomes when compared with services without peer staff.
- Peer Support workers tend to produce specific improvements in patients' feelings of empowerment, self-esteem, and confidence.
- In some studies, the presence of peer workers in teams also seems to be associated with improvements in self-reported physical and emotional health and in clinician-assessed global functioning.
- In some studies, they also bring about improvements in satisfaction with services and quality of life, although with regard to the latter the findings are mixed.
- In both cross-sectional and longitudinal studies, patients receiving peer support have shown improvements in community integration and social functioning.
- The introduction of Peer Support workers has been associated with a reduction of alcohol and drug use among patients with co-occurring substance abuse problems.
- In some studies, when patients are in frequent contact with Peer Support workers, their stability in employment, education, and training has been shown to increase.

As indicated above, some of these findings are not replicated across all studies, and there is also significant variability in the nature of the intervention evaluated (e.g., the amount of training peers receive prior to placement, the nature and frequency of the interactions between peers and service users, and the degree of integration of peers into the professional teams). This makes some inconsistency in the findings not surprising and, as with Recovery Colleges, highlights the need for further work before replicable interventions can be evaluated in control group designs. Nevertheless, Repper (2013b) has described some of the key features necessary to "standardize" the peer worker interventions. These include open recruitment, with clear job descriptions and "person specifications"; high-quality training; careful preparation of teams before placement; good supervision and support for peers once placed; and clear job roles, with appropriate payment, on recognized pay scales, and terms and conditions like other workers. Most of all Repper stresses the importance of organizational commitment to support their introduction and ensure that their integrity is maintained.

Again, as with Recovery Colleges, in addition to the direct benefits for those receiving the service, there is also evidence of benefits for the peer workers themselves. They feel more empowered in their own recovery journey, have greater confidence and self-esteem, feel more valued and less stigmatized, and have a more positive sense of identity (Repper and Carter 2011). Just as peer workers provide hope and inspiration for service users, so they can challenge negative attitudes of staff and provide an inspiration for all members of the team. Their example demonstrates to everyone that people with mental health problems can make a valued contribution to their own and others' recovery if they are given the opportunity. In our experience, this observation of cultural change is common in services where peer workers have become established, but to our knowledge it has not been formally investigated.

9.6.3   Cost-Effectiveness

In relation to Recovery Colleges, in the review by Shepherd et al. (in press), they noted that attendance at Recovery Colleges can reduce the use of hospital and/or community services leading to significant cost savings (Rinaldi and Wybourn 2011; Mid-Essex Recovery College 2014).[1] For example, in the case of South West London and St. George's for students attending more than 70 % of their chosen courses, this amounted to approximately £800 per student per year. For a College with a thousand students on the books (not uncommon), this amounts to a substantial saving. Similarly, in relation to Peer Support workers, Trachtenberg et al. (2013) examined a small sample of outcome studies ($n = 6$) which aimed to evaluate whether the introduction of Peer Support workers into community crisis teams or acute inpatient wards reduced the use of hospital beds (either by preventing or delaying admissions to hospital or by shortening the length of inpatient stays). Across the studies, the average benefit to cost ratio (taking into account sample size) was more than 4:1. Thus, the estimated value of the reduction in hospital bed use achieved by introducing peer workers far exceeded the cost of employing them. There are methodological limitations with this study due to the small sample size, but the results provide preliminary support for the proposition that adding Peer Support workers to existing mental health teams may result in significant cost savings in terms of inpatient bed days. This conclusion is echoed in a recent review commissioned by the UK charity Rethink (2014) from the Personal Social Services Research Unit, led by Professor Martin Knapp, at the London School of Economics. They suggest, *"An approach which may also in time offer the biggest scope for cost savings in mental health care is to promote and expand co-production, drawing on the resources of people who are currently using mental health services, for example in peer support roles"* (p. 6).

These studies therefore support the case for the cost-effectiveness of developments like Recovery Colleges and Peer Workers. There are also other potential savings which have not yet been factored into these calculations. For example, both of these developments depend on the employment of peer workers, and we know from the IPS literature that, in the long term, there are considerable cost savings for people who enter the employment market as they make less use of mental health services and become less dependent on public subsistence (Sainsbury Centre for Mental Health 2009). In addition, there is anecdotal evidence that adopting more recovery-oriented ways of working can have dramatic effects on reducing staff sickness and absence.[2] Since it is estimated that mental health problems account for more than a third of sickness absence in the NHS workforce (Health Service Journal

---

[1] There is also anecdotal evidence that a minority of students (around 20–25 %) actually *increase* service use in the first few months of attending, probably due to increased awareness of support options (Barton, Southwest Yorkshire Foundation Trust, *personal communication*, 2014).

[2] For example, in the study cited above on reducing levels of physical restraint and forcible medication on acute wards, the 50 % reduction in these incidents was accompanied by a more than 90 % reduction in staff sickness and absence (King et al. 2014).

2013) costing about £500 million, there is also huge potential for additional cost savings through this route.

To summarize, there is evidence that *both Recovery Colleges and Peer Workers* may not only deliver a wide range of benefits, but can also be highly cost-effective. Specifically in relation to peer workers – whether in Recovery Colleges or working alongside staff in teams – *adding* them to the existing workforce seems likely to reduce, rather than increase, costs, particularly if they are targeted on those people at highest risk of repeated admissions to hospital (e.g., many people with psychosis). On the other hand, if Peer Support workers are *substituted* for a proportion of traditional mental health workers, then, assuming broadly similar rates of pay, any benefits in health or quality of life for service users is sufficient to justify their use as it is, in effect, a costless improvement.

Conclusions

To conclude, there is good evidence that attempts to provide support for "recovery" – in the sense of helping people with psychotic conditions pursue their chosen life goals – can be delivered *both effectively and cost-effectively*. To do so, it requires the implementation of a set of approaches and interventions at the level of individual care, supported by key organizational (service) developments which will maintain these changes over time. *These changes do not require huge increases in staff time, but they may require fundamental changes in staff attitudes.* Staff need to believe in the capacity of people to find and construct – sometimes with some help – new meanings to their experiences and new solutions to their problems. This means sharing power and respecting each other's expertise. If this is combined with practical help in the area of key social goals like housing, occupation, and financial stability, then it maximizes the opportunities for service users to live the kinds of "ordinary lives" that everyone else aspires to whether or not they have continue to experience residual symptoms. Simply existing in these valued roles will go a long way to minimizing symptoms and maintaining progress. Genuine collaboration and real partnerships, between consumers and professionals, also mean that burdens are lifted on both sides and services will be both more valued *and* more cost-effective.

Of course, there is still much to do before this can be achieved. We need to know more about exactly *which* individual-level interventions are most effective. Similarly, we need to know more about the effectiveness of key service developments (Recovery Colleges, Peer Workers) where it is clear that, currently, developments in practice seem a long way ahead of service evaluation. This may mean making greater user of quasi-experimental designs, in addition to randomized controlled trials. This would be facilitated if there was clearer agreement on routine outcome and "input" measurements ("who" was getting "what"?). We could then begin to summate findings across studies. We also need to know more about the process of care, what are the mechanisms underlying change in these new interventions? What do these changes in feelings of "hope" and "empowerment" tell us about what is happening in the psychology of the individuals concerned? Can the interventions be fine-tuned to particularly focus on achieving these kinds of changes? Finally, we still need to know much more about how to help organizations change so as to most effectively support these changes in practice. How do we get professionally led, health-oriented organizations to focus on non-health (social) goals and make these as much a priority as the alleviation of symptoms? How do we get health and non-health organizations to work more effectively together, respecting each other's unique contribution, while recognizing the need to collaborate? These are the big questions that we need to address if we are to get the maximum value out of investment in mental health and social care services and solve some of the pressing capacity problems raised at the outset.

References

Alakeson V, Perkins R (2012) Personalisation and personal budgets, vol 2, ImROC Briefing paper. Centre for Mental Health, London, Retrieved from http://www.imroc.org/wp-content/uploads/Recovery_personalisation_and_personal_budgets1.pdf

Anthony WA (1993) Recovery from mental illness: the guiding vision of the mental health service system in the 1990s. Psychosoc Rehabil J 16(4):11–23

Ashcraft L, Anthony WA (2005) A story of transformation. An agency fully embraces recovery. Behav Healthc Tomorrow 14(6):12–21

Ashcraft L, Bloss M, Anthony WA (2012) The development and implementation of "no force first" as a best practice. Psychiatr Serv 63(5):415–417

Baker E, Fee J, Bovingdon L, Campbell T, Hewis E, Lewis D, Mahoney L, Roberts G (2013) From taking to using medication: recovery-focussed prescribing and medication management. Adv Psychiatr Treat 19(1):2–10

Becker DR, Drake RE, Concord NH (1994) Individual placement and support: a community mental health center approach to vocational rehabilitation. Community Ment Health J 30(2):193–206

Berwick D (2008) The science of improvement. JAMA 299(10):1182–1184

Bird V, Leamy M, Le Boutillier C, Williams J, Slade M (2011) REFOCUS: promoting recovery in community mental health services. RETHINK Registered Office 89 Albert Embankment, London, SE1 7TP

Boardman J, Roberts G (2014) Risk, safety and recovery, vol 9, ImROC Briefing Paper. Centre for Mental Health and Mental Health Network, NHS Confederation, London, Retrieved from http://www.imroc.org/latest-news/publications/imroc/

Bond GR, Drake RE, Becker D (2008) An update on randomized controlled trials of evidence-based supported employment. Psychiatr Rehabil J 31(4):280–290

Bora R, Leaning S, Moores A, Roberts G (2010) Life coaching for mental health recovery: the emerging practice of recovery coaching. Adv Psychiatr Treat 16:459–467

Borg M, Kristiansen K (2004) Recovery-oriented professionals: helping relationships in mental health services. J Ment Health 13(5):493–505

Boyle D, Harris M (2009) The challenge of co-production: how equal partnerships between professionals and the public are crucial to improving public services. Retrieved from: http://b.3cdn.net/nefoundation/312ac8ce93a00d5973_3im6i6t0e.pdf

Burns T, Catty J, Becker T, Drake R, Fioritti A, Knapp M, Lauber C, Tomov T, Busschbach J v, White S, Wiersma D (2007) The effectiveness of supported employment for people with severe mental illness: a randomised controlled trial. Lancet 370(9593):1146–1152

Cahn E (2001) No more throwaway people: the co-production imperative. Essential Books, Washington, DC

Cook J, Russell C, Grey DD, Jonikas JA (2008) A self-directed care model for mental health recovery. Psychiatr Serv 59(6):600–602

Copeland ME (2015) Wellness Recovery Action Plan (WRAP). http://mentalhealthrecovery.com/store/wrap.html

Davidson L, Bellamy C, Guy K, Miller R (2012) Peer support among persons with severe mental illnesses: a review of evidence and experience. World Psychiatry 11(2):123–128

De Silva D (2011) Helping people help themselves. The Health Foundation, London, http://www.health.org.uk/publications/evidence-helping-people-help-themselves/

Deegan PE, Drake RE (2006) Shared decision-making and medication management in the recovery process. Psychiatr Serv 57(11):1636–1639

Department of Health (2007) Independence, choice and risk: a guide to best practice in supported decision-making. http://webarchive.nationalarchives.gov.uk/20130107105354/http://www.dh.gov.uk/en/Publicationsandstatistics/Publications/PublicationsPolicyAndGuidance/DH_074773

Drake RE, Deegan PE, Rapp C (2010) The promise of shared decision making in mental health. Psychiatr Rehabil J 34(1):7–13

Foster G, Taylor SJ, Eldridge SE, Ramsay J, Griffiths CJ (2007) Self-management education programmes by lay leaders for people with chronic conditions. Cochrane Database Syst Rev 17(4):CD005108. Retrieved from http://www.ncbi.nlm.nih.gov/pubmed/17943839

Francis R (2013) The Mid Staffordshire NHS Foundation Trust Public Inquiry final report. http://www.midstaffspublicinquiry.com/report

Greenhalgh T, Hurwitz M (1999) Narrative based medicine: why study narratives? Br Med J 318(7175):48–50

Harding CM, Brooks GW, Ashikaga T, Strauss JS, Breier A (1987) The Vermont longitudinal study of persons with severe mental illness, II: long-term outcome of subjects who retrospectively Met *DSM-III* criteria for schizophrenia. Am J Psychiatry 144(6):727–735

Hasson-Ohayon I, Roe D, Kravetz S (2007) A randomized controlled trial of the effectiveness of the illness management and recovery program. Psychiatr Serv 58(11):1461–1466

Health Foundation (2013) Quality improvement made simple. Retrieved from http://www.health.org.uk/sites/default/files/QualityImprovementMadeSimple.pdf

Health Services Journal (2013) Why it's time to help the helpers. Mental Health Supplement, 6 Dec, pp 2–3

Henderson C, Flood C, Leese M, Thornicroft G, Sutherby K, Szmukler G (2004) Effect of joint crisis plans on use of compulsory treatment in psychiatry: a single blind randomised controlled trial. Br Med J 329(7458):136–138

Henderson C, Flood C, Leese M, Thornicroft G, Sutherby K, Szmukler G (2008) Views of service users and providers on joint crisis plans. Soc Psychiatry Psychiatr Epidemiol. doi:10.1007/s00127-008-0442-x, Published online 4 October 2008

Howard LM, Heslin M, Leese M, McCrone P, Rice C, Jarrett M, Spokes T (2010) Supported employment: randomised controlled trial. Br J Psychiatry 196(5):404–411

Iles V, Sutherland K (2001) Organisational change – a review for health care managers, professionals and researchers. National Co-ordinating Centre for NHS Service Delivery and Organisation (NCCSDO), London School of Hygiene and Tropical Medicine, Keppel Street, London WC1E 7HT, England

Killaspy H, White S, Taylor T, King M (2012) Psychometric properties of the mental health recovery star. Br J Psychiatry 201(1):65–70

King L, Robb J, Riley D, Benson I, Tyrer K (2013) NO FORCE FIRST – changing the culture to create coercion-free environments. Presentation to ImROC Learning Set, 11/12/13, Manchester, England. London: www.ImROC.org

Kirusek TJ, Sherman RE (1968) Goal attainment scaling: a general method for evaluating comprehensive community mental health programs. Community Ment Health J 4(6):443–453

Latimer E (2010) An effective intervention delivered at sub-therapeutic does becomes an ineffective intervention. Br J Psychiatry 196(5):341–342

Le Boutillier C, Leamy M, Bird V, Davidson L, Williams J, Slade M (2011) What does recovery mean in practice? A qualitative analysis of international recovery-oriented practice. Psychiatr Serv 62(12):1470–1476

Leamy M, Bird V, Le Boutillier C, Williams J, Slade M (2011) Conceptual framework for personal recovery in mental health: systematic review and narrative synthesis. Br J Psychiatry 199(6):445–462

Lloyd-Evans B, Mayo-Wilson E, Harrison B, Istead H, Brown E, Pilling S, Johnson S, Kendall T (2014) Systematic review and meta-analysis of randomized controlled trials of peer support for people with severe mental illness. BMC Psychiatry 14:39. doi:10.1186/1471-244X-14-39

McGregor J, Repper J, Brown H (2014) The college is so different from anything I have done. A study of the characteristics of Nottingham Recovery College. J Ment Health Educ Train Pract 9(1):3–15

McKeith J, Burns S (2010) The recovery star: user guide, 2nd edn. Mental Health Providers Forum, London, www.mhpf.org.uk

Mead S, Hilton D, Curtis L (2001) Peer support: a theoretical perspective. Psychiatr Rehabil J 25(2):134–141

Meddings S, Guglietti S, Lambe H, Byrne D (2014) Student perspectives: recovery college experience. Ment Health Soc Incl 18(3):142–150

Meddings S, Campbell E, Guglietti S, Lambe H, Locks L, Byrne D, Whittington A (2015) From service user to student – the benefits of recovery college. Soc Clin Forum 268:32–37, http://www.bps.org.uk/networks-and-communities/member-microsite/division-clinical-psychology/clinical-psychology-forum

Mid-Essex Recovery College (2014) Hope health, opportunity and purpose for everyone. Evaluation report. North Essex Partnership University NHS Foundation Trust, Trust Headquarters, 103 Stapleford Close, Stapleford House, Chelmsford, Essex, CM2 0QX, England

Mueser KT, Corrigan PW, Hilton DW, Tanzman B, Schaub A, Gingerich S, Essock SM, Tarrier N, Morey B, Vogel-Scibilia S, Herz MI (2002) Illness, management and recovery: a review of the research. Psychiatr Serv 53(10):1272–1284

Mueser KT, Meyer PS, Penn DL, Clancy R, Clancy DM, Salyers M (2006) The illness, management and recovery program: rationale, development, and preliminary findings. Schizophr Bull 32(Suppl 1):S32–S43

National Institute for Health and Care Excellence (2014) Psychosis and schizophrenia in adults: treatment and management. Retrieved from http://www.nice.org.uk/guidance/cg178/chapter/1-recommendations#first-episode-psychosis-2

Nesta/Innovation Unit/nef (2012) People powered health co-production catalogue. Retrieved from: http://www.nesta.org.uk/sites/default/files/co-production_catalogue.pdf

NHS Confederation/Centre for Mental Health (2012) Supporting recovery in mental health, vol 244, Briefing paper. NHS Confederation, London, Retrieved from http://www.mentalhealthrecoverystories.hscni.net/wp-content/uploads/2014/01/Supporting-recovery-in-mental-health.pdf

North Essex Research Network with South Essex Service User Research Group (2014) Evaluation of the Mid Essex Recovery College October–December 2013. Anglia Ruskin University. Retrieved from http://hdl.hand.lenet/10540/347125

O'Connor AM, Stacey D, Legere F (2008) Coaching to support patients in making decisions. Br Med J 336(7638):228–229

Olstrom E (1973) Community organization and the provision of police services. Sage Publications, Beverley Hills

Padgett D, Gulcur L, Tsemberis S (2006) Housing first services for people who are homeless with co-concurring serious mental illness and substance abuse'. Res Soc Work Pract 16(1):74–83

Parsonage M (2013) Welfare advice for people who use mental health services. Centre for Mental Health, London, Retrieved from http://www.centreformentalhealth.org.uk/welfare-advice-report

Perkins R, Rinaldi M (2007) Taking back control: a guide to planning your recovery. Southwest London & St. George's Mental Health NHS Trust, Trust Headquarters, Springfield University Hospital, 61 Glenburnie Road, London SW17 7DJ, England

Perkins R, Repper J, Rinaldi M, Brown H (2012) Recovery colleges, ImROC, briefing 1. Centre for Mental Health (online). Retrieved from http://www.centreformentalhealth.org.uk/pdfs/Recovery_Colleges.pdf

Pitt V, Lowe D, Hill S et al (2013) Consumer providers of care for adult clients of statutory mental health services. Cochrane Database Syst Rev (3)

Rapp CA (1998) The strengths model: case management with people suffering from severe and persistent mental illness. Oxford University Press, New York

Rennison J, Skinner S, Bailey A (2014) CNWL recovery college annual report. Central and North West London NHS Foundation, 2nd Floor, Stephenson House, 75 Hampstead Road, London, NW1 2PL, England

Repper J (2013a) Peer support workers: theory and practice, vol 5, ImROC Briefing Paper. Centre for Mental Health and Mental Health Network, NHS Confederation, London, Retrieved from http://www.centreformentalhealth.org.uk/peer-support-workers-theory-and-practice

Repper J (2013b) Peer support workers: a practical guide to implementation, vol 7, ImROC Briefing Paper. Centre for Mental Health and Mental Health Network, NHS Confederation, London, Retrieved from http://www.centreformentalhealth.org.uk/peer-support-a-practical-guide

Repper J, Carter T (2011) A review of the literature on peer support in mental health services. J Ment Health 20(4):392–411

Repper J, Perkins R (2003) Social inclusion and recovery. Baillière Tindall, London

Rethink (2014) Investing in recovery – making the business case for effective interventions for people with schizophrenia and psychosis. Retrieved from http://www.rethink.org/?gclid=CJyCsMmmjcYCFYnJtAodHnsAbg

Revans R (1998) ABC of action learning. Lemon and Crane, London

Rinaldi M, Wybourn S (2011) The recovery college pilot in Merton and Sutton: longer term individual and service level outcomes. South West London and St. Georges Mental Health NHS Trust, Building 15, Second Floor, Springfield University Hospital, 61 Glenburnie Road, London, SW17 7DJ, England

Roberts G (2000) Narrative and severe mental illness: what place do stories have in an evidence-based world? Adv Psychiatr Treat 6:432–441

Royal College of Psychiatrists (2014) Improving the lives of people with mental illness: antipsychotics. Retrieved from http://www.rcpsych.ac.uk/healthadvice/treatmentswellbeing/antipsychoticmedication.aspx

Ryle A, Kerr IB (2002) Introducing cognitive analytic therapy: principles and practice. Wiley, Chichester

Sainsbury Centre for Mental Health (2009) Commissioning what works: the economic and financial case for supported employment, Briefing paper. Sainsbury Centre for Mental Health, London, Retrieved from http://www.centreformentalhealth.org.uk/briefing-41-commissioning-what-works

Salyers MP, Godfrey JL, McGuire AB, Gearhart T, Rollins AL, Boyle C (2009) Implementing the illness management and recovery program for consumers with severe mental illness. Psychiatr Serv 60(4):483–491

SAMSHA (2011) Shared decision-making in mental health care: practice. Research and future directions, HHS Publication No. SMA-09-4371. Centre for Mental Health Services, Substance Abuse and Mental Health Services Administration, Rockville, http://store.samhsa.gov/product/Shared-Decision-Making-in-Mental-Health-Care/SMA09-4371

Shelter (2008) Housing first. www.shelter.org.uk/goodpracticebriefings

Shepherd G, Macpherson R (2011) Residential care. In: Thornicroft G, Szmukler KG, Mueser T, Drake RE (eds) Oxford textbook of community mental health. Oxford University Press, Oxford

Shepherd G, Boardman J, Slade M (2008) Making recovery a reality. Centre for Mental Health (online). Retrieved from: http://www.centreformentalhealth.org.uk/pdfs/Making_recovery_a_reality_policy_paper.pdf

Shepherd G, Boardman J, Burns M (2010) Implementing recovery: a methodology for organisational change. Centre for Mental Health, London, Retrieved from http://www.centreformental-health.org.uk/implementing-recovery-paper

Shepherd G, Boardman J, Rinaldi M, Roberts G (2014) Supporting recovery in mental health services: quality and outcomes. ImROC Briefing Paper 8. Centre for Mental Health (online). Retrieved from http://www.centreformentalhealth.org.uk/pdfs/ImROC_briefing8_quality_and_outcomes.pdf

Shepherd G, McGregor J, Meddings S, Roeg W (in press) Recovery colleges and co-production. In: Slade M, Oades L, Jarden A (eds) To appear in 'Wellbeing, Recovery and Mental Health'. Cambridge University Press, Cambridge

Simon D, Willis CE, Harter M (2009) Shared decision-making in mental health. In: Edwards A, Elwyn G (eds) Shared decision-making in health care: achieving evidence-based patient choice, 2nd edn. Oxford University Press, Oxford, pp 269–276

Slade M (2009) Personal recovery and mental illness. Cambridge University Press, Cambridge

Stergiopoulos V, Hwang SW, Godzik A, Nisenbaum R et al (2015) Effect of scattered-site housing using rent supplements and intensive case management on housing stability among homeless adults with mental illness – a randomized trial. JAMA 313:905–915. doi:10.1001/jama.2015.1163

Strauss JS, Carpenter WT (1977) Prediction of outcome in schizophrenia. III. Five-year outcome and its predictors. Arch Gen Psychiatry 34(2):159–163

Thornicroft G, Farrelly S, Szmukler G, Birchwood M, Waheed W et al (2013) Clinical outcomes of Joint Crisis Plans to reduce compulsory treatment for people with psychosis: a randomised controlled trial. Br J Psychiatry 381:1634–1641

Torrey WC, Drake R (2009) Practicing shared decision making in the outpatient psychiatric care of adults with severe mental illnesses: redesigning care in the future. Community Ment Health J. doi:10.1007/s10597-009-9265-9, Published online: 08 November 2009

Trachtenberg M, Parsonage M, Shepherd G, Boardman J (2013) Peer support in mental health care: is it good value for money? Centre for Mental Health, London, Retrieved from www.centreformentalhealth.org.uk/peer-support-value-for-money

Warner (2009) Recovery from schizophrenia and the recovery model. Curr Opin Psychiatry 22(3):374–380

Whitley R, Gingerich S, Lutz WJ, Mueser KT (2009) Implementing the illness management and recovery program in community mental health settings: facilitators and barriers. Psychiatr Serv 60(2):202–209

World Health Organization (2008) Global burden of disease report. Retrieved from http://www.who.int/healthinfo/global_burden_disease/estimates_country/en/index.html

Wunderink L, Nieboer RM, Wiersma D, Sytema S, Nienhuis FJ (2013) Recovery in remitted first-episode psychosis at 7-years of follow-up of an early dose reduction/discontinuation or maintenance treatment strategy: long-term follow-up of a 2-year randomised clinical trial. JAMA Psychiatry 70(9):913–920. doi:10.1001/jamapsychiatry.2013.19

Employment Support for People with Psychosis

10

Andy Bell

10.1 Introduction

For most of us, having paid work is essential for well-being and financial security. But for many people who require some support to get into work, especially those with mental health problems, the right to employment is often not upheld. This chapter explores ways in which support with employment can be a part of a personal recovery journey for many more people than it is today. It focuses on interventions that can be provided by services to improve the support people with mental health conditions including psychosis receive to gain and retain employment.

10.2 Evidence About Employment for People with Psychosis

Research indicates that work is good for our physical and mental health (Waddell and Burton 2006), and many people who are using specialist mental health services want to work (Secker et al. 2001) and would like more help to get back into employment. Psychosis is considered as a severe mental illness and, hence compared to other mental illnesses, results in more disruption to employment status of individuals suffering from psychosis. The costs of lost employment due to mental health problems are substantial. In England in 2007, it was estimated that these amounted to nearly £20 billion (McCrone et al. 2008). There is persuasive evidence that being in employment is an important part of recovery for someone living with psychosis and indeed for most mental health conditions (Drake 2008). Gaining and retaining competitive employment has been demonstrated to achieve improved mental health outcomes and to sustain them over long periods. In a review of four

A. Bell
Deputy Chief Executive, Centre for Mental Health, Borough High Street, London, UK
e-mail: Andy.Bell@centreformentalhealth.org.uk

© Springer International Publishing Switzerland 2016
B. Pradhan et al. (eds.), *Brief Interventions for Psychosis:*
A Clinical Compendium, DOI 10.1007/978-3-319-30521-9_10

163

models of psychiatric rehabilitation in people with psychosis, Baronet and Gerber (1998) concluded that being in employment was associated with an increase in independence, an improved sense of self-worth, and an improved family atmosphere. Similarly, Mueser et al. (1997) found that compared to those who were unemployed, participants who were in employment, after a period of 18 months, tended to have lower symptoms (particularly thought disorder), higher global assessment scores, better self-esteem, and more satisfaction with their finances and vocational services. Lysakar and Bell (1995) found a significant improvement in social skills after 17 weeks of job placement. Despite the evidence of its benefits, in the UK, the 2014 Care Quality Commission survey of community mental health service users found that 44 % of the 3,329 respondents said they would have liked support to find or keep a job but did not receive any (Care Quality Commission 2014): a finding that has been consistent each year this survey has taken place. Unemployment and mental health problems appear to have a causal link in both directions. People with mental health problems are much less likely than average to be in paid employment (Marwaha and Johnson 2004; Rinaldi et al. 2011, and people who have been unemployed for at least 6 months are more likely to develop depression or other mental health conditions (Paul and Moser 2009; Diette et al. 2012). McManus et al. (2012) found that one third of the new Jobseeker's Allowance claimants in the UK reported that their mental health deteriorated over a period of 4 months in this study, while those who entered work noted improved mental health. The employment rate of people with severe and enduring mental health problems is the lowest of all disability groups in England, at less than 10 %, and yet the research evidence on what works in supported employment for this group is particularly strong (Centre for Mental Health 2013). This finding is consistent with other countries like Australia (Frost et al. 2002). However some middle-income countries have shown high rates of employment for people with a severe mental illness. For example, Suresh et al. studied the work functioning of a cohort of 201 people who received community-based treatment in a rural south Indian community, and two thirds of individuals were employed at 3-year follow-up (Gudlavalleti et al. 2014). There may be lessons that can be shared in this area from developing countries.

10.3   Individual Placement and Support (IPS)

Research shows that the most effective method of supported employment for people with severe and enduring mental health problems is Individual Placement and Support (IPS). IPS was developed in the USA in the 1990s and has been replicated and successfully demonstrated in many other places including the UK, Norway, Denmark, Hong Kong, Canada, New Zealand, and Australia. A six-center randomized controlled trial (Burns et al. 2007) found that IPS was around twice as effective as the best alternative vocational rehabilitation service at achieving paid work outcomes in all sites. This study also revealed that people entering work did so more quickly and could sustain their employment for longer in the IPS services than in the alternatives. IPS has been found to be significantly better on all employment outcome measures in people with first-episode psychosis than various control conditions, and patients receiving IPS gain significantly more jobs, earn significantly more money, and work longer (Crowther et al. 2001). To date there are at least 15 randomized controlled trials that demonstrate the efficacy of IPS (Drake and Bond 2011). Evidence on efficacy has emerged from randomized trials of IPS from many other countries, e.g., Canada (Latimer et al. 2006), Europe and the UK (Burns et al. 2007), Australia Killackey et al. (2008), The Netherlands (Michon et al. 2011), Switzerland (Hoffmann et al. 2012), and Hong Kong (Kin Wong et al. 2008). A briefer form of IPS (IPS–LITE) has also been tested and found to be equally effective to IPS (Burns et al. 2015).

As described below, IPS has *eight principles* and to be effective, supported employment services have to work faithfully to these principles:

1. *Competitive employment is the primary goal.*
   The fundamental assumption should be that paid employment (part-time or full-time) is a realistic goal for everyone who wants a job. Placement in education and training may provide a "stepping stone" for younger people and other forms of training might help some people, but the central goal of the service must always be paid employment.
2. *Everyone is eligible.*
   There are no "eligibility criteria" for entry into IPS programs beyond an expressed motivation to "give it a try." This should be irrespective of issues such as job readiness, symptoms, substance use, social skills, or a history of violent behavior. If a person believes paid employment is possible, and they receive the help they think they need, then their prospects are good. If they are subject to lengthy assessments to determine their "job readiness" and endless preparation of CVs and interview practice, then they will soon lose heart. People are "job ready" when they say they are and that is the time to start.
3. *Job search is consistent with individual preferences.*
   Working closely with someone's personal interests and experience significantly increases the chances of them enjoying and retaining a job. *"Do you want to work?"* and *"What do you want to do?"* are therefore the key – and indeed often the only – important assessment questions.
4. *Job search is rapid.*
   The job search should be started early (preferably within 1 month of referral to an employment specialist). A positive, "can-do" attitude should be cultivated in both staff and service users. Clear targets with dates for action need to be agreed and adhered to. Preparation should be concurrent with job search.
5. *Employment specialists and clinical teams work and are located together.*
   One of the most crucial aspects of the IPS approach is the quality of joint working between employment specialists and mental health teams. Employment specialists should be integrated, and preferably colocated, with clinical teams, irrespective of who employs them. They should actively take part in assessment meetings, influence referrals, and share in the decision-making process. The ideal scenario is that of a team wherein the employment specialist is part of the

team and is involved in developing with the client a care plan reflecting the personal preferences of the client. The employment specialist in collaboration with the client and the team is responsible for providing interventions that support employment as part of the client's recovery goals as, for example, in assertive community treatment teams (Schmidt et al. 1995). This may present a challenge to services that are more used to working separately, one after the other, i.e., "in a series," rather than "in parallel" together. It means that employment specialists must be central and equal members of the team, not peripheral "add-ons." In this way, the whole caseload of the clinical team is automatically the caseload of the employment specialist.

6. *Support is time unlimited and individualized to both the employer and employee.*
   The IPS approach makes getting a job the *start* of the process rather than the end point (it is "place then train," rather than "train then place"). Thus, support must bridge this crucial transition and continue in work for as long as is necessary. This means that individuals receive support that is based on their individual needs in relation to their jobs, skills, and preferences. Support is provided by a variety of ways by a variety of people including but not limited to employment specialists and clinicians (e.g., to help people to manage their mental health in the workplace) (Frydecka et al. 2015). Efforts should be made to include family members and close friends in the team to support people in their working lives, if they wish. Employment specialists may also provide support to the employer in line with the individual's wishes. Employment specialists should not require people to disclose their mental health problems to employers. Their role is to discuss the benefits and risks of disclosure and nondisclosure with the individual and support them in their decision.

7. *Welfare benefit counseling supports the person through the transition from benefits to work.*
   It is essential that employment specialists or clinicians offer assistance in obtaining individualized counseling services to understand the financial implications of starting work. This should include the process of managing the transition from welfare benefits to work and advice on in-work benefits such as Working Tax Credit, which is being replaced by Universal Credit. It is essential to have good relationships with specialist experts in the Jobcentre Plus and other welfare benefit agencies, such as Citizen's Advice.

8. *Jobs are developed with local employers.*
   This is a crucial aspect. The role of the employment specialists includes reaching out to local employers to identify potential jobs that fit well with an individual's skills, interests, and preferences.

10.4   Current Availability of IPS

The spread of IPS is still patchy, but it is growing. In 2009 only 2.1 % of US mental health clients had access to evidence-based vocational services (2009) but in 2011, IPS was offered by mental health agencies in at least 13 states. The Johnson & Johnson – Dartmouth Community Mental Health Program was created to further the dissemination of IPS by providing a structure for supporting implementation of the various elements of IPS at the state level. This program has resulted in the formation of a national learning collaborative that supports the implementation of IPS services (Becker et al. 2011). In the UK, the Centre for Mental Health has recognized 14 sites as IPS Centers of Excellence, where fidelity to the evidence-based model, including excellent employer engagement strategies and effective partnership working between employment support workers and health professionals, is evident. But even in most of those high-performing areas, not all clinical teams have an assigned IPS worker, and therefore there are still large numbers of people who are denied access to an IPS service. The evidence base for IPS is predicated on trials within secondary care settings. There are, however, promising examples of the success of using the IPS model with primary care mental health teams. In the UK, there are IPS workers in some IAPT (Improving Access to Psychological Therapy) services, including Wolverhampton Healthy Minds and Wellbeing Service. Extending and adapting IPS to primary care for people with common mental health problems was among the major recommendations of a government-commissioned report by RAND Europe (van Stolk et al. 2014) which is, at the time of this writing, being piloted in four areas of England. There is also evidence from a pilot scheme run by the Central and North West London NHS Foundation Trust that IPS can be successfully adapted to people with drug or alcohol addictions (Centre for Mental Health 2014). In addition, another pilot project on IPS is currently under way in the West Midlands (UK) that intends to provide employment support to people with mental health problems who are leaving prison.

10.5 The Impact of Employment: An Example from Practice

From the narrative accounts of people's journeys through supported employment in Central and North West London, Miller et al. (2014) have identified the benefits of being in work and the unique path each person takes to gain and retain employment. One service user described his journey, which began with him wanting to work and contacting an employment specialist (ES) as: "When I met my ES, she discussed what my motivations were and whether I wanted to work. I felt at last there was someone to help…" (Miller et al. 2014). He describes a process that began with rapid job search based on his interests and skills and which included help in preparing for interviews. The ES then *proactively* sought a suitable role for him and offered both him and his employer ongoing advice and support. "I am now in part time work as a cleaner. I cannot believe I have finally got a job. It has changed my life. I feel happy within myself, the bad thoughts from my head have disappeared" (Miller et al. 2014).

10.6 Barriers to Employment and Suggestions to Address the Barriers

There are numerous barriers to people with mental health problems getting paid work. Limited availability of IPS is a major barrier, but there are other obstacles, as discussed below.

10.6.1 Stigma and Discrimination

The fear of being stigmatized and discriminated against either in the process of job seeking or within the employment itself is common among people with mental health problems. A study of 949 people with mental health problems found that 53 % reported some experience of discrimination. The areas in which this discrimination most frequently occurred included employment, housing, and criminal justice system interactions (Corrigan et al. 2003). A Mental Health Foundation study looking at return to work after sickness absence found that almost half of employees off sick with physical health problems also experienced mild to moderate depression, but were more worried about telling their employer about their mental health issues than about their cancer or heart disease Loughborough University/Mental Health Foundation 2009). Danson and Gilmore (2009) found that employers are wary of employing people with a health condition. They found that while employers had sympathy toward people with disabilities, mental health problems, or those who had recovered from serious illness, they were also concerned that, as employees, their disability or illness might lead to future difficulties and financial pressures for the business.

The continuing existence of stigmatizing attitudes toward people with a mental illness remains a significant barrier for people seeking work. The *Time to Change* campaign in England, which has run since 2007, is aimed at both the general population and at specific target groups, such as employers and health professionals. The campaign has made use of social marketing, advertising campaigns, and events designed to deliver social contact between people with experience of mental health problems and various target groups. Between 2006 and 2010, *Time to Change* measured encouraging reductions in discrimination in five areas of life, including finding a job and keeping a job (Corker et al. 2013). Henderson et al. (2013) found that employers' attitudes toward potential employees with mental health problems improved during *Time to Change*. There are similar campaigns and initiatives in a number of other states, including Scotland, Australia, and New Zealand. These need to be sustained in order to create the lasting change in attitudes and improvements in knowledge that are vital to reduce experiences of discrimination over time. Whereas Biggs et al. (2010) had noted that employers were concerned that people with mental health conditions would need additional supervision and would be less likely to use initiative or to deal confidently and appropriately with the public, Henderson et al. (2013) found employers had become less likely to perceive people with mental health problems as a risk with respect to their reliability, working directly with customers, or in terms of their colleagues' reactions to them. In contrast to the above examples of stigma and discrimination, many rural areas in low- and middle-income countries seem to provide a community that is accepting of individuals with psychosis and provide them a variety of opportunities to engage in meaningful employment (Yang et al. 2013).

10.6.2 Low Expectations

When people with mental health conditions experience discrimination and therefore difficulty in finding and keeping work, it can reduce expectations that future employment experiences will be happier and more successful. Identification with the personal experiences of others may also spread a feeling of pessimism about the real possibility of work among job seekers with mental health problems. Employers with no direct experience of employing someone with a mental health condition themselves may also be influenced by the experiences of other employers, which, if negatively described, can dissuade them from giving a chance to anyone with a mental illness.

Low expectations can be reinforced by health professionals. Many people with mental health conditions report that their doctor, psychiatrist, or nurse saw their illness as a genuine barrier to employment (Marwaha et al. 2009). Bevan et al. (2013) found that clinicians tend to believe that people with schizophrenia who want to work would probably be capable only of noncompetitive work (i.e., voluntary or sheltered work). Yet suggesting that people put their employment aspirations "on the back burner" during months or even years of experiencing a range of therapies, drug treatments, and social support (through day service attendance or participation in vocational training or sheltered work units) has been shown to result not only in lower levels of employment, which would be expected, but also in higher levels of psychiatric illness demonstrated by more frequent and longer hospital admissions over time (Bush et al. 2009). Even when mental health professionals do believe that the people they are supporting are capable of work, this does not necessarily translate into encouragement to find work or referrals to employment services. For example, a study of the employment status of clients using a London community mental health service found that while mental health staff rated 18.9 % of their clients as capable of open-market employment, the percentage actually in work was only 5.5 % (Lloyd-Evans et al. 2012). In the area under review, mental health service users did not have access to a supported employment service providing high-fidelity Individual Placement and Support, although some other forms of employment support were available including voluntary sector employment services and Jobcentre Plus disability employment advisors.

Health and social care staff have regular opportunities to discuss employment with people using their services. It is vital that these opportunities are taken and that a person's motivation and sense of hope are encouraged rather than dampened in the interactions they have with professionals.

10.7 Government Policy

In the UK, welfare benefit caps and the changes to benefit rules in recent times mean that anyone with a mental health condition who is unemployed and claiming the benefits is highly likely to increase their income by entering paid employment, even where this is part-time. Government policies over many years have dis-incentivized a life on benefits and vilified anyone considered to be capable of work for remaining unemployed. Patrick (2012) discusses the "determined focus" of the three main political parties on work as the central duty of all "good" citizens.

Universal Credit, introduced in 2013, was designed to simplify the benefits system by replacing the six main out-of-work benefits and Working Tax Credit.

The earnings disregard, changed to an annual amount, depending on personal circumstances, tapering the amount of Universal Credit received as earnings increase. Disability Living Allowance, a benefit payable to people with mobility and care needs, regardless of employment status or income, was replaced by Personal Independence Payment (PIP), with most existing claimants likely to be reassessed in 2015. In the UK, anyone found fit for work through the Work Capability Assessment or those put into the Work-Related Activity Group (WRAG) of Employment and Support Allowance and people who have claimed Jobseeker's Allowance for 3 months are usually mandated to the Work Programme. People with additional needs, including people in the Support Group of Employment and Support Allowance, meanwhile, are able to engage voluntarily with the Work Programme or to use the Work Choice, the specialist employment program for disabled people. The Work Programme gives providers wide scope to find their own creative and individualized support options for people with any disability or need which may place them at a disadvantage in the labor market. Employment support is funded through staged payments which the Work Programme provider draws down at engagement, job entry, and successive points of job retention. A person previously claiming disability-related benefits such as Employment and Support Allowance (ESA) attracts a higher rate of payment to the provider when they become employed and maintains that employment, than a person who had been claiming Jobseeker's Allowance. Unfortunately the figures to date for the Work Programme describe the lack of success that providers have had in helping people on disability benefits into work (House of Commons Committee of Public Accounts 2013). Critics of the Work Programme say that people with additional support needs are not receiving the individualized support package they require and that easier-to-help clients are being "creamed" and helped quickly and successfully into work, while those who need more intensive or specialist support are being "parked" with very little expectation that they will ever find work.

Work Choice, the DWP program designed for people with additional needs, has been able to support only 650 people with a severe mental illness during the 42 months from April 2011 to September 2014. In this program although an encouraging 37 % of these people have achieved a job outcome, this is only 240 across the whole country (Department for Work and Pensions 2014). This figure looks all the more paltry when compared with the 403 people with severe and enduring mental health problems who could be supported into jobs by just one IPS service (Southdown, in Sussex) in the 20 months between April 2011 and November 2012 (Centre for Mental Health 2012). Unfortunately the DWP schemes are not succeeding in improving the current levels of employment of people with mental health conditions nor are they able to address the huge inequality in employment rates between people with mental health problems and those with other disabilities, other health conditions, or no disability. Thus a better targeted and evidence-based approach to supported employment is indeed necessary to meet the needs of this group of job seekers.

10.8   Funding for Supported Employment

In some locations, mainstream health and social care funding has established IPS services. However, provision is being cut back where budget reductions make this necessary, and in some areas, supported employment is only funded by short-term grants to voluntary sector services. The local need for IPS services should be recognized by Clinical Commissioning Groups and local authorities because employment for people with mental health problems is an expected outcome in the NHS, public health, and adult social care outcomes frameworks. Usually local authority social care services prioritize the care needs of people, including those with mental health problems, according to the criteria of the Fair Access to Care Services (FACS) framework. Someone who, without intervention, would not sustain their involvement in many aspects of work, education, or learning is considered to have a substantial social care need in this area and is likely to be eligible for support.

A possible option for funding the IPS where there is currently no established service could be through a personal budget. The Community Care (Direct Payments) Act 1996 gave local authorities the power to make direct cash payments to individuals instead of providing the community care services they have assessed those individuals as needing. People who receive the payments use the money for the purchase of support, services, or equipment which will meet the assessed need. Many local areas have trialed the use of Personal Health Budgets which identify, through a similar process, the amount of funding available to be spent on an intervention for a healthcare need. A Personal Health Budget is the provision of this funding to the individual to use in a way which suits their personal circumstances and aspirations better than the standard or "mainstream" service on offer. Personal budgets through health or social care (or possibly a pooled health *and* care budget) could enable an individual to buy the services of an IPS employment specialist with a proven track record in successful work outcomes for people with mental health problems. However this model may require additional funding to become viable. At present there are few areas where personal budgets for employment support are being used or indeed could be used. This may be because either there are no local IPS services to purchase or because the costs would have to be set at a relatively high level per person to cover the overheads of keeping the service viable, i.e., running with a minimum number of staff, and the amount of personal budget awarded may not be sufficient to cover the cost of employment support (which may be needed for at least a year).

Craig et al. (2014) have published findings from their study of local authority and NHS spending on supported employment. They asked a specific question about personal budgets, i.e., whether people are allowed to spend their personal budgets on employment support and, if so, whether they do. In this study, 76 % of respondents stated that people are allowed to use personal budgets for employment support, 12 % responded that they were not, and 11 % did not respond. Only 28 % of respondents actually knew that people were using their personal budgets for employment support, 17 % knew that they were not, and 35 % did not know either way. The remainder did not respond. For mental health service users, the breakdown of personal budget spend on employment support was as below:

- Specific work preparation activity in day services: 36 %
- Support into paid work: 30 %
- Support into self-employment or microenterprise: 8 %
- College courses: 7 %
- Volunteering with an end focus on paid work: 7 %
- Support into unpaid work: 2 %
- Not specified: 10 %

10.9   Access to Work

The Access to Work scheme provides government funding to employers to make "reasonable adjustments" at work to enable them to employ a disabled person. The Sayce Report *Getting In, Staying In and Getting On* (Sayce 2011) reviewed some of the specialist provision aiming to increase the employability of disabled people which was available to them at the time. The report noted that Access to Work was underused, largely unknown, and yet had the potential to provide a tailored package of support which could enable people with disabilities, including those with mental health needs, to overcome their own barriers to work. Similarly, Biggs et al. (2010) investigated employers' attitudes toward making reasonable adjustments to support employees with mental health needs. They commented that Access to Work could have been used more effectively for transport to and within work since they found that a significant number of employers stated that they would be prepared to allow flexible working hours, job sharing, and temporary assignment of duties to other colleagues and to accommodate sick leave, but few were prepared to provide or pay for transport to get to work, to get to meetings, or to visit clients.

In recognition of the different needs of people with a mental health condition and the disproportionately low take-up of Access to Work by this group, the government tendered a contract to provide a specific Mental Health Access to Work service, for which Remploy was the successful bidder, and the service became operational in 2012. The Remploy service is able to meet needs such as:

(i) Advice and personal support to manage a mental health condition at work
(ii) Mediation with employers regarding reasonable adjustments and human resource processes
(iii) Information about ongoing sources of support
(iv) Signposting to other services

The support generally takes the form of a number of face-to-face or telephone support meetings over a period of time, not exceeding 26 weeks. At present, just 4 % of Access to Work funding is used to support people with mental health conditions in work (Work and Pensions Committee 2014).

10.10 Conclusion

For many people, having a psychosis means losing work and multiple individual, family, and societal barriers to regaining employment. The costs of lost employment due to mental health problems are enormous. The good news is that attitudes are beginning to change with professionals recognizing that competitive work is possible and beneficial for people with psychosis and health systems and governments trying to create programs to help people to find employment. However, the provision of effective support for people with a range of mental health problems to stay in work or get a new job is patchy and burdened by significant limitation of available resources. What we need is interdisciplinary and concerted action from government, health services, local authorities, and employment services to offer support that works, building on the evidence we have and exploring opportunities for further learning, for people with mental health problems who want to work.

10.11 More Information

More information on supporting people with mental health problems into employment is available at www.centreformentalhealth.org.uk.

References

Baronet A, Gerber GJ (1998) Psychiatric rehabilitation: efficacy of four models. Clin Rev Psychol 18:189–228

Becker D, Drake R, Bond G, Nawaz S, Haslett W, Martinez R (2011) Best practices: a national mental health learning collaborative on supported employment. Psychiatr Serv 62(7):704–706. doi:10.1176/appi.ps.62.7.704

Bevan S, Gulliford J, Steadman K, Taskila T, Thomas R, Moise A (2013) Working with schizophrenia: pathways to employment, recovery & inclusion. The Work Foundation, London

Biggs D, Hovey N, Tyson P, MacDonald S (2010) Employer and employment agency attitudes towards employing individuals with mental health needs. J Ment Health 19(6):505–516

Burns T, Catty J, Becker T, Drake R, Fioritti A, Knapp M (2007) The effectiveness of supported employment for people with severe mental illness: a randomized controlled trial in six european countries. Lancet 370:1146–1152

Burns T, Yeeles K, Langford O, Montes M, Burgess J, Anderson C (2015) A randomised controlled trial of time-limited individual placement and support: IPS-LITE trial. Br J Psychiatry. doi:10.1192/bjp.bp.114.152082

Bush P, Drake R, Xie H, McHugo G, Haslett W (2009) The long-term impact of employment on mental health service use and costs for persons with severe mental illness. Psychiatr Serv 60(8):1024–1031

Care Quality Commission (2014): www.cqc.org.uk

Centre for Mental Health (2012) Briefing 44: implementing what works. Centre for Mental Health, London

Centre for Mental Health (2013) Barriers to employment: what works for people with mental health problems. Centre for Mental Health, London

Centre for Mental Health (2014) Employment support and addiction: what works

Corker E, Hamilton S, Henderson C, Weeks C, Pinfold V, Rose D, Williams P, Flach C, Gill V, Lewis-Holmes E, Thornicroft G (2013) Experiences of discrimination among people using mental health services in England 2008–2011. Br J Psychiatry 202:s58–s63

Corrigan P, Thompson V, Lambert D, Sangster Y, Noel J, Campbell J (2003) Perceptions of discrimination among persons with serious mental illness. Psychiatr Serv 54(8):1105–1110

Craig T, Shepherd G, Rinaldi G, Smith J, Carr S, Preston F, Singh S (2014) Vocational rehabilitation in early psychosis: cluster randomised trial. Br J Psychiatry 205(2):145–150. doi:10.1192/bjp.bp.113.136283

Crowther R, Marshall M, Bond GR, Huxley P (2001) Vocational rehabilitation for people with severe mental illness. Cochrane Database Syst Rev (2):CD003080. doi:10.1002/14651858. CD003080

Danson M, Gilmore K (2009) Evidence on employer attitudes and EQUAL opportunities for the disadvantaged in a flexible and open economy. Environ Plan C: Gov Policy 27(6):991–1007

Department for Work and Pensions (2014) Work choice: official statistics November 2014 https://www.gov.uk/government/uploads/system/uploads/attachment_data/file/373185/work-choice-official-statistics-nov-2014.pdf

Diette T, Goldsmith A, Hamilton D, Darity W (2012) Causality in the relationship between mental health and unemployment. In: Appelbaum L (ed) Reconnecting to work: policies to mitigate long-term unemployment and its consequences. WE Upjohn Institute for Employment Research, Michigan

Drake R (2008) The centre for mental health lecture, 2008. Available at http://www.centreformentalhealth.org.uk/pdfs/BobDrake_FutureOfSupportedEmployment_Transcript.pdf. Accessed 5 Jan 2015

Drake R, Bond G (2011) IPS supported employment: a 20-year update. Am J Psychiatr Rehabil 14(3):155–164. doi:10.1080/15487768.2011.598090

Frost B, Carr V, Halpin S (2002) On behalf of the low prevalence disorders study group. Employment and psychosis: a bulletin of the low prevalence disorders study. National survey of mental health and wellbeing

Frydecka D, Beszłej JA, Gościmski P, Kiejna A, Misiak B (2015) Profiling cognitive impairment in treatment-resistant schizophrenia patients. Psychiatry Research. https://www.researchgate.net/deref/http%3A%2F%2Fdx.doi.org%2F10.1016%2Fj.psychres.2015.11.028

Gudlavalleti MVS, John N, Allagh K, Sagar J, Kamalakannan S, Ramachandra S (2014). Access to health care and employment status of people with disabilities in South India, the SIDE (South India Disability Evidence) study. Available from: https://www.researchgate.net/publication/267734959_Access_to_health_care_and_employment_status_of_people_with_disabilities_in_South_India_the_SIDE_South_India_Disability_Evidence_study. Accessed Mar 26, 2016

Henderson C, Williams P, Little K, Thornicroft G (2013) Mental health problems in the workplace: changes in employers' knowledge, attitudes and practices in England 2006–2010. Br J Psychiatry 202:s70–s76

Hoffmann H, Jäckel D, Glauser S, Kupper Z (2012) A randomised controlled trial of the efficacy of supported employment. Acta Psychiatr Scand 125(2):157–167

House of Commons Committee of Public Accounts (2013) Department for work and pensions: work programme outcome statistics. The Stationery Office, London

Killackey E, Jackson HJ, McGorry PD (2008) Vocational intervention in first-episode psychosis: individual placement and support v. treatment as usual. Br J Psychiatry 193(2):114–120. doi:10.1192/bjp.bp.107.043109

Kin Wong K, Chiu R, Tang B, Mak D, Liu J, Chiu SN (2008) A randomized controlled trial of a supported employment program for persons with long-term mental illness in Hong Kong. Psychiatr Serv 59(1):84–90. doi:10.1176/appi.ps.59.1.84

Latimer EA, Lecomte T, Becker DR, Drake RE, Duclos I, Piat M, Lahaie N, St-Pierre M-S, Therrien C, Xie H (2006) Generalisability of the individual placement and support model of supported employment: results of a Canadian randomised controlled trial. Br J Psychiatry 189:65–73. doi:10.1192/bjp.bp.105.012641

Lloyd-Evans B, Marwaha S, Burns T, Secker J, Latimer E, Blizard R, Killaspy H, Totman J, Tanskanen S, Johnson S (2012) The nature and correlates of paid and unpaid work among service users of London community mental health teams. Epidemiol Psychiatr Sci. doi:http://dx.doi.org/10.1017/S2045796012000534

Loughborough University/Mental Health Foundation (2009) Returning to work: the role of depression. Mental Health Foundation, London

Lysaker P, Bell M (1995) Work performance over time for people with schizophrenia. Psychosoc Rehabil J 18:141–145

Marwaha S, Johnson S (2004) Schizophrenia and employment – a review. Soc Psychiatry Psychiatr Epidemiol 39(5):337–349

Marwaha S, Balachandra S, Johnson S (2009) Clinicians' attitudes to the employment of people with psychosis. Soc Psychiatry Psychiatr Epidemiol 44(5):349–360

McCrone P, Dhanasiri S, Patel A, Knapp M, Lawton-Smith S (2008) Paying the price: the cost of mental health care in England to 2026 (PDF). The King's Fund, London

McManus S, Mowlam A, Dorsett R, Stansfeld S, Clark C, Brown V, Wollny I, Rahim N, Morrell G, Graham J, Whalley R, Lee L, Meltzer H (2012) Mental health in context: the national study of work-search and wellbeing. DWP Research Report No 810. Available at: http://research.dwp.gov.uk/asd/asd5/rports2011-2012/rrep810.pdf

Michon Harry, van Vugt M, van Busschbach J (2011) Effectiveness of individual placement and support; 18 & 30 months follow-up. Paper presented at the Enmesh Conference, Ulm, Germany

Miller L, Clinton-Davis S, Meegan T (2014) Journeys to work: the perspective of client and employment specialist of 'individual placement and Support' in action. Ment Health Soc Incl 18(4):198–202

Mueser KT, Becker DR, Torrey WC et al (1997) Work and nonvocational domains of functioning in persons with severe mental illness: a longitudinal analysis. J Nerv Ment Dis 185(7): 419–426

Patrick R (2012) Work as the primary 'Duty' of the responsible citizen: a critique of this work-centric approach. People Place Policy Online 6(1):5–15

Paul K, Moser K (2009) Unemployment impairs mental health: meta-analyses. J Vocat Behav 74(3):264–282

Rinaldi M, Montibeller T, Perkins R (2011) Increasing the employment rate for people with longer-term mental health problems. Psychiatrist 35:339–343

Sayce L (2011) Getting in, staying in and getting on. Department for Work and Pensions, The Stationery Office, London

Schmidt MJ, Allscheid SP (1995) Employee attitudes and customer satisfaction: Making theoretical and empirical connection. Personal Psychology 48:521–536

Secker J, Grove B, Seebohm P (2001) Challenging barriers to employment, training and education for mental health service users: the service users perspective. J Ment Health 10:395–404

Van Stolk C, Hofman J, Hafner M, Janta B (2014) Psychological wellbeing and work: improving service provision and outcomes. Department for Work and Pensions and Department of Health, London

Waddell G, Burton AK (2006) Is work good for your health and wellbeing? The Stationery Office, Norwich

Work and Pensions Committee (2014) Improving access to work for disabled people. Available at http://www.publications.parliament.uk/pa/cm201415/cmselect/cmworpen/481/48105.htm#a4

Yang LH, Anglin DM, Wonpat-Borja AJ, Opler MG, Greenspoon M, Corcoran CM (2013) Public stigma associated with psychosis risk syndrome in a college population: Implications for peer intervention. Psychiatric Services 64(3):284–288. doi: 10.1176/appi.ps.003782011

Further Reading

2009 CMHS Uniform Reporting System Output Tables. Substance abuse and mental health services administration. Retrieved 30 December 2011. http://www2.pr.gov/agencias/assmca/Documents/EstudiosyEstadisticas.pdf

Bulletin 3. Commonwealth of Australia. http://www.abs.gov.au/AUSSTATS/abs@.nsf/DetailsPage/2110.01933?

Care Quality Commission (2012) Community mental health survey 2012. http://www.cqc.org.uk/content/cqc-annual-report-201213

Greig R, Chapman P, Eley A, Watts R, Love B, Bourlet, G (2014) The cost effectiveness of employment support for people with disabilities NDTi available from http://www.ndti.org.uk/uploads/files/SSCR_The_cost_effectiveness_of_Employment_Support_for_People_with_Disabilities,_NDTi,_March_2014_final.pdf. Accessed 6 Jan 2015

Layard R, Clark D, Knapp M, Mayraz G (2007) Cost-benefit analysis of psychological therapy. National Institute Economic Review 202(1):90–98. doi: 10.1177/0027950107086171

Mental Health Today (online) (2013) Individual placement and support approach delivers more than 50% employment in Nottinghamshire available at: https://www.mentalhealthtoday.co.uk. Accessed 13 Apr 2014

Secker J, Margrove KL (2014) Employment support workers' experiences of motivational interviewing: results from an exploratory study. Psychiatr Rehabil J 37(1):65–67. doi:10.1037/prj0000034. Epub 2014 Jan 13

Cultural Factors in the Treatment of Psychosis

11

Andres J. Pumariega

11.1   Culture and Mental Health/Illness

Culture has been defined as an integrated pattern of human behaviors including thoughts, communication, actions, customs, beliefs, values, and institutions of a racial, ethnic, religious, or social nature (Pumariega et al. 2013). Hughes (1993) further defined culture as a socially transmitted system of ideas that (1) shapes behavior, (2) categorizes perceptions, (3) names selected aspects of experience, (4) is widely shared by members of a particular society or social group, (5) is an orientating framework to coordinate and sanction behavior, and (6) conveys values across the generations. Most societies define normality and deviance in human behavior within the context of culture, including the acceptable range of affective expressiveness, idioms and threshold of distress, and expressed beliefs and actions.

The overt expression of illnesses, with both physical and mental components, is also expressed and understood within the context of culture. Cultural values and beliefs influence the emphasis and expression of particular symptoms and idioms of distress. Many cultures have cultural syndromes which are variations of symptom clusters that bear some similarity to medical or psychiatric diagnostic criteria but deviate in culturally specific manners. Cultures also include explanatory models of illness, which reflect the values or beliefs of the culture. In traditional cultures, these often involve spiritual, supernatural, interpersonal, and relational factors that go beyond biological or psychological models. These explanatory models influence symptom expression as well as healing models, even when the underlying pathophysiology may be invariant. Explanatory models and syndromes are adopted and modified as cultural beliefs evolve and are handed down through generations and across cultures (e.g., the belief in the "evil eye," which has variations in Turkey,

A.J. Pumariega
Department of Psychiatry, Cooper Medical School of Rowan University and
Cooper Health System, Camden, NJ, USA
e-mail: Pumariega-Andres@Cooperhealth.edu

© Springer International Publishing Switzerland 2016
B. Pradhan et al. (eds.), *Brief Interventions for Psychosis:
A Clinical Compendium*, DOI 10.1007/978-3-319-30521-9_11

Italy, and Hispanic countries) (American Psychiatric Association 2013; Lewis-Fernández et al. 2014; Pumariega et al. 2013). As people emigrate to new nations and are exposed to different prevailing host cultures, their symptom expression and explanatory models will change as they adopt host culture beliefs and behavioral patterns. However, many immigrants and children of immigrants hold both prevailing culture and culture of origin beliefs and explanatory models in parallel. They may believe that medical treatments help but at the same time blame their illness on forces beyond human control or influence and engage in traditional spiritual practices from their culture of origin. The latter beliefs and practices are often called upon more frequently during times of distress. Therefore, it is not unusual that first-, second-, and even third-generation immigrants undergoing psychological or psychiatric distress will jointly use formal mental health services as well as engage in traditional rituals and healing practices (Rothe et al. 2010; Pumariega et al. 2013).

11.2 Psychosis in Cultural Context

Diverse cultures have based explanatory models for psychosis or reality disturbance on spiritual, supernatural, and social-interpersonal beliefs. These explanatory models affect how psychosis is viewed and addressed in different cultural contexts, especially by believers in traditional folk culture. For example, McCabe and Priebe (2004) studied explanatory models of psychosis in samples of Whites, Bangladeshis, Afro-Caribbean, and West Africans diagnosed with schizophrenia in the UK. They found that Whites cited biological causes more frequently than the three non-White groups, who cited supernatural and social causes more frequently. A biological explanatory model was related to enhanced treatment satisfaction and therapeutic relationships but not treatment compliance. Those groups who endorsed supernatural or social causation preferred counseling and natural/spiritual healing practices. These differences clearly influence how psychosis is viewed by families and society, the degree of stigma associated with mental illness associated with psychotic symptoms, and the help-seeking behaviors and interventions sought by affected individuals and their families (see Sect. III below).

The intersection of culture and psychosis may be best understood in the context of the continuum of experiences of psychotic symptoms. On one end of the spectrum are brief isolated psychotic symptoms experienced by otherwise "normal" individuals, which in studies have been identified at relatively high rates (Myers 2011). The other end of the spectrum includes severe mental illnesses, including psychotic symptoms associated with severe episodes of mood disorders and psychotic relapses or chronic functional thought disorders such as schizophrenia. In the middle of the spectrum, there is now recognition of what are called "traumatic psychoses," which are psychotic reactions associated with traumatic experiences (e.g., hallucinations based on a perpetrator's reappearance) and can occur in people with and without serious mental illnesses (Kingdon and Turkington 2005). Some scholars have proposed that the common denominator in this continuum is that of dissociative experiences, which are relatively common cognitive-emotional reactions in humans

(Castillo 2003). The differentiators across this continuum are the severity of the acute precipitating stress and the perpetuating psychological and biological factors associated with the experiences. Culture provides the belief system and explanatory model that interprets human emotional and behavioral experiences, including psychotic experiences, both for the sufferer and for the family and community they live within (Spiegel 1971; Castillo 2003).

Many diverse cultures have culturally syntonic experiences associated with psychotic symptoms. Some of these are reactive to stressors, such as the process of grief and loss (hallucinations based on the presence of the lost loved one), and many cultural syndromes which are associated with significant stress-related psychotic symptoms focus on disturbances of reality testing. For example, in the classic Japanese syndrome termed Koro, a male can hallucinate that their penis is physically shrinking (Durst and Rosca-Rebaudendo 1991). Some psychotic symptoms are based on religious-spiritual experiences (such as experiencing apparitions of religious figures), which are reactive or adaptive to stressors. It is important to recognize such experiences so as to not over-interpret or inappropriately patholo-gize them and distinguish them from true indicators of serious psychopathology. Consultation with cultural consultants, spiritual healers, or family members who understand or share the patient's explanatory model and can place the patient's experience within outside of the range of expected cultural experiences can be helpful to effectively evaluate their context and pathological significance (Pumariega et al. 2013).

Differences in the expression of psychiatric symptomatology across different cultural groups and populations will also lead to misdiagnosis and mistreatment associated with psychosis. Epidemiological differences and diagnostic biases have been identified in the diagnosis of psychosis across cultures (Myers 2011). In developing nations and non-Western cultures, brief transient psychoses have been found to be far more common than in Western cultures and identified as being related to social stress and often self-remitting, with an unclear relationship to chronic psychotic illness (Jilek and Jilek-Aall 1970; Jillek 2000; Mamah et al. 2012). A classic finding of diagnostic bias is the overdiagnosis of schizophrenia versus bipolar disorder in certain nations (e.g., in the USA versus Europe) and the overdiagnosis of schizophrenia in African-origin people both in Western nations and in Africa (Kilgus et al. 1995; Myers 2011).

Another impact that culture can have on psychotic symptoms is in the context of immigration. Acculturation stress can be one of the major stressors precipitating psychosis, particularly when that stress of encountering a very different culture and language is sudden or acute (otherwise known as "culture shock"). Other complicating traumatic factors associated with immigration include pre-migratory experiences that led to the emigration (war, natural disaster, terrorism), treacherous emigration journeys (dangerous travel, abuse and victimization, losses of loved ones), and traumatic stressors involved in resettlement (uncertain and insecure residence, loss of contact with family, and social supports) (Bhugra 2004; Rothe et al. 2010). Many studies have pointed to a higher rate of psychotic symptoms and illness among first-generation immigrants. This effect has also been linked to the degree of ethnic density, or ethnic-cultural isolation, that the new immigrant finds themselves in; thus, settlement in an ethnic enclave is a protective factor (Bhugra and Jones 2010; Myers 2011).

11.3 Culture and Traditional Interventions for Psychosis

There is a long history of the use of culturally prescribed rituals and ceremonies to treat psychotic symptoms among traditional and indigenous cultures, occurring for centuries before the medicalization of mental illness. Most such interventions have been directed at addressing spiritual/supernatural factors (such as exorcisms of evil spirits or addressing the relationship between the individual and responsible deities). These interventions have often been combined with the use of herbal remedies or even the use of psychoactive agents in ceremonies. The latter are intended to facilitate or induce altered states of consciousness to better commune with responsible spirits. There is some evidence that traditional healing interventions have value in the management of psychotic symptoms and illnesses, and functionally such interventions address the dissociative experiences and symptoms associated with traumatic psychoses. Collaboration with traditional healers who can perform such rituals can enhance services for individuals with psychosis, especially in minority communities and resource-limited environments (Abbo et al. 2012).

Another important component of how traditional cultures have addressed psychosis has been through social rehabilitation and integration. The psychotic symptom itself is viewed as expression of special supernatural or spiritual abilities or insight. The psychotic person is thereby assigned special "spiritual roles" where their "special powers" have special spiritual meaning and value for the community (Halifax 1979; Myers 2011). These practices, which some have termed "protective stigma," became an interesting way to integrate people with mental illness and reduced the stigma they might have experienced among their family members and neighbors.

11.4 Cultural Influences on Psychological Interventions

More formal psychological therapeutic models based on cultural beliefs have been developed in recent history. These are also infused with the values/beliefs of the predominant culture and informed by its explanatory models.

Yoga and meditation are perhaps the oldest psychotherapeutic interventions. Buddha as the integrative theorist used Pali and Hindu teachings and explanations to develop a model oriented to address distress and enhance human potential. Parallels have been between Kundalini awakening (a Tantric tradioton of Yoga) and psychosis. Kundalini, a spiritual concept, is a powerful energy that resides at the base of the tail bone, often represented by a snake twisting up the spine. In most people, this energy is dormant until something causes it to awaken. This can be induced through specific types of yoga, breathing exercises, or chanting. In some cases the causes of awakening are unclear – it can be totally spontaneous. When the Kundalini awakens, it may stir up a lot of repressed feelings and traumas from the unconscious and cause considerable anguish and pain in the individual. A premature Kundalini awakening may cause psychotic episodes in individuals with severe early traumas. Such traumas are usually associated with serious organic or biological disturbances. Some people with psychotic symptoms tend to show low-amplitude alpha mixed with moderate- to high-amplitude fast beta waves, often predominating in the frontal and perhaps in the temporal lobes of the brain. This may indicate a partial Kundalini arousal on a fragmented and fragile basis. This fast EEG frequency pattern, which lacks the slow-frequency, high-amplitude components, indicates a lack of grounding and a dissociation between levels of consciousness. On the other hand, there are also yogic techniques oriented to reducing Kundalini, and recent applications with schizophrenia have addressed negative symptomatology and social cognition (Sannella 1987; Arias et al. 2006).

Morita therapy is a systematic psychotherapy based on Eastern psychology, named in 1919 after Shoma Morita, a Japanese psychiatrist. It is a behavioral, structured program and tries to lead patients from preoccupation with somatic symptoms and attempts to eliminate neurotic symptoms through four phases by accepting them as natural while engaging an outward perspective on life and increased social functioning, with an emphasis on moral teachings. It has had some recent application in the treatment of schizophrenia with some positive results (Li and He 2008).

Psychoanalysis as an explanatory and therapeutic model is based on the values of Western European culture and attempted to explain human psychological distress and disorder as resulting from early developmental failures and the impact of unresolved psychological conflict overwhelming the rational mind. Psychosis is addressed in psychoanalytic psychotherapy through strengthening defense mechanisms to better address internal distress and conflict that may fuel psychotic symptoms and improve insight to strengthen reality testing. In current day practice, psychoanalytic psychotherapy is seen as complimentary or adjunctive to the use of pharmacotherapy to treat psychotic symptoms (Fenton 2000).

Cognitive behavioral therapy (CBT) developed as a late twentieth-century Western model that focuses on distortions of rational thoughts and behaviors and their resulting emotions as the main explanatory model for psychiatric disturbance, as well as the development of functional cognitive and behavioral skills for daily living and functioning. It applies this explanatory model and the resulting structured therapeutic techniques to address such distortions for a growing range of psychiatric disorders. It was initially applied to address depression and anxiety, with significant efficacy and effectiveness, but progressively has been applied to more serious disorders such as bipolar disorder and schizophrenia and even disorders with a neurological basis such as Tourette's disorder. This is again not surprising due to the relationship between psychotic symptoms (especially traumatic psychoses) and dissociative experiences driven by anxiety as previously discussed (Castillo 2003; Kingdon and Turkington 2005), with the early work on CBT and anxiety informing this work. It has had recent significant application to the treatment of psychosis (associated with schizophrenia and mood disorders) through similarly assisting the individual in identifying and addressing reality distortions as thought distortions. It has a primarily Western cultural bent, though it has recently been the focus of work on cultural modification to address diverse cultural orientations (see Sect. V).

Family therapy is a mid-twentieth-century Western model that initially focused on family dysfunction as being causative of psychosis, influenced by the work of the communication theorists, who hypothesized that disturbed communication within social contexts that placed vulnerable individuals in highly conflicted situations (such as within distressed families) was causative in the onset and perpetuation of psychosis. There were even attempts to treat schizophrenia through intensive family therapy in long-term experimental inpatient settings (Watzlawick 1963). The hypothesis of communication and relationship dysfunction as causative was found to be fallacious, but the role of disturbed communication leading to increased distress and vulnerability toward psychotic relapse was supported empirically (McFarlane and Cook 2007). This led to the concept of high "expressed emotion" (EE) being a significant mediating factor in symptom stability and reduction and a target for intervention. However, it has also been found that high EE is actually normative among many cultural groups, and in those contexts, EE is less significant in precipitating or exacerbating psychotic symptoms (Karno et al. 1987). In addition, the role of families in supporting cognitive and functional rehabilitation has been supported by many studies (McFarlane et al. 2003). Family therapy has also progressively been adopted in different cultural contexts and also been increasingly informed by cultural adaptations.

11.5   Cultural Adaptation of Western Evidence-Based Interventions

As CBT and other forms of evidence-based psychotherapies have evolved, there has been greater emphasis on its cultural adaptation to enhance effectiveness with more diverse populations, especially non-European-origin groups.

Griner and Smith (2006) conducted a meta-analysis of 80 publications on culturally adapted psychotherapies and found three levels of cultural adaptations (in order of extensiveness): Level 1, translation of therapeutic materials into the language of the client; Level 2, incorporation of cultural values/beliefs and contextual variables (unique stressors and challenges) into the psychotherapy; and Level 3, incorporation of cultural theories of problem formation and therapeutic change. Falicov (2009) identified other levels of cultural adaptation of psychotherapies, which included (1) incorporation of cultural values/beliefs and contextual variables (including stressors and challenges unique to that cultural group); (2) implementation by professionals of the same race, ethnicity, and language as clients; (3) addressing accessibility and flexibility of scheduling to fit cultural values and needs; and (4) clinician collaboration with natural resources (extended family, spiritual traditions, and community) and engagement strategies.

One of the most comprehensive frameworks for the cultural adaptation of psychotherapy was proposed by Tseng et al. (2005) that outlines four levels of adjustment to the therapy and adapted for psychosis by Rathod and colleagues (2015): (1) Philosophical reorientation or reexamination and orientation of the fundamental view of life which affects the direction and goal of therapy, e.g., acceptance or conquering, normality, and maturity. This domain includes level of acculturation, beliefs and attributions of illness, and cultural orientation toward psychotherapy. (2) Practical considerations of societal factors that impact on the performance of therapy (e.g., racism, legal status, economic conditions, health systems and reputation, funding arrangements, level of stigma associated with mental illness, etc.), all of which impact on the patient's experiences and often determine their trust or lack of it in the system of care. (3) Technical adjustments of methods and skill in providing psychotherapy, including the mode and manner of therapy and various clinical issues within the therapy for clients of various backgrounds. This incorporates understanding of the setting and environment of therapy, therapeutic relationship, choice of therapy, family structures and goals, and role of religion and spirituality. (4) Theoretical modifications of concepts need to be made for a best fit for the individual and their cultural strength (including views on mind-body relations, self and ego boundaries, individuality vs. collectiveness, personality development, parent-child relations, and preferred defense mechanisms and coping styles).

The evidence for culturally adapted psychotherapies has been mixed but promising. Griner and Smith (2006), conducting a meta-analysis of 76 studies, demonstrated an effect size of 0.45 for culturally adapted evidence-based interventions in comparison to nonculturally adapted treatments. Huey and Polo (2008), using a meta-analysis of 38 studies of interventions for minority youth, was inconclusive insofar as comparative effectiveness, but demostrated significantly stronger treatment adherence to culturally adapted interventions. The ultimate challenge faced by culturally adapted interventions is making the necessary adaptations while retaining fidelity to the original concepts and methodology of interventions.

Conceptually, cultural adaptations of psychological interventions for psychosis and psychotic symptoms need to include and address the following key elements: (a) demystification and psychoeducation (culturally relative explanatory models of psychosis, cultural framework around reality testing), including stigma; (b) cultural idioms around psychotic experiences; (c) the role of the family in efforts for rehabilitation and recovery, including the culturally relative nature of EE; and (d) cultural role expectations for rehabilitation. Kingdon and Turkington (2005) discuss early intervention techniques used in working with traumatic psychoses, chiefly identification of relevant stressors and context, reattribution of hallucinations, dealing with patient's beliefs and attitudes about key events, and (in cases where borderline personality characteristics are present) the use of dialectic behavioral techniques (p.40–41). They first recommend ethnic and gender matching (in therapist or even in supervisor) – may be ideal, but not always feasible. They go on to recommend attention to therapist style (language, tone of voice, and areas of emphasis), eliciting basic beliefs and considering spiritual or cultural explanations for inclusion in the therapeutic work.

Rathod et al. (2010) conducted a qualitative study in ethnic minority groups that concluded that CBT would be acceptable for minority patients with psychosis and may be more effective if it was culturally adapted to meet their needs. Based on the principles outlined by Tseng (2005) for cultural adaptation of psychotherapy, Rathod et al. (2013) pursued a randomized controlled trial of a culturally adapted cognitive behavioral therapy for psychosis (CaCBTp). This trial was conducted in two centers in the UK ($n = 33$) with culturally diverse participants with a diagnosis of a schizophrenic disorder, including Black British, African Caribbean/Black African, and South Asian Muslim participants. Assessors blind to randomization and treatment allocation conducted administration of outcome measures. Participants in the CaCBTp group achieved statistically significant results posttreatment compared to those in the treatment as usual arm, with some gains maintained at follow-up. High levels of satisfaction with the CaCBTp were reported.

Mausbach et al. (2008) pursued the comparative evaluation of a group-based manualized behavioral itnervention targeting areas of everyday functioning (managing medications, improving social and commmunication skills, organizing and planning daily life, using tramsportation, and managing finances). The culturally adapted version of this program included (a) translation of interrvention and assessment materials from English to Spanish, (b) inclusion of bicultural/ bilingual group faciltiators, (c) integrating culturally specific icons and idioms in the materials, and (d) basing the format, content, and treatment goals on Mexican cultural values such as *simpatia* (the use of polite social relations) and *personalismo* (emphasizing warm relationships). Fifty-nine Latino participants diagnosed with persistent psychotic disorders were assigned to either the culturally tailored skills-training intervention ($n = 21$), the equivalent non-tailored intervention ($n = 15$), or a community-based support group ($n = 23$). Participants receiving the culturally tailored intervention showed significant improvement in several outcomes, particularly significant improvement in the ability to role-play a variety of complex daily functional situations, significantly fewer medication errors, and higher quality of well-being scores at 6 months. Rathod et al. (2015) present the most up-to-date research on CBT in ethnic minority groups and present the cultural adaptation of core CBT techniques including reattribution, normalization, explanation development and formulation, reality testing, inference chaining, and resetting expectations.

Acceptance and commitment therapy (ACT) is a newer behavioral treatment that promotes radical acceptance of unavoidable psychological distress in the service of pursuing valued goals and actions. Patients are encouraged to accept unavoidable events, to acknowledge but let go of symptoms without treating them as either true or false, and to identify and work toward goals that were consistent with their broader life values. Bach and Hayes (2002) first demonstrated the effectiveness of ACT in a small randomized trial with brief treatment of psychotic inpatients. The ACT group showed a 50 % reduction in re-hospitalization rates by 4-month follow-up and reported less distress from and believability in their psychotic symptoms. Paradoxically, patients receiving ACT simultaneously reported a higher frequency of psychotic symptoms at follow-up, possibly demonstrating increased acceptance of the symptoms. Guadiano and Herbert (2006) replicated the Bach and Hayes (2002) study with a predominantly (80 %) poor African-American population, with better measures and a better control condition that controlled for experimental contact. They found significant results, especially on measures of overt psychotic behavior such as the Brief Psychiatric Rating Scale.

Some models of evidence-based culturally adapted interventions have focused on families to address these key elements. Koppelowicz et al. (2003) developed a family intervention for Latinos with schizophrenia that focused on behavioral, conflict resolution, and cognitive skills training for patients and family members. It had significant impact on re-hospitalization, symptoms, function; no difference in caregiver burden or quality of life. Barrio and Yamada (2010) pursued an iterative intervention development process guided by a cultural exchange framework, based on findings from an ethnographic study of Latino families with members with schizophrenia. They piloted this multifamily group 16-session intervention with 59 Latino families in a randomized control trial. The preliminary data from family- and client-level outcomes and post-study focus groups indicate that the intervention is effective by increasing illness knowledge and reducing family burden. Yang et al. (2014) developed and piloted an anti-stigma intervention based on a peer-family group format, co-led by a clinician and a trained family caregiver, to counter stigma among Chinese immigrants. The intervention provides psychoeducation, strategies to counter experienced discrimination, and techniques to resist internalized stigma. Results suggest preliminary efficacy in reducing internalized stigma for caregivers who evidenced at least some prior internalized stigma.

Some of the work on cultural adaptation of psychotherapy of psychosis has involved further investigation of the application of the concept of *expressed emotions* (EE). Mexican Americans have been found to have lower rates of high EE than other ethnic and national groups (Jenkins and Karno 1992). In the USA, and relative to European-Americans, Mexican American caregivers have been found to be less critical of their ill relatives (Kopelowicz et al. 2006), as well as more likely to live with and spend more time with them (Lopez et al. 2004; Ramirez Garcia et al. 2004). The relation between expressed emotion (EE) and caregiver acceptance was tested with the use of video-recorded interactions between 31 Mexican American family caregivers and their relatives with schizophrenia. Acceptance was defined as the family caregiver's engagement with the ill relative along with low levels of expectations for behavioral change. Three aspects of caregiver acceptance were measured: global acceptance of the patient, unified detachment (i.e., non-blaming but engaged problem discussion), and low aversive responses to patient behavior (e.g., criticisms and demanding change). Relative to high EE caregivers, low EE caregivers were consistently more accepting of their ill relatives across the three measures of acceptance. Unified detachment was negatively associated with emotional overinvolvement, and aversive responses were positively related to criticism. Warmth was not related to acceptance. Such findings can guide the development of cultural adaptations that address family EE effectively within a cultural context and improve the prognosis for the patient and the caregiving environment (Vaughn and Leff 1981).

The pharmacotherapy of psychosis also requires cultural adaptations to address both biological and psychological factors. Increasing evidence points to differential pharmacogenetics based on ethnically and racially specific polymorphisms of metabolic enzymes and postsynaptic receptors. Many of these polymorphisms have been handed down multiple generations via population migrations. These polymorphisms include D2 receptor sensitivity in African origin (which increase risk for extrapyramidal symptoms and tardive dyskinesia), CPY2D6 slow metabolism with Asian origin and indigenous American populations (which increase risk of side effects and potency with lower doses), and CPY2D6 slow metabolism in dietary context with Latinos (through the use of corn and citrus). Clinicians have to be alert to these polymorphisms when prescribing psychiatric medications, especially antipsychotics. They also need to be alert to ethnic/racial/cultural biases around diagnosis, which can lead to inappropriate treatment. Patients and families, especially from ethnic minority groups, also experience specific stigma through the use of pharmacotherapy for psychiatric disorders, feeling that these have at times been misused for cultural oppression. Psychoeducation needs to demystify pharmacotherapy and empower patients and families from diverse backgrounds by the process of informed consent and therapeutic choice (Lin and Finder 1983; Lin et al. 1995; Malik et al. 2010).

11.6   Impact of Globalization

Concern has been voiced by some critics of globalization in mental health, such as Watters (2010), that this may lead to the Westernization of mental health, with a greater emphasis on standardization of assessment and treatment that would minimize cultural factors such as explanatory models, treatment acceptability, and culturally specific interventions. Watters identifies these explanatory models, accompanied by symptom expression and idioms of distress unique to the cultural context, as important in the prevention of alienation and stigma and the maintenance of the bond between the affected individual and their families and communities. He cites various examples of studies that have shown that the Western scientific model may have the opposite effect than intended around stigma and social integration, possibly serving to alienate those affected with mental illness from their families and communities. There is also danger in excessive reductionism adversely impacting the rich diversity in understanding and interventions of psychotic experiences.

However, globalization could lead to a healthy exchange and mutual learning of approaches to treat psychotic disorders. The use of culturally based interventions and of natural supports such as families and spiritual institutions may provide solutions to one of the main challenges in serving those people with these illnesses: overcoming their socio-cognitive impairments in order to sustain their connections to their families and communities. Such social connections are critical in enhancing function and recovery from psychotic illnesses. Western psychiatric service systems have often failed in providing such social connectedness and rehabilitation while spending large sums per capita in the treatment of psychotic relapses (in hospitalization, residential treatment, and pharmacotherapy). Naturalistic, community-based models of care in low-resource nations may be important exemplars to reform our service systems for these vulnerable citizens.

Even with this greater openness to culturally based interventions and care models, access to such approaches still poses a major challenge. This lack of access particularly impacts some of our most vulnerable populations (minorities, immigrants) who tend to utilize traditional mental health services at much lower rates due to these being less acceptable and culturally relevant (Pumariega et al. 2013). We cannot count on ethnic matching of mental health providers as a solution since these are in lower relative numbers among the overall pool of professionals compared to the overall population. Additionally, mental health professionals from minority and immigrant backgrounds are themselves not often trained in culturally informed models. The best approach to address this major access gap is training all mental health providers in principles of culturally informed care and evidence-based culturally based interventions, especially those for psychoses. Such training and standard setting efforts are underway by some professional organizations and some public mental health providers (Pumariega et al. 2013), but they need to be far broader if we are to catch-up with the increasing cultural diversity of our populations and their needs.

Additionally, mainstream mental health providers can collaborate with culturally specific healers in providing parallel care, particularly sharing their mutual understanding of the management of psychotic symptoms and experiences. An early example of this is provided by Pedro Ruiz, well-known leader in world psychiatry, who found, as a young attending heading a partial hospitalization program for Latinos with serious mental illness in New York City, that many of his patients were dropping out of the program at high rates. He attempted to make the ambiance of the program more culturally welcoming, but this did not yield results. It was only after he discovered that the patients instead were attending an Espiritismo center-church (Puerto Rican Afro-Caribbean religion) for their spiritual healing needs that he then was able to establish a successful collaboration with the church based on mutual support of each others' explanatory model and interventions that led to more comprehensive care (Ruiz 1977).

Conclusions

The cultural adaptation and tailoring of psychiatric treatment in general and of schizophrenia and other psychotic disorders in particular is an area that will witness continued growth in interest and application. This will occur as there is greater emphasis on mental health care and services worldwide and greater exchange in knowledge and treatment models as a result of globalization and improving socioeconomic conditions in emerging nations.

References

Abbo C, Okello ES, Musisi S, Waako P, Ekblad S (2012) Naturalistic outcome of treatment of psychosis by traditional healers in Jinja and Iganga districts, Eastern Uganda – a 3- and 6 months follow up. Int J Ment Health Syst 6(1):13

American Psychiatric Association (2013) Diagnostic and statistical manual of mental disorders, 5th edn. American Psychiatric Association, Washington, DC

Arias A, Steinberg K, Banga A, Trestman R (2006) Systematic review of the efficacy of meditation techniques as treatments for medical illness. J Altern Complement Med 12(8):817–832

Bach P, Hayes S (2002) The use of acceptance and commitment therapy to prevent the rehospitalization of psychotic patients: a randomized controlled trial. J Consult Clin Psychol 70:1129–1139

Barrio C, Yamada A (2010) Culturally based intervention development: the case of latino families dealing with schizophrenia. Res Soc Work Pract 20(5):483—492

Bhugra D (2004) Migration and mental health. Acta Psychiat Scand 109(4):243–258

Bhugra D, Jones P (2010) Migration and mental illness. In: Rahul Bhattacharya R, Cross S, Bhugra D (eds) Clinical topics in cultural psychiatry. The Royal College of Psychiatrists, London, pp 15–26, Chapter 2

Castillo RJ (2003) Trance, functional psychosis, and culture. Psychiatry 66:9–21

Durst R, Rosca-Rebaudendo P (1991) The disorder named Koro. Behav Neurol 4:1–14

Falicov (2009) Commentary: On the wisdom and challenges of culturally attuned treatmetns for Latinos. Family Process; 48(2): 292–309.

Fenton WS (2000) Evolving perspectives on individual psychotherapy for schizophrenia. Schizophr Bull 46:47–72

Gaudiano BA, Herbert JD (2006) Acute treatment of inpatients with psychotic symptoms using acceptance and commitment therapy. Behav Res Ther 44:415–437

Griner D, Smith T (2006) Culturally adapted mental health interventions: a meta-analytic review. Psychotherapy (Chic) 43:531–548

Halifax J (1979) Shamanic voices. Dutton, New York

Huey S, Polo A (2008) Evidence-based psychosocial treatments for ethnic minority youth. J Clin Child Adoles Psychol 37:262–301

Hughes C (1993) Culture in clinical psychiatry. In: Gaw A (ed) Culture ethnicity and mental illness. American Psychiatric Press, Washington, DC, pp 3–42

Jenkins JH, Karno M (1992) The meaning of expressed emotion: theoretical issues raised by cross-cultural research. Am J Psychiat 149:9–21

Jilek WG (2000) Culturally related syndromes. Chapter 4.16. In: Gelder MG, Lopez-lbor JJ, Andreasen N (eds) New Oxford textbook of psychiatry, vol 1. Oxford University Press, Oxford, pp 1061–1066

Jilek WG, Jilek-Aall L (1970) Transient psychoses in Africans. Psychiatr Clin 3:337–364

Karno M, Jenkins J, de la Selva A, Santana F, Telles C, Lopez S, Mintz J (1987) Expressed emotion and schizophrenic outcome among Mexican-American families. J Nerv Ment Dis 175(2):142–151

Kilgus MD, Pumariega AJ, Cuffe S (1995) Race and diagnosis in adolescent psychiatric inpatients. J Am Acad Child Adol Psychiat 34(1):67–72

Kingdon DG, Turkington D (2005) Cognitive-behavioral therapy of schizophrenia. Guilford Publications) New York-London. pp 40–41 and 52–53

Kopelowicz A, López SR, Zarate R et al (2006) Expressed emotion and family interactions in Mexican-Americans with schizophrenia. J Nerv Ment Dis 194:330–334

Kopelowicz, A., Zarate, C., Gonzalez-Smith, V., Liberman, R. (2003) Disease management in Latinos with schizophrenia: A family-assisted, skills, training approach. Schizophrenia Bulletin, 29(2): 211–227.

Lewis-Fernández R, Aggarwal N, Bäärnhielm S, Rohlof H, Kirmayer L et al (2014) Culture and psychiatric evaluation: operationalizing cultural formulation for DSM-5. Psychiatry 77(2): 130–154

Li C, He Y (2008) Morita therapy for schizophrenia. Schizophr Bull 34(6):1021–1023. doi:10.1093/schbul/sbn124

Lin K-M, Finder E (1983) Neuroleptic dosage for Asians. Am J Psychiatry 140:490–491

Lin K, Anderson D, Poland R (1995) Ethnicity and psychopharmacology: bridging the gap. Psychiatr Clin N Am 18(3):635–647

López SR, Hipke KN, Polo JA, Jenkins JH et al (2004) Ethnicity, expressed emotion, attributions, and course of schizophrenia: family warmth matters. J Abnorm Psychol 113:428–439

Malik M, Lawson W, Lake J, Joshi S (2010) Culturally adapted pharmacotherapy and the integrative formulation. Child Adolesc Psychiatric Clin N Am 19:791–814. doi:10.1016/j.chc.2010.08.003

Mamah D, Mbwayo A, Mutiso V, Barch D, Constantino J, Nsofor T, Khasakhala L, Ndetei D (2012) A survey of psychosis-risk symptoms in Kenya. Compr Psychiatry 53(5):516–524. doi:10.1016/j.comppsych.2011.08.003

Mausbach B, Bucardo J, Cardenas V, McKibbin C, Barrio C, Goldman S, Jeste D, Patterson T (2008) Evaluation of a culturally tailored skills intervention for Latinos with Persistent Psychotic Disorders. Am J Psychiatr Rehabil 11(1):61–75

McCabe R, Priebe S (2004) Explanatory models of illness in schizophrenia: comparison of four ethnic groups. Br J Psychiatry 185:25–30

McFarlane W, Cook W (2007) Family expressed emotion prior to the onset of psychosis. Fam Process 46(2):185–197

McFarlane W, Dixon L, Lukens E, Lucksted A (2003) Family psychoeducation and schizophrenia: a review of the literature. J Marital Fam Ther 29(2):223–245

Myers N (2011) Update: schizophrenia across cultures. Curr Psychiat Rep 13:305–311

Pumariega AJ, Rothe E, Mian A, Carlisle L, Toppelberg C, Harris T, Gogineni R, Webb S, Smith J, the Committee on Quality Issues (2013) Practice parameter for cultural competence in child and adolescent psychiatric practice. J Am Acad Child Adolesc Psychiatry 52(10):1101–1115

Ramírez García JI, Wood JM, Hosch HM, Meyer LM (2004) Predicting psychiatric rehospitalizations: the role of Latino versus European American ethnicity. Psychol Serv 1:147–157

Rathod S, Kingdon D, Phiri P, Gobbi M (2010) Developing culturally sensitive cognitive behaviour therapy for psychosis for ethnic minority patients by exploration and incorporation of service users' and health professionals' views and opinions, Behavioural and Cognitive Psychotherapy 38(5):511–533

Rathod S, Phiri P, Harris S, Underwood C, Thagadur M, Padmanabi U, Kingdon D (2013) Cognitive behaviour therapy for psychosis can be adapted for minority ethnic groups: a randomised controlled trial. Schizophr Res 143(2–3):319–326

Rathod S, Kingdon D, Pinninti N, Turkington D, Phiri P (2015) Cultural adaptation of CBT for serious mental illness: a guide for training and practice. Wiley-Blackwell, New York, p 352

Rothe E, Tzuang D, Pumariega AJ (2010) Acculturation, development, and adaptation. Child Adolesc Psychiatr Clin N Am 19(4):681–696

Ruiz P (1977) Culture and mental health: a Hispanic perspective. J Contemp Psychother 9(1):24–27

Sannella L (1987) The Kundalini experience: psychosis or transcendence. Integral Publishers, San Francisco

Spiegel J (1971) Transactions: the interplay between individual, family, and society. Science House, New York

Tseng W-S (1999) Culture and psychotherapy: review and practical guidelines. Transcult Psychiatry 36:131

Tseng W-S, Chang S-C, Nishizono M (eds) (2005) Asian culture and psychotherapy: implications for East and West. University of Hawaii Press, Honolulu

Vaughn CE, Leff JP (1981) Patterns of emotional response in relatives of schizophrenic patients. Schizophr Bull 7(1):43–44

Watters E (2010) The Americanization of mental illness. New York Times, 10th January

Watzlawick PA (1963) A review of the double bind theory. Fam Process 2:132–153

Yang L, Lai G, Tu M, Luo M, Wonpat-Borja A, Jackson V, Lewis-Fernandez R, Dixon L (2014) A brief anti-stigma intervention for Chinese immigrant caregivers of individuals with psychosis: adaptation and initial findings. Transcult Psychiatry 51:139–157

Brief Intervention Models in Psychosis for Developing Countries (Asia and Africa)

12

Muhammad Irfan, Lydia Stone, Nusrat Husain, and Peter Phiri

12.1 Introduction

Low- and middle-income countries (LAMIC) have enormous burden of psychotic disorders with prevalence of schizophrenia between 1.4 and 4.6 per 1,000 (Jablensky 2000). While the burden is very heavy, the resources available to treat them are very limited. "For example, per 100,000 population, Psychiatrists working in the mental health sector in the most populous developing countries of Asia and Africa i.e., India, Pakistan, Nigeria and Ethiopia are 0.301, 0.185, 0.06 and 0.04 respectively" (World Health Organization 2011). A combination of limited access and cultural belief systems leads to many individuals' first accessing help from complimentary or alternate practitioners or spiritual healers. Additionally,

M. Irfan (✉)
Department of Psychiatry & Behavioral Sciences, Peshawar Medical College,
Peshawar, Pakistan

Provincial Chapter Chief, Pakistan Psychiatric Society Council Member, Committee on
Publication Ethics General Secretary, Pakistan Association of Cognitive Therapists
e-mail: mirfan78@yahoo.com

L. Stone
Chartered Principal Clinical Psychologist, Oxfordshire County Council, The ATTACH team, Nash
Court 4440 John Smith Drive Oxford Business Park South COWLEY, Oxford OX4, NJ, USA

N. Husain
Reader in Psychiatry Lead, Global Mental Health Institute of Brain, Behaviour & Mental
Health, University of Manchester

Director Research Global Health, Manchester Academic Health Sciences Centre (MAHSC)
Honorary Consultant Psychiatrist, Lead Culture & International Mental Health Research
Group, Lancashire Care NHS Foundation Trust

P. Phiri
R&D Manager, Southern Health NHS Foundation Trust Research & Development, Clinical
Trials Facility Tom Rudd Unit, Moorgreen Hospital, Botley Rd, West End, Southampton

© Springer International Publishing Switzerland 2016
B. Pradhan et al. (eds.), *Brief Interventions for Psychosis:
A Clinical Compendium*, DOI 10.1007/978-3-319-30521-9_12

there is an inverse relationship between GDP and duration of untreated psychosis (Large et al. 2008), and duration of untreated psychosis is shown to be correlated with adverse outcomes of poorer response to treatment and increased disability (Farooq et al. 2009).

12.2 Epidemiology and Outcomes of Psychotic Disorders in Developing Countries

Research data on epidemiology of severe mental disorders is limited from LAMIC (Jablensky et al. 2000). However, the small number of studies available paints a gray picture (Mahy et al. 1999; Menezes et al. 2007; Bhugra 2005; Saha et al. 2005). For example, Adams et al. (2006) estimated that in Bihar, one of most economically deprived states in India, the number of people suffering from schizophrenia is larger than in the whole North America. Similarly, these countries have large populations living in the age range which is high risk for psychotic disorders such as schizophrenia, e.g., 21.5 % of Pakistan population is in the age range of 15–24 years (Pakistan Demographic Profile 2014).

Strikingly, as far as outcomes are concerned, schizophrenia might have better outcomes in LAMIC (Isaac et al. 2007). The International Pilot Study of Schizophrenia (World Health Organization 1976) and later the International Study on Schizophrenia (ISoS) (Harrison et al. 2001) suggested better outcomes in the LAMICs. Kulhara and Chakrabarti (2001) reported that sociocultural factors might contribute to the better outcome of schizophrenia in LAMICs. However, in recent years Patel and his colleagues (2006) questioned this strongly held belief about better outcomes of schizophrenia in such countries. Calls for more research into this unexpected differential in outcome for psychosis between developed and developing countries continue (Hopper and Wanderling 2000).

12.3 Treatment of Psychosis in Lamic

There is very little evidence, if any, on the effectiveness of typical pharmacological and psychological interventions in these populations, although favorable outcome is reported by large studies (Jablensky et al. 2000; Leff et al. 1992). This is in contrast to voluminous literature on the epidemiology of schizophrenia in these countries. Evidence for the effectiveness of psychosocial interventions in psychosis is reasonably robust in high-income countries (NICE 2014) but differences in sociocultural factors and health systems may limit the generalizability of this evidence to LAMICs (Patel et al. 2006). In LAMICs the treatment gap for psychotic disorders is large because of the scarcity of resources to offer evidence-based interventions (Kohn et al. 2004). There is evidence for a significant delay in seeking treatment for people with psychotic disorders from LAMICs. Therefore the delivery of evidence-based interventions is a challenge in such countries and a global mental health priority (Lancet Global Mental Health Group 2007).

12.3.1 Psychosocial Interventions for Psychosis in LAMIC

12.3.1.1 Research on Beliefs About the Illness

It is important in this aspect to consider the concepts about the illness and its causes, as these lead to help-seeking behaviors. Our group has conducted research in both Pakistan and the UK to explore the beliefs about psychosis among Muslim South Asians in the UK and the local population in Pakistan. There is evidence to suggest that some Asian clients use a bio-psycho-social-spiritual model of understanding of illness (Table 12.1). Saravanan et al. (2007), for example, considered the dissonance of belief models about first-episode psychosis between patients and professionals in South India and reported that the majority of patients prioritized spiritual and mystical factors as the cause of the disorder, and this affected their pattern of help seeking. Looking at the same region, Joel et al. (2003) examined the beliefs of community health workers about psychosis and found a variety of indigenous beliefs which contradicted the biomedical model and so led to the conclusions that medical doctors could not help; clearly, this would have a significant impact on referral to and general accessibility of psychiatric treatment, including brief interventions.

12.3.1.2 Help-Seeking Behaviors

Beliefs about mental illness are likely to affect the way we seek help. They are also likely to have an effect on professionals' assessment of whether the individual may benefit from different treatments. Saravanan and colleagues (2007) reported that those patients who held a more conventional biomedical model of psychosis were scored as having greater insight; as we know, this concept is strongly linked to assessment of individuals as suitable for talking therapy, including brief therapy.

A study of clinicians' attitudes to cognitive behavior therapy (CBT) in Tanzania (Stone and Warren 2011) indicated more positive beliefs about the utility of this particular type of brief intervention, but this was not specific to psychosis. Unpublished qualitative data from this cohort identified key themes which influenced clinicians' views about CBT (and its effectiveness), including the medical model's dominance among trained professionals, the novelty of a talking therapy approach, the practicalities of implementing it, and the personal cultural influence the individual therapist brought. Interestingly, it seems that local views of psychotherapeutic interventions may depend very much on the degree to which the culture is interpersonally attuned and syntonic and therefore able to benefit from an interpersonal form of treatment. In Tanzania, psychotherapeutic interventions appear to be gaining in popularity (despite the scarcity of providers) and may not suffer from the same stigma that traditional psychiatric treatments have.

12.3.1.3 Examples of Tried Interventions

There are not many published studies in this area. The limited work so far has focused on effectiveness of short but practical interventions that tested cost-effective strategies to improve outcomes in schizophrenia. For example, Farooq and colleagues (2011) conducted a RCT including 110 patients with schizophrenia or schizoaffective disorder to evaluate the effectiveness of an intervention that involves a family member in

Table 12.1 Bio-psycho-social-spiritual model

Pakistan (Naeem et al. 2014c)	UK (Rathod et al. 2010)	UK (Bhikha et al. 2012)	Pakistan (Awan 2015)
Psychosocial	*Previous wrongdoing* +++++	*Spiritual/religious causes* (55 %)	*Psychosocial*
Stress or worry (25)			Stress (24)
Poverty (22)			
Loss of balance of mind (2)	*Supernatural beliefs* +++++	*Psychosocial*	Interpersonal (11)
Too much thinking (1)		Stress (18 %)	
Personality (1)		Interpersonal causes (20 %)	
Biological	*Social factors* ++++		*Spiritual/religious*
Hereditary (4)	*Biological* +++	*Biological* (4.4 %)	Spiritual (17)
Chemicals in brain (6)	*Being arrested* +++*		Taweez/jadoo (17)
Childbirth (1)	*Drug induced* +++*	*Dual explanatory models of psychosis* [combining prescribed medication and seeing a traditional faith healer as a treatment method] (77.7 %)	Supernatural (3)
Phlegm (1)			
Increased heat in the liver (1)	*For African Caribbean only. The rest are similar for both Asians and African Caribbeans		*Biological*
Spiritual/religious and cultural			
Spirits, magic, taweez, fear of Hawaii things (like ghosts) (8)			
Learning of spiritualism (2)			
Evil eye (1)			Hereditary (2)
Gods will (1)			Physical illness, e.g., fever (6)
Other causes			
Masturbation (1)			
Don't know (6)			*Don't know* (11)
			Others [THC, head injury, sleep deprivation, suspiciousness, side effect of other medicines] (22)

supervising treatment in outpatients for schizophrenia (STOPS) compared with treatment as usual (TAU). Following assessment, it was concluded that supervised treatment can play a useful role in enhancing adherence to treatment in LAMI countries. Others have tested the impact of psychoeducation on the burden of schizophrenia on the family (Nasr and Kausar 2009) and culturally adapted CBT for psychosis for inpatients (Habib et al. 2015). In India, Hegde and colleagues (2012) studied the effectiveness of cognitive retraining program in a RCT for 45 patients with first-episode schizophrenia, on neuropsychological functions, psychopathology, global functioning, psychological health, and perception of level of family distress in their caregivers. Patients and one of their caregivers were assessed at baseline, post-assessment (2 months), and follow-up assessment (6 months). The addition of home-based cognitive retraining along with TAU led to significant improvement in neuropsychological functions.

12.3.2 Development and Testing of a Brief Culturally Adapted CBT for Psychosis (CBTp) Intervention in a LAMI Country

12.3.2.1 Rationale and Background for Developing Brief CBTp

There is evidence to suggest that for nonpsychotic disorders, many cognitive behavior therapy (CBT) treatments delivered in a brief format lead to significant clinical improvement and symptom reduction, relative to other forms of psychotherapy (Bond and Dryden 2005). Various approaches have been tried to increase the efficiency of CBT treatments including adapting individual treatments to a group format and develop self-help resources, bibliotherapy, and eMedia-assisted therapy program (Hofmann et al. 2012; Hazlett-Stevens et al. 2002). The most common approach for efficiency enhancement is to make existing CBT treatments brief by reducing the number of treatment sessions.

Our group has culturally adapted CBT for psychosis both in the UK and Pakistan (Rathod et al. 2015 and Naeem et al. 2015b). In our previous work in Pakistan to culturally adapt CBT for depression, open-ended interviews were conducted by a psychiatrist trained in CBT and qualitative methods. We further developed semi-structured questionnaires that could be used by psychology graduates, thus reducing the cost and further standardizing the process of interviews (Naeem et al. 2009a, b, 2010, 2012, 2015a; Naeem and Ayub 2013). In order to do this, interview transcripts were repeatedly read from previous studies and their results. This exercise focused on the topics and the questions used in our past work and formed the basis of the semi-structured interview guide. These semi-structured interviews consisted of open-ended questions, with prompts and guidance on exploratory questions. A total of 92 interviews were conducted by 3 psychologists. We conducted qualitative interviews with mental health professionals ($n=29$), patients ($n=33$), and their carers ($n=30$). The results of the mentioned studies highlighted the barriers in therapy (e.g., lack of awareness of therapy, family's involvement, traveling distance and expenses, and uncooperative family caregivers) as well as strengths while working with this patient group. Patients and their carers in Pakistan use a bio-psycho-social-spiritual model of illness (Table 12.1). They seek help from various sources, including faith healers. Therapists make minor adjustments in therapy. Findings from these studies have been described in separate papers (Naeem et al. 2014a, b, c).

12.3.2.2 Development and Testing of CaCBTp Intervention

Adaptations were made to reflect the views of therapists and carers by our group in Pakistan. However, the major issue to be tackled was overcoming resources related barriers-finances, therapy time, transport, distance from the service facility, etc. We had numerous discussions among the group members and contacted the patients who had either received therapy or had shown an interest. Finally, the consensus was built that therapy should be time limited and brief for it to be acceptable. We therefore used a brief version of this therapy that we had culturally adapted. This therapy was provided according to a manualized treatment protocol (Kingdon and Turkington 1994) by psychology graduates with more than 5 years of experience of working in mental health, trained by an expert and supervisions. Although therapy was provided flexibly, the sessions typically focused on formulation and psycho-education; normalization and introduction to stress vulnerability model; working with delusions, hallucinations, and negative symptoms; and termination work and relapse prevention. In addition a spiritual dimension was included in formulation, understanding, and therapy plan; Urdu equivalents of CBT jargons were used in the therapy; culturally appropriate homework assignments were selected and participants were encouraged to attend even if they were unable to complete their homework; and folk stories and examples relevant to the religious beliefs of the local population were used to clarify issues. Families are heavily involved in patient's care and serve as the main caregivers to psychiatric patients in Pakistan. Also, through our experience of adaptation of CBT for Pakistan, it is understandable that their involvement can enhance the acceptability of treatment. Therefore, this brief version consisted of 6 sessions for the participant plus one session for the family/carer. During this session, a key carer was identified (acting as a co-therapist) with whom the therapist worked closely. The carer attended the sessions with the patient's consent and helped in therapy (e.g., with homework, if required).

This brief version was found to be effective in the first trial of CBT for psychosis from outside the western world. A total of 116 participants with schizophrenia were recruited to this RCT from 2 hospitals in Karachi, Pakistan. A brief version of CaCBTp was provided over 4 months. Participants in treatment group showed statistically significant improvement in all measures of psychopathology at the end of the study compared with control group (Naeem et al. 2015b). These findings, though highly encouraging, need replicating in other low- and middle-income countries.

12.3.2.3 Focus of Adaptation

The process of adapting CBT for specific groups should focus on three major areas of therapy, rather than simple translation of therapy manuals. These are related to the barriers in delivering therapy. These include:

(a) Awareness of relevant cultural issues and preparation for therapy:
  (i) *Culture and related issues* (*culture, religion, and spirituality*; *language and communication*; *family-related issues*)
  (ii) *Capacity and circumstances* (*individual issues, systems of support and treatment, and pathways to care and help-seeking behavior*)

(iii) *Cognitive errors and dysfunctional beliefs which are directly related to the problem and its treatment*

(b) Assessment and engagement

(c) Adjustments in therapy

12.4 Barriers to Psychosocial Interventions in LAMIC

There are a wide range of factors that act as barriers to any type of psychotherapeutic intervention in LAMIC.

12.4.1 Engagement Issues

Often people with psychosis struggle to engage with treatment as their predominant model of illness might be based in spiritual and religious explanations. They seek help from faith healers. If the mental health professionals are not respectful of their views, they are less likely to engage.

(a) Gender

Gender roles are widely understood to affect different social behaviors across different countries, including LAMIC. Assertiveness is often not encouraged in some diverse cultures among women which clearly has implications for treatment seeking both in initial (or prodromal) phases of psychosis and ongoing engagement in interventions in acute or chronic stages.

(b) Collectivist cultures

In collectivist cultures, the self is defined in terms of group identity and interdependence with group members (Owusu-Bemph 2002). As such, group goals have supremacy over individual goals and individuals suppress their own needs for the communal needs. The emphasis is on the group need rather than individual needs, in stark contrast to individualistic western cultures. Individuals from collectivist cultures tend to oscillate between the culture of the country of origin, culture of host country, and communal culture (Rathod and Kingdon 2009).

(c) *Guru-Chela* (*student*) versus *Socratic method of teaching*

There are wide differences between Asian and eastern clients in their views of the therapists. While CBT uses a Socratic method and is based in collaborative empiricism, the Asian model of learning is usually more like a Guru-Chela relationship. In Asian clients like sermons and didactic teaching, therefore it is not surprising that they prefer a more structured and prescriptive approach to therapy (Iwamasa 1993).

(d) *Spirituality/religion*

Spiritual development is a vital part of many different cultures (Laungani 2004). In Western countries, a clinician's ignorance or interpretation of spiritual experiences as manifestations of psychopathology and lack of confidence may result in this not being addressed. The influence of religion and spirituality remains strong in non-Western cultures despite westernization and acculturation when they immigrate (Williams et al. 2006) and, rather than a barrier, could be an asset when offering brief interventions in LAMIC. Spiritual healers may play a constructive role if collaborations are developed with them (Ramakrishnan et al. 2014).

12.4.2 Social Behaviors

Social validity (acceptability and viability of the intervention) by the community is vital in negating barriers to the effectiveness of interventions for psychosis. For many groups in LAMIC, the community trusts its network and prefers it to mainstream services initially. Reliance on word of mouth has been emphasized by members of South Asian Muslim communities and both the Pakistani and Bangladeshi participants in a study by Rathod and colleagues (2010) reported that often individuals would go to their general practitioners and request that they be prescribed the same medication as "that person" because they have been told that it works. They would also act on informal information to see a particular "faith healer" because a member of the community has recommended them. Ball and Vincent (1998) emphasized that in order for psychological interventions to be accessible and acceptable to LAMIC, individual communities would need to see the benefits that are revealed through "word of mouth" to other community members.

(a) Racism
   Racial discrimination is common in many cultures, e.g., across ethnic, caste, and tribal groups, and may affect treatment seeking and engagement in psychological treatment for psychosis. Vulnerable individuals often find it difficult to talk about this with clinicians, while clinicians may similarly avoid discussing or addressing anything that could be considered as discriminatory. Therapist should be aware of stereotypical assumptions of the groups they are working with and ensure that these are addressed so that they do not impact on therapy process.
(b) Stigma
   Stigma of mental illness affects populations across the world, leading to delays in help seeking and other difficulties with therapeutic interventions, but for LAMIC may need greater attention due to the possible likelihood of misinformation about psychosis. In LAMIC, the subject of mental illness is frequently seen as a taboo and therefore not talked about openly. Acceptance of psychosis in some LAMI countries is varied; some view people with psychosis as "spiritually" and will respect them, whereas others will stigmatize them and label them as "insane." The shame associated with stigma that mental illness brings to individuals and their immediate families adds on to the existing problem (Phiri 2012).
   Often, dealing with somatic presentations common across cultures of LAMIC (e.g., South Asian groups) is emphasized in therapy. Tsai and Chenston-Dutton

(2002) argue that somatic presentations were common among Chinese psychiatric patients. Rathod and colleagues (2010) reported that South Asian Muslim participants preferred expressing somatic complaints, as they were less embarrassing and feared being stigmatized as holding bizarre beliefs. Chinese groups share a similar belief on somatization.

12.4.3 Access and Referrals

A systemic barrier to effective treatment for psychosis in LAMIC is the issue of access to services and providers offering appropriate interventions and difficulties with the referral process. In places where investment in and resources for mental health services are scant, services may not actively seek referrals and their role may in fact include "gate keeping" due to overwhelming demand. In rural areas, geography plays a significant challenge for access to healthcare services and appropriate interventions; for instance, villagers may need to travel long distances to the city areas to seek psychological input, travel costs will impact on limited resources, and where income depends on individuals tilling the land, they may decide against traveling to the city in order to ensure other needs are met.

(a) *Referrer's perceptions*

We learned through our qualitative studies in Pakistan that psychiatrists are psychopharmacologically oriented and therefore less likely to refer their patients for psychotherapy to psychologists. They are also not convinced that the therapy works. This can be a major barrier in access to psychological therapies.

(b) *Communication and Interpreters*

The populations of LAMICs may often entail groups speaking diverse languages, meaning service users and clinicians may not hold the same first language or share any language in common at all. For example, as India is such a large country, it is very likely that there is a linguistic mismatch between the therapist and client. Language barriers account for an increase in healthcare costs (Bischoff and Denhaerynck 2010) which of course are already a significant issue in many LAMICs. Meanwhile, all clinicians are well aware that "Language is the principle investigative tool in mental health. Without it we cannot assess a patient effectively" (Farooq and Fear 2003). Therapists may vary in their degree of experience or confidence in using an interpreter (Phiri 2012). Farooq and Fear (2003) have identified key factors to consider for an appropriate interpreter which is helpful in aiming for a gold standard.

(c) *Expectations of treatment*

There may be discrepancies between the individual's or family's ultimate aims and those of the service provider. Goals for treatment that are seen as appropriate in West, such as improved quality of life, self-determination, and independence (Pinninti et al. 2005), may not be those that patients, families, and

Table 12.2 Barriers and possible solutions to psychosocial interventions in LAMIC

Barriers	Possible solutions
1. Lack of resources (trained therapists, distance from hospital, transport, etc.)	1. Developing low-cost interventions, use of technology (e.g., Skype) for supervision, etc.
2. Mistrust of services/practitioners	2. Understanding local norms
3. Worries about confidentiality/breach	3. Confidentiality has different meaning in different cultures. Therapist should be aware of these issues
4. Poor information on psychological therapies/accessibility	4. Psychoeducation is normally a major part of culturally adapted interventions
5. Language and terminology	5. Culturally sensitive language and terms, rather than literal translations
6. Fear of being stigmatized	6. Reattributing illness to a bio-psycho-social spiritual model and understanding of stigma (e.g., stigma might be due to genetic causes of illness)
7. Doubt regarding CBT being empowering enough	7. Offer tester sessions and choosing initial interventions that provide an experience of improvement.
8. Cultural incompetence or Eurocentric approach	8. Use of culturally adapted CBT manuals
9. Clinician's beliefs in the power of drugs	9. Working with medical professionals
10. Faith/spirituality and religion	10. Better understanding of these issues, as well as working together with clients' families and religious scholars
11. Gender issues	11. Trying to help family understand the cost of the illness (e.g., impact of mothers' illness on children's education)
12. Financial implication	12. Focus on low-intensity, brief, and guided self-help or self-help

clinicians would be satisfied with in LAMI countries. Thus, clinicians working in LAMIC may need to adapt the typical examples of therapeutic goals they find in the literature and evidence-based writing in order to meet the needs of those individuals they offer interventions to.

Table 12.2 gives a quick overview of the barriers as well as suggesting possible solution to overcome these barriers.

12.5   Key Skills, Clinical Approaches, and Training Implications

In considering brief intervention models for the treatment of psychosis in LAMIC, important issues for reducing barriers to access and adapting existing approaches have already been highlighted. Brief interventions may be more successful in LAMIC due to a variety of reasons, including but not limited to therapists' factors (e.g., limited number and time), patient factors (e.g., having to travel long distances to bigger cities and to return to work as there is no financial support for disability), and system factors (e.g., too many patients). Further to these, we would like to draw attention to some additional key skills for providing clinically effective therapies:

- In order to increase the social validity of brief interventions, user acceptability and satisfaction must be given priority.
- Behavioral or environmental change may offer a tangible route to prevention in either prodromal stages or when working on relapse prevention. Therefore patients, clinicians, and researchers should advocate and explore the notion that social factors play an important role in mental disorders such as psychotic phenomenon (Van Os and McGuffin 2003) and use this within brief therapies.
- Clinicians working in LAMIC face unique challenges through having limited access to relevant literature, training, and supervision/support in their practice. Initial education and ongoing professional development should be focused on ensuring that professionals are aware of those factors pertinent to cultural adaptations of brief therapies as well as to wider issues of treatment seeking and the reduction of DUP.
- Clinicians should be mindful of the importance of language in delivering interventions. For example, where issues of stigma are prominent and clients present with a focus on somatic complaints, re-labeling or reframing of organic symptoms into psychological terminology may become acceptable only as the therapeutic relationship develops.
- Barriers to seeking treatment, accepting brief interventions, and engaging fully in the therapeutic process could be reduced through new advances in development and technology – such as the use of mobile phone communication and apps. Likewise, new approaches to integrating CBT models with other approaches (e.g., family-focused therapies, motivational interviewing) could also play a role in overcoming obstacles common to populations in LAMIC
- When considering cultural adaptations, we would promote the idea of cultural sensitivity, i.e., flexible consideration of a diverse balance between numerous factors affecting definitions of culture, including religion, ethnicity, class, gender roles, socioeconomy, etc. We can now acknowledge that the way in which culture influences the course of psychosis through specific patterns and timing is complex; and much closer, on-the-ground documentation of local contingencies is required (Hopper and Wanderling 2000).
- Role of religion in psychological well-being can act as coping strategy, e.g., when an orthodox follower of a particular religion refrains from unhelpful behaviors and believes that in following God's teaching, they will go to heaven. Spirituality can enable one to strive to create a meaningful and purposeful life, thereby promoting a sense of well-being. One may maintain a personal relationship with one's deity and gain mental strength to see one through stressful periods.
- When addressing issues of religion and spirituality, consulting religious experts where appropriate can help understand how far an individual may be deviating from cultural norms and how much distress this is causing them; working with religious experts can also serve to recruit a co-therapist who may have a uniquely therapeutic relationship with the patient, relatives, and others.
- Given that culture and religion are entwined in LAMIC, use of culturally relevant explanations sensitive to the individual's beliefs, norms, and values is essential to fostering engagement.

- At the outset we would recommend that clinicians emphasize that trust will be earned and use examples of situations where the individual implies trust as leverage to engaging in a therapeutic relationship.

Conclusion

Although the epidemiological data are insufficient, there are reasons to believe that a high number of individuals in LAMIC are affected by psychotic disorders. There are also reasons to believe that the outcomes are not as positive as we once believed. Treatment strategies are at a very preliminary stage, with a focus on psycho pharmacological interventions. It is therefore not surprising that psychosocial interventions are not often reported from LAMIC. There is an underlying assumption that psychosocial interventions need to be culturally adapted for use in non-western cultures. There are significant barriers in providing psychosocial interventions in LMIC. The most notable of these barriers include time, distance, and resources. The limited work so far highlights many barriers to promote psychosocial interventions for this population and one way these might be overcome is by developing brief interventions for psychosis for these countries.

References

Adams CE, Tharyan P, Coutinho ES, Stroup TS (2006) The schizophrenia drug-treatment paradox: pharmacological treatment based on best possible evidence may be hardest to practice in high-income countries. Br J Psychiatry 189(5):391–392

Awan NR (2015) Explanatory model of illness of patients with schizophrenia and the role of educational intervention. Shaheed Benazir Bhutto Women University Peshawar, Peshawar

Ball SJ, Vincent C (1998) I heard it on the grapevine: hot knowledge and school choice. Br J Sociol Educ 19(3):377–400

Bhikha AG, Farooq S, Chaudhry N, Husain N (2012) A systematic review of explanatory models of illness for psychosis in developing countries. Int Rev Psychiatry 24(5):450–462. doi:10.310 9/09540261.2012.711746

Bhugra D (2005) The global prevalence of schizophrenia. PLoS Med 2(5):e151–e152

Bischoff A, Denhaerynck K (2010) What do language barriers cost? An exploratory study among asylum seekers in Switzerland. BMC Health Serv Res 10(1):248–254

Bond FW, Dryden W (2005) Handbook of brief cognitive behaviour therapy. Wiley, Chichester

Farooq S, Fear C (2003) Working through interpreters. Adv Psychiatr Treat 9:104–109

Farooq S, Large M, Nielsson O, Waheed W (2009) The relationship between the duration of untreated psychosis and outcome in low-and-middle income countries: a systematic review and meta analysis. Schizophr Res 109(1-3):15–23

Farooq S, Nazar Z, Irfan M, Akhter J, Gul E, Irfan U, Naeem F (2011) Schizophrenia medication adherence in a resource-poor setting: randomised controlled trial of supervised treatment in out-patients for schizophrenia (STOPS). Br J Psychiatry 199(6):467–472. doi:10.1192/bjp.bp.110.085340

Habib N, Dawood S, Kingdon D, Naeem F (2015) Preliminary evaluation of culturally adapted CBT for psychosis (CA-CBTp): findings from developing culturally-sensitive CBT project (DCCP). Behav Cogn Psychother 43(2):1–9

Harrison G, Hopper K, Craig T, Laska E, Siegel C, Wanderling J, Wiersma D (2001) Recovery from psychotic illness: a 15-and 25-year international follow-up study. Br J Psychiatry 178(6):506–517

Hazlett-Stevens H, Craske MG, Roy-Byrne PP, Sherbourne CD, Stein MB, Bystritsky A (2002) Predictors of willingness to consider medication and psychosocial treatment for panic disorder in primary care patients. Gen Hosp Psychiatry 24(5):316–321

Hegde S, Rao SL, Raguram A, Gangadhar BN (2012) Addition of home-based cognitive retraining to treatment as usual in first episode schizophrenia patients: a randomized controlled study. Indian J Psychiatry 54(1):15–22

Hofmann SG, Asnaani A, Vonk IJJ, Sawyer AT, Fang A (2012) The efficacy of cognitive behavioral therapy: a review of meta-analyses. Cogn Ther Res 36(5):427–440

Hopper K, Wanderling J (2000) Revisiting the developed versus developing country distinction in course and outcome in schizophrenia: results from ISoS, the WHO collaborative followup project. Schizophr Bull 26(4):835–846

Isaac M, Chand P, Murthy P (2007) Schizophrenia outcome measures in the wider international community. Br J Psychiatry 191(50):71–77

Iwamasa GY (1993) Asian Americans and cognitive behaviour therapy. Behav Ther 16:233–235

Jablensky A (2000) Epidemiology of schizophrenia: the global burden of disease and disability. Eur Arch Psychiatry Clin Neurosci 250(6):274–285

Jablensky A, McGrath J, Herrman H, Castle D, Gureje O, Evans M et al (2000) Psychotic disorders in urban areas: an overview of the study on low prevalence disorders. Aust N Z J Psychiatry 34:221–236

Joel D, Sathyaseelan M, Jayakaran R, Vijayakumar C, Muthurathnam S, Jacob KS (2003) Explanatory models of psychosis among community health workers in South India. Acta Psychiatr Scand 108(1):66–69

Kingdon D, Turkington D (1994) Cognitive behavioral therapy of schizophrenia. Lawrence Erlbaum Associates, Hove

Kohn R, Saxena S, Levav I, Saraceno B (2004) The treatment gap in mental health care. Bull World Health Organ 82(11):858–866

Kulhara P, Chakrabarti S (2001) Culture and schizophrenia and other psychotic disorders. Psychiatr Clin N Am 24(3):449–464

Lancet Global Mental Health Group (2007) Scale up services for mental disorders: a call for action. Lancet 370(9594):1241–1252

Large M, Farooq S, Nielssen O, Slade T (2008) Relationship between gross domestic product and duration of untreated psychosis in low-and middle-income countries. Br J Psychiatry 193(4):272–278

Laungani P (2004) Asian perspectives in counselling and psychotherapy. Brunner-Routledge, New York

Leff J, Sartorius N, Jablensky A, Korten A, Ernberg G (1992) The international pilot study of schizophrenia: five-year follow-up findings. Psychol Med 22(01):131–145

Mahy GE, Mallett R, Leff J, Bhugra D (1999) First-contact incidence rate of schizophrenia on Barbados. Br J Psychiatry 175(1):28–33

Menezes PR, Scazufca M, Busatto GF, Coutinho LM, Mcguire PK, Murray RM (2007) Incidence of first-contact psychosis in So Paulo, Brazil. Br J Psychiatry 191(51):102–106

Naeem F, Ayub M (2013) Culturally adapted CBT (CaCBT) for depression, Therapy manual for use with South Asian Muslims. Pakistan Association of Cognitive Therapists, Pakistan (Kindle Ed).

Naeem F, Gobbi M, Ayub M, Kingdon D (2009a) University students' views about compatibility of cognitive behaviour therapy (CBT) with their personal, social and religious values (a study from Pakistan). Ment Health Rel Cult 12(8):847–855. doi:10.1080/13674670903115226

Naeem F, Ayub M, Gobbi M, Kingdon D (2009b) Development of Southampton adaptation framework for CBT (SAF-CBT): a framework for adaptation of CBT in non-western culture. J Pak Psychiatr Soc 6(2):79–84

Naeem F, Gobbi M, Ayub M, Kingdon D (2010) Psychologists experience of cognitive behaviour therapy in a developing country: a qualitative study from Pakistan. Int J Ment Heal Syst 4(2):1–9

Naeem F, Ayub M, Kingdon D, Gobbi M (2012) Views of depressed patients in Pakistan concerning theirillness,itscausesandtreatments.QualHealthRes22:1083–1093.doi:10.1177/1049732312450212

Naeem F, Sarhandi I, Gul M, Khalid M, Aslam M, Anbrin A, Saeed S, Noor M, Fatima G, Minhas F, Husain N, Ayub M (2014a) A multicentre randomised controlled trial of a carer supervised culturally adapted CBT (CaCBT) based self-help for depression in Pakistan. J Affect Disord 156:224–227. doi:10.1016/j.jad.2013.10.051

Naeem F, Farooq S, Kingdon D (2014b) Cognitive behavioural therapy (brief versus standard duration) for schizophrenia. Cochrane Database Syst Rev 4:CD010646, http://dx.doi.org/10.1002/14651858.CD010646.pub2

Naeem F, Habib N, Gul M, Khalid M, Saeed S, Farooq S, Munshi T, Gobbi M, Husain N, Ayub M, Kingdon D (2014c) A qualitative study to explore patients', carers' and health professionals' views to culturally adapt CBT for psychosis (CBTp) in Pakistan. Behav Cogn Psychother 2:1–13, http://dx.doi.org/10.1017/S1352465814000332

Naeem F, Gul M, Irfan M, Munshi T, Asif A, Rashid S et al (2015a) Brief culturally adapted CBT(CaCBT) for depression: a randomized controlled trial from Pakistan. J Affect Disord 177:101–107

Naeem F, Saeed S, Irfan M, Kiran T, Mehmood N, Gul M et al (2015b) Brief culturally adapted CBT for psychosis (CaCBTp): a randomized controlled trial from a low income country. Schizophr Res 164(1-3):143–148

Nasr T, Kausar R (2009) Psycho education and the family burden in schizophrenia: a randomized controlled trial. Ann Gen Psychiatry 8(17):1–6

National Collaborating Centre for Mental Health UK (2014) Psychosis and schizophrenia in adults: treatment and management. National Clin Guidel 178, http://www.nice.org.uk/guidance/cg178

Owusu-Bempah K (2002) Culture, self and cross-ethnic therapy. In: Mason B, Sawyer A (eds) Exploring the unsaid: creativity, risks and dilemmas in working cross-culturally. Karnac, London

Pakistan Demographic Profile 2014, (2015, Nov 10). Retrieved from http://www.indexmundi.com/pakistan/demographics_profile.html

Patel V, Cohen A, Thara R, Gureje O (2006) Is the outcome of schizophrenia really better in developing countries? Rev Bras Psiquiatr 28(2):149–152

Phiri P (2012) Adapting cognitive behaviour therapy for psychosis for black and minority ethnic communities. University of Southampton, Southampton

Pinninti NR, Stolar N, Scott T (2005) 5-minute first aid for psychosis. Defuse crises; help patients solve problems with brief cognitive therapy. Curr Psychiatry 4:36–48

Ramakrishnan P, Rane A, Dias A, Bhat J, Shukla A, Lakshmi S et al (2014) Indian health care professionals' attitude towards spiritual healing and its role in alleviating stigma of psychiatric services. J Relig Health 53(6):1800–1814

Rathod S, Kingdon D (2009) Cognitive behaviour therapy across cultures. Psychiatry 8(9):370–371

Rathod S, Kingdon D, Pinninti N, Turkington D, Phiri P (2015) Cultural adaptation of CBT for serious mental illness: a guide for training and practice. Wiley-Blackwell, Chichester

Rathod S, Kingdon D, Phiri P, Gobbi M (2010) Developing culturally sensitive cognitive behaviour therapy for psychosis for ethnic minority groups by exploration and incorporation of Service User's and Health Professionals views and opinions. Behav Cogn Psychother 38(5):511–533

Saha S, Chant D, Welham J, Mcgrath J (2005) A systematic review of the prevalence of schizophrenia. PLoS Med 2(5):e141–e161

Saravanan B, Jacob KS, Johnson S, Prince M, Bhugra D, David AS (2007) Belief models in first episode schizophrenia in *World Psychiatry* South India. Soc Psychiatry Psychiatr Epidemiol 42(6):446–451

Stone L, Warren F (2011) Cognitive behaviour therapy training in a developing country: a pilot study in Tanzania. Cogn Behav Ther 4(4):139–151

Tsai JL, Chentsova-Dutton Y (2002) Understanding depression across cultures. In: Gotlib IH, Hammen CL (eds) Handbook of depression. Guildford, New York, pp 467–491

van Os J, McGuffin P (2003) Can the social environment cause schizophrenia? Br J Psychiatry 182:291–292

Williams PE, Turpin G, Hardy G (2006) Clinical psychology service provision and ethnic diversity within the UK: a review of the literature. Clin Psychol Psychother 13:324–338

World Health Organization (1976) Schizophrenia. An international follow-up study. Wiley, New York

World Health Organization. Mental Health Atlas (2011) Available from URL: http://www.who.int/mental_health/evidence/atlas/profiles/en/

Policy Implications in Psychosis

13

Narsimha R. Pinninti and Shanaya Rathod

In this book, we have thus far reviewed the current effective psychosocial interventions for psychosis adapted for a brief format at an individual or microlevel. The overarching theme has been providing these effective interventions within the context of constant resource constraints and imperfect systems of care. Interventions at the microlevel are dependent on the agenda set by macrolevel policies, priorities, and practices. In this chapter, we describe the scenarios at a macrolevel, looking at systems of care; we examine the current limitations in the systems of care and suggest steps to address these limitations. We do recognize that the health-care systems of the USA, most European countries, and low- and middle-income countries (LAMI) differ significantly but share the same common goals of providing effective evidence-based interventions for most people in the most efficient way. The discussion will be initially global and relevant for all systems followed by more specific discussion about the different systems.

13.1 History of Services for Psychosis

Individuals with psychosis and their families need access to effective comprehensive biopsychosocial interventions and ongoing monitoring aimed at achieving recovery. The health systems and/or commissioners of mental health services require information on the effectiveness of various interventions that allow them to

N.R. Pinninti, MD (✉)
Department of Psychiatry, Rowan University SOM,
Suite 100, 2250 Chapel Avenue East, Cherry Hill, NJ 08034, USA
e-mail: Narsimha.Pinninti@twinoakscs.org; narsimhanrp@gmail.com

S. Rathod, MD
Antelope House, Southern Health NHS Foundation Trust,
Southampton, SO14 0YG, UK
e-mail: Shanaya.rathod@southernhealth.nhs.uk; shanayarathod@nhs.net

© Springer International Publishing Switzerland 2016
B. Pradhan et al. (eds.), *Brief Interventions for Psychosis:*
A Clinical Compendium, DOI 10.1007/978-3-319-30521-9_13

make meaningful decisions to allocate limited available resources. Historically, mental health systems have taken a custodial role focused on protecting the society from the burden of dealing with seriously mentally ill while those with minor problems were not serviced. They did this by seperating those who were dangerous and or disruptive to the families, seperating them from society by institutionalizing them (Chow and Priebe 2013). From the 1950s onward, there has been a shift in the provision of care, with the locus of care of mentally ill moving from institutions to communities. For example, in the USA, in 1955, the number of persons in state hospitals reached its peak at 339 per 100,000, while in 1998, the inpatient census declined to 21 per 100,000 on any given day (Lamb and Bachrach 2001). The deinstitutionalization of individuals with serious mental illness was driven by four factors: public revelations regarding the state of public mental hospitals, the introduction of antipsychotic medications, the introduction of federal programs to fund patients who had been discharged, and civil libertarian lawyers. Unfortunately, this has resulted in approximately 3.2 million individuals with untreated serious mental illness living in the community (Fuller Torrey 2015). In addition, many individuals ended up either homeless or in prisons. According to a report published by Fuller Torrey, there are ten times as many individuals with mental illnesses in jails and prisons as they are in psychiatric beds (Rubinow 2014). Until very recently, the expectations for individuals with psychosis were low and focused on symptom control and preventing hospitalization, while recovery, improvement in functioning (Zipursky et al. 2013) and reintegration into community a priority.

The introduction of various psychotropic medications since the 1950s gradually moved the focus of psychosis from a biopsychosocial perspective to one of biological reductionism. The discovery of various antipsychotic agents starting with chlorpromazine in 1952 created a sense of optimism and excitement that psychotic disorders could be understood on biological basis and that medications would be found that would resolve the disorders. The aggressive marketing of medication as a solution to psychotic disorders by profit pharmaceutical industry and the nexus of relationship between academic psychiatry and the industry provided strength to the narrative that a single biological solution will be found for treatment of psychotic disorders. However, that expectation and hope that we would find a biological cause and treatment for psychotic disorders including schizophrenia is unrealized. For a long time, psychotropic medication was considered critical and mainstay in the treatment of psychotic disorders. However, we are more aware of the significant limitations of psychotropic medications including their limited efficacy and risk for side effects. Medications are effective in reducing acute symptoms and reducing the likelihood of relapses. Also, medications are only partially effective in reducing positive psychotic symptoms, are relatively ineffective in negative and cognitive symptoms, and are associated with significant side effect burden and high rate of nonadherence (Leucht et al. 2013; Ragins 2005, 2012; Waterreus et al. 2012). There is evidence that long-term use of antipsychotic medication may impede recovery and evidence that less medication sometimes is better (Mosher and Bola 2013).

A variety of factors in the past two decades have led to a focus on recovery for psychotic disorders as a realistic goal and expectation. In the USA, recovery as a desirable and attainable goal for all mentally ill was enunciated as a policy statement by US government for the first time in 2003 (health 2003). The NHS (national health services) in the UK incorporated recovery-oriented thinking into their service models before the USA. There is strong evidence that significant social stress due to environmental risk factors such as migration, social marginalization, urbanity, childhood trauma, social defeat, and other adverse experiences increases the risk of psychosis (Mizrahi 2015), and medication alone is inadequate to address the vulnerabilities from these factors. In the USA, an empowerment model of dealing with psychosis is proposed that focuses on instillation of hope, exposure to recovered individuals who act as role models, developing the person's internal resources, and strengthening the social supports while relegating the role of medication to that of a tool that is needed for periods of time and not necessarily indefinitely. Similar treatment approaches that specifically aim to minimize the use of medication such as open dialog are showing better social and vocational outcomes, thereby questioning our basic paradigm that medication is critical part of treatment (Seikkula and Olson 2003). Better outcome in rural areas of low- and middle-income countries (LMIC) is an established observation and is thought to be due to supportive systems that are available for individuals with psychosis. A closer look at these studies also shows that individuals had less exposure to traditional treatments, and this may in part explain the results of better symptomatic and vocational outcomes (Yang et al. 2013).

Societal attitudes toward psychosis and the available treatments determine engagement with services. For many years, while the illness model was reported as the prevalent one for psychosis, in different countries including the UK (Furnham and Bower 1992), Germany (Angermeyer and Matschinger 1999), India (Srinivasan and Thara 2001), Mongolia, and Russia (Dietrich et al. 2004), the funding for research in psychosocial interventions was neglected. Consequently, we have systems of care that are not designed to provide effective psychosocial interventions for individuals with psychosis. The efficacy and effectiveness of various psychosocial interventions for treatment of psychotic disorders is well established for some interventions including cognitive behavior therapy (Wykes et al.2008), vocational rehabilitation (Mueser and McGurk 2014), family interventions (Mueser et al. 2013), and motivational interviewing (Bradley et al. 2007), and it is promising for psychodynamic therapy (Brus et al. 2012) and avatar therapy (Leff et al. 2013). There are some innovative and merging treatments such as Yoga mindfulness based cognitive therapy (YMBCT) described in chapter five.

13.2   Current Status of Services for Psychosis

There are two main issues to address when discussing psychosocial interventions for individuals with psychotic disorders. First one is that care delivered in routine settings does not include evidence-based psychosocial interventions in any consistent or coherent manner. This gap between what is known to be effective and the actual delivery of care is due to problems of access, limited resources and training, insurance coverage, fragmentation of care and financial responsibility, and the lack of requirement that evidence-based interventions be provided as part of routine care.

There is no standard system in place to ensure that the psychosocial interventions delivered to patients/consumers are adequately reviewed and effective (IOM 2015). A second major drawback in incorporating psychosocial treatments in routine settings is the lack of a knowledge and coherent methodology to incorporate them in the care of an individual appropriate to their level of symptoms and stage of illness. Also, there are no clear guidelines on whether the various interventions should be delivered simultaneously or successively, the dosage of various interventions, and how the various interventions fit together. It is known that recovery from psychosis is an active process, and no single psychosocial intervention alone addresses the unique strengths, weaknesses, aspirations, and goals of the individual and helps them to create a personal narrative about their past and a plan for the future. Hence, some authors recommend integrative psychotherapy as the way forward to address the different needs of individuals with psychosis (Lysaker and Roe 2015). The elements of integrative psychotherapy are an active role in the process played by the client, the therapist showing vulnerability in terms of not having all knowledge and understanding and along with the client cocreating a personal narrative to explain the illness, its impact on their life, and a future actionable plan. The concept of integrative psychosocial interventions is still emerging, and much work needs to be done in this area.

13.3 Global View

Effective mental health services are based on financing, organizational, and delivery systems that work seamlessly and are driven by a coherent policy with clearly laid-out priorities. In a world where medicine is forever progressing and the needs and expectations of the people serviced are evolving, the interplay between the three critical systems is dynamic and should be constantly evaluated to provide optimal services for the population the system serves. Financing is first and the most critical element in provision of mental health services and probably remains the single-most important factor in determining the nature and type of interventions provided for people with psychotic disorders. Health-care spending varies very widely in different countries with the USA spending about 17.2 % of GDP on health in 2012 (Centers for Medicare and Medicaid Services 2012); in the UK, total health-care expenditure accounted for 8.8 % of GDP in 2013 (ONS 2013). The total health-care expenditure as a percentage of GDP in the UK rose sharply between 2008 and 2009, but has decreased since 2009. Compared to these figures, a middle-income country such as India spends 4.6 % on health. In India, neuropsychiatric problems are estimated to contribute to 11.8 % of global burden of disease, but the funding for mental health is 0.06 % of the health-care budget (http://www.who.int/mental_health/evidence/atlas/profiles/ind_mh_profile.pdf). Cost is a significant barrier to access in health care with duration of untreated psychosis in low- and middle-income countries (LAMI) being twice as long as high-income countries (Large et al. 2008). Usually, longer duration of untreated psychosis is associated with poor outcomes, and contrary to the expectation, outcomes for these disorders are better in LAMI countries per two prior WHO studies (Jablensky et al. 1992).

Mental illness is the second leading cause of disability and premature mortality internationally (Newcomer and Hennekens 2007). In the USA, severe mental illnesses (SMIs) collectively account for more than 15 % of the overall burden of disease from all causes (Kessler et al. 2005). Despite this high degree of prevalence, mental health disorders are not treated as equal to the physical health disorders. The problem is compounded by new advances in the treatments of various physical disorders that increase the expenses for treating these disorders and limit the funding available for mental disorders even further. Second element of mental health funding is tied into the organizational and delivery systems. In the USA, health-care dollars are distributed by the federal government, but many health-care service decisions are made at the level of the state. As a result, there is a wide variation in the planning, organization, and delivery of mental health services (NAMI 2009). Similarly, variations are seen in the UK due to the fragmented commissioning provider interface with a reduction in mental health funding and increasing demand due to the impact of the economic downturn on employment, housing, etc. (Rathod 2015).

Next to funding, organizational and delivery systems are nearly as important in providing good care, and they will be discussed together. Health systems across the world remain significantly fragmented, affecting access, quality, and costs of the care delivered. Strengthening health systems is a global health challenge for all countries, and these issues are addressed very differently by different countries as discussed below.

13.4   Scenario in the USA

The problems in US mental health fall into fiscal and organizational categories. The USA spends a very small percent (5.6 % of the health budget on mental health needs), and there is a shortage of qualified personnel to provide a vast array of necessary services except in few urban and suburban areas (Weil 2015). The state has responsibility for health of the population, but a significant proportion of the cost for health care comes from the federal government, and it comes with strings attached. As a result, the state governments decide the extent they want to take the federal dollars, and hence there is a wide variation in the nature, type, and extent of services provided for the mentally ill. The NAMI (National Alliance for Mentally Ill) reviewed the services provided in all 50 states in the USA and graded them based on four categories: health promotion and measurement, financing and core treatment and recovery services, consumer and family empowerment, and community integration and social inclusion. None of the states got an A grade and only 6 got a B, while 18 got C, 21 D, and 6 an F showing the wide disparity that exists between states in the provision of mental health services (NAMI 2009). Delving a little deeper into the grades, most parts of the country, it is well recognized that we do not have a coherent system of care but a number of fragmented ineffective services that are rejected by most individuals with schizophrenia. As a result, 95 % of individuals with schizophrenia (psychotic disorders) do not receive the appropriate range of EB services (Drake and Essock 2009). The challenge in trying to improve a system where 50 states individually control how the mental health services are organized and delivered is enormous. However, there is hope and expectation that two recent laws, Mental Health Parity and Addiction Equity Act of 2008 and the Patient Protection and Affordable Care Act of 2010 (ACA), will significantly expand access to high-quality interventions for mental health/substance use disorders. In anticipation of that, the Institute of Medicine produced a report addressing the role of psychosocial interventions in the treatment of mental health disorders with recommendations to strengthen the evidence base for psychosocial interventions and establish methods for successfully implementing and sustaining these interventions in regular practice, including the training of workforce. The bedrock of this entire process is consumer perspective (IOM 2015). The three pillars of health-care delivery are access, quality, and cost, and usually there can be a change in one to bring about improvements in the entire system. ACA promised to improve both access and quality, and that is a tall undertaking and would lead to increases in cost. In order to make it politically acceptable, the federal government promised that the ACA would improve access and quality without increase in cost. The reality is that health-care costs are rising and expected to do so placing a tremendous burden on existing systems (Gabel et al. 2015).

13.5   Scenarios in the UK and Europe

Over the course of the last half century, across UK, Europe, and Australasia, as well as the USA, the focus of care of severely mentally ill has moved from hospitals to community. In the UK, there has been a steady reduction from a maximum of 155,000 beds in 1954 to 27,000 in 2008 (Tyrer 2011). Services have seen a fragmentation of care with the introduction of the functional model. This has meant different teams looking after the person in different phases of illness, thereby compromising continuity of care during acute phases, crisis and rehabilitation, and recovery phases. And above all, there is a marked disparity between the level of funding for mental health services and the impact that mental health problems have at a population level, and there has been a notable reduction in funding to NHS since 2010/2011 (Kingsfund 2015). Then, compared to the funding schemes for physical health conditions by "payment by results" scheme, the differential deflator on block contracts for mental health has confounded the problem institutionalizing the perennial vulnerability of mental health budgets to being raided (NHS Providers 2015) by physical health conditions and organizations. Therefore, mental health organizations are struggling to balance the quality versus financial agenda that is impacting on care people receive from services.

As discussed in Chap. 2, early intervention in psychosis services was set up with additional funding across the UK, Europe, and Australia in the early 2000s, but a recent survey of 96 of the 125 early intervention in psychosis services in the UK found that 53 % reported a decrease in the quality of their services in the past year, and 58 % of early intervention in psychosis services had lost staff in the previous year (Rethink Mental Illness 2014).

Political commitment to achieving parity of esteem between mental and physical health services by 2020 promises additional funding for the access and waiting time standards, but whether it can deliver is yet to be seen as funding is not ring fenced, and secondly, reporting to targets does not necessarily change the quality of patient care. There is insufficient staff numbers and limited skill mix in provider organizations, and no service currently has the capacity to deliver NICE-concordant services to more than 50 % of new first-episode cases by 2016 (Khan and Brabham 2015).

Yet better access and delivery of mental health care could have an impact across the system. As discussed in detail in Chap. 2, an integrated care pathway called TRIumPH (Treatment and Recovery In PsycHosis) – which prescribes time frames around access and clinical interventions – has been developed and evaluated in the UK (Rathod et al. 2015) for the first time in mental health. The work has used a similar approach to that taken to improve stroke care, where there has been a demonstrable improvement in outcomes for patients and carers. This approach aims to achieve a culture change and social movement in the care of psychosis.

13.6   Scenarios in the Low- and Middle-Income (LAMI) Countries

The low- and middle-income countries face very different kind of challenges when dealing with mental illnesses in general and psychosis in particular. India is taken as an example of LAMI country and the issues in India reflect those that similar other LAMI countries face. The challenges facing mental health services in India are financial and organizational. India has a federal government with its budget and individual states have their own budgets. The federal budget allocated 4.6 % of the GDP for health which works out to per capita paltry sum of ($ 0.22). The lack of funding is compounded by low priority afforded to mental health as evidenced by 0.06 % of the general health budget being spent on mental health. Mental health services are integrated into primary health services with support and supervision from a mental health team at the district level. However, not all districts are covered under this program, and many primary health-care physicians have not received any training in mental health issues for over 5 years. Referral services are available for individuals who cannot be treated at the primary care physician level, and the referral is to mental health outpatient facilities, psychiatric wings of general hospitals, or the dedicated psychiatric facilities. There is an acute shortage of mental health personnel in India wherein, for example, for 100,000 populations we have 0.3 % psychiatrists, 0.04 % psychologists, and 0.03 social workers. While the mental health resources are limited, on the positive side, the family support systems are fairly strong particularly in rural areas. As a general rule, mentally ill live with their families. In addition, the larger community is more open and accepting of individuals with psychosis, and systemically there are vocational opportunities for these individuals. In the affluent countries, the user and family groups are very well organized and a strong force. They influence public and government debate and policy about mental illness. National Alliance for Mentally Ill (NAMI) has influenced public debate on mental illness, fought for parity in mental health coverage that eventually led to a legislative action and has also supported research into mental illness by fund raising and providing grants for innovative treatments. As opposed to this, the family and user associations are present in LAMI countries but are not strong and do not participate in the development of policy and procedures. Community-based rehabilitation is a feasible and acceptable intervention with a beneficial impact on disability for the majority of people with psychotic disorders in **low**-resource settings. The impact on disability is influenced by a combination of clinical, program and social determinants. In this study of community-based rehab, lower baseline disability scores, family engagement with the program, medication adherence, and being a member of a self-help group were independent determinants of good outcomes (Chatterjee et al. 2009).

13.7   Recommendations to Improve Current Systems of Care

Recommendations to improve existing systems of care can be discussed under the following headings.

13.7.1 Government Policy and Priorities

Mental health has to be afforded the same importance as physical health when planning and delivering services, but this parity does not occur even in high-income countries. In the USA, after decades of inequity, the Mental Health Parity and Addiction Equity (MHPAE) Act (P.L. 110–343) was passed into law in 2008 that aimed to create "parity" by eliminating historical differences in group health insurance coverage for mental health and substance abuse (MH/SA) benefits and medical/surgical benefits (Barry et al. 2010). Funding is primarily provided for treatment of diseases, and rehabilitative work is not paid adequate attention. In psychotic disorder, significant support for rehabilitative work is essential to help individuals regain lost life roles. One such important area is competitive work environment. Current disability policies support people with disabilities but also impose major constraints. Critics argue that the policies often lead to lifelong poverty and dependency and are antithetical to the values expressed in the Americans with Disabilities Act (ADA). The majority of beneficiaries live below the federal poverty level, and very few (less than 1 % of people with disabilities on SSI or SSDI each year) leave the programs for reasons other than aging out or death. There are strong disincentives to return to work including risk of losing health insurance, becoming psychologically disabled by the often lengthy process of applying for and receiving benefits, unrealistic income replacement formulas (a person loses too much income support immediately upon return to work), and inability to understand the complicated regulations (Drake et al. 2009). With current evidence of the effectiveness of supported employment programs, the government policies have to catch up to help individuals to get into competitive work environment.

In the UK, the Health and Social Care Act 2012 created a new legal responsibility for the NHS to deliver "parity of esteem" between mental and physical health, and the government has pledged to achieve this by 2020. Parity of esteem involves ensuring that there is as much focus on improving mental as physical health and that people with mental health problems receive an equal standard of care (Ref). According to King's fund report, there have been specific steps taken, but the challenges to provide equal standard of care for both mental health and physical health are enormous and require ongoing commitment from the government (http://www.kingsfund.org.uk/projects/verdict/has-government-put-mental-health-equal-footing-physical-health).

In LAMI countries with low budgets for health and multiple seemingly urgent priorities such as infectious diseases and high maternal and infant mortality, it is not realistic to expect mental health parity in near future. However, instead, there can be increased education and awareness of mental health issues and to find ways to integrate mental health into existing system of care delivery. Many LAMI countries do not have adequate outpatient services as focus is on providing inpatient care. However, this is being addressed, and in a survey of 36 countries, 90 % of LAMI countries' mental health plans included a goal of developing community services (Saxena et al. 2011). In addition to the funding, government policies should address existing stigma against mental illness instead of inadvertently causing stigma. One area the government policies can address stigma is addressing structural stigma. There are structural stigmas built into policy and procedures of individual countries. A 1999 survey of state laws in the USA revealed that 44 states imposed some restrictions on the rights of mentally ill individuals to serve on a jury, 37 imposed restrictions on their voting, 23 imposed restrictions on their holding elective office, and 27 imposed restrictions on their parental rights (Hemmens et al. 2002).

13.7.2 Organization of Services

According to clients, in an ideal health-care system, appropriate and timely health-care access is of paramount importance. Continuity and coordinated care, patient-centered care, and affordability were equally the second most important health-care priorities (Sav et al. 2015). For individuals with psychosis, it is important to provide access to evaluation and educational services at the earliest point in the development of psychotic experiences. As mentioned in Chap. 2, most psychotic experiences are transient and do not adversely impact the functioning of the individual. This fact is not well known in health-care provider community let alone the general public who view all psychotic experiences are pathological requiring treatment. Conceptualization of psychotic experiences as pathological medicalizes these symptoms, increases stigma, adds to the stress level, and reduces the possibility of recovery. The community should be educated that psychotic expereinces are benign and self limiting in a majority of cases (Jonas and Markon 2013). There cannot be more effective antidote for stigma than the recognition that psychotic experiences are common and do not mean that a person is "mentally ill or crazy." It is sometimes very difficult to distinguish spiritually evolved individuals from those with diagnosis of schizophrenia (Bhargav et al. 2015). The education can be at the community level or individual level, and the primary care setting is the best place to engage and educate clients with psychosis at an individual level. Gunn and Blount et al. in a recent review found that primary care providers are probably the number one gateway for mental health services as evidenced by the following: (a) primary care providers prescribe 60–70 % of psychotropic medications in the USA; (b) 45 % of individuals who commit suicide had contact with a primary care provider; and (c) "68 % of patients with diagnosable mental health conditions will seek care from a primary care medical professional" (p. 236). It offers a significant opportunity to screen, engage, and address the needs of individuals with psychotic experiences (Gunn and Blount 2009). In addition to the primary care, individual who deal with mentally ill can facilitate engagement in traditional mental health services by being open to the alternate, complimentary, and spiritual interventions that many clients from LAMI countries engage with. In a study, a quarter of allopaths (24.4 %) and 38 % of traditional and complementary medicine (TCAM) physicians reportedly cross-refer their grieving patients to religious/TCAM healer and *psychiatrist*/psychologist, respectively (Ramakrishnan et al. 2014).

There should be a paradigm shift in conceptualization and provision of services for individuals with psychotic disorders. This shift should look at the entire process of psychosis from the earliest experience to complete recovery and plan services across the entire spectrum of psychosis and the life span of an individual. Services should be client centered, integrated, and involve the client's universe of social support and should help in the pursuit of three aims: improving the experience of health care, improving the health of populations, and reducing per capita costs of health care. The portal of providing this type of care can vary depending on the country and their existing systems of care. In the USA that is undergoing transformational changes due to the affordable care act, the primary care medical homes serve this purpose. The PCMHs (primary care medical homes) in Affordable Care Act are the local systems to deliver efficient, cost-effective, and quality health-care services (Orszag and Emanuel 2010). The ACA is expected to move the provision of US health care from its current episodic, fragmented, and problem-oriented type to longitudinal care that is integrated and promoting health and wellness in a proactive manner. In addition to this, the initiative from National Institute of Mental Health to evaluate psychosocial interventions for psychotic disorders is further discussed under the research section.

The UK is making changes to the NHS to provide more equitable coverage for mental health. An example of a shift in organization of services is the ImROC (Implementing Recovery through Organizational Change) program. The ImROC program was launched by the Secretary of State for Health in England in April 2010 and described in detail in Chap. 10 and hence not covered here. LAMI countries offer a different challenge in terms of organization of services. In a study of over 36 LAMI countries, mental health services were predominantly provided in inpatient setting with less than one community contact (0.70) per inpatient day. Hospitals consumed 80 % of the mental health budget and outpatient services were extremely limited (Saxena et al. 2011). Enhancing the capacity of outpatient services within the limitations of budget is mentioned as a priority by these countries. One way to do this is to understand the social context of the particular country and attempt to integrate the services into the health care and social service fabric. In a randomized controlled trial of 282 patients, community-based collaborative care with psychiatric facility as a backup was found to be modestly more effective in reducing the symptoms and disability from psychosis compared to the facility-based care. This positive effect for community-based collaborative care model was more pronounced in rural areas (Chatterjee et al. 2014). Individuals are likely to do well when the communities of which they are a part accept them and provide opportunities to be meaningfully engaged. In a study of 393 individuals with psychosis in China, those in rural areas were three times more likely to be employed and also did better symptomatically. The authors conclude that social and contextual factors promote accommodations for work and allow individuals to thrive in low-skilled and low-stress jobs (Yang et al. 2013). In a survey, 90 % of LAMI countries' mental health plans included a goal of developing community services (Saxena et al. 2011).

13.7.3 Workforce Issues: Training and Development

As mentioned earlier in the chapter, limited workforce remains a significant barrier in providing psychosocial interventions for individuals with psychosis, and there is recognition that the situation is not likely to improve. On the other hand, there is evidence to suggest that psychosocial interventions would allow targeted postponement of antipsychotic medication, and the outcomes are better than with early medication management (Bola et al. 2009). However, psychosocial interventions are labor intensive, and training staff in the various treatments and helping them maintain their skill set remain a significant barrier in widespread uptake and delivery of these services. The challenges of training adequate workforce are compounded by limited resources available to hire, train, and retain staff (Clark and Samnaliev 2005). As a result, medication management becomes the mainstay of treatment, and evidence-based psychosocial interventions have been unavailable for most individuals with psychosis (Ben-Zeev et al. 2015; Drake and Essock 2009). There are several ways in which the issue of qualified workforce shortage can be addressed and detailed below.

The issues of workforce shortage unique to each country and hence the solutions also wary depending on the particular country. In LAMI countries, the workforce issues are magnified manifold, and there are ways in which the impact of available psychiatrists can be increased. The role of psychiatrist can be shifted from direct service provision that impacts finite number of individuals to a more public health approach of designing mental health-care programs that can be delivered by non-specialists, building their health system's capacity for delivering care, including supporting frontline health workers through support supervision, raising awareness on mental health and patients' rights in addition to promoting essential research (Kigozi and Ssebunnya 2014). Another solution is to utilize informal providers who are part of the communities in identifying cases in the community and directing them to the appropriate agencies to obtain help. The informal providers can also be incorporated into the care pathway to augment the limited skilled providers

(Burns 2015). A third solution is the utilization of peers with lived experience of illness. Peers help fight the stigma of mental illness, instill hope, and help individuals to navigate the experiences of psychosis and promote recovery. Peer outreach to families has been shown to lower distress, enhance coping skills, and improve functioning. These results were sustained at follow-up of three months (Lucksted et al. 2013). Utilization of peers also serves the added purpose of creating vocational opportunities for individuals with mental illnesses. One of the recommendations by IOM is that US Department of Health and Human Services and other public and private funding agencies should ensure that clients are active participants in the development of practice guidelines, quality measures, policies, and implementation strategies for, as well as research on, psychosocial interventions for people with mental health and substance use disorders and that systems of care as well as government should provide appropriate incentives to that end. In addition, it is recommended that family members of consumers should be provided with opportunities to participate in such activities (IOM 2015).

Another way to address manpower shortage is utilizing existing technology to expand the services that are provided. These include web-based cognitive behavioral interventions for coping with auditory hallucinations, online peer support, and social therapy for first-episode psychosis, Internet-based family intervention programs, computerized "relational agents" designed to enhance medication adherence and physical activity, clinic-based computerized patient kiosks for self-assessment, virtual-reality paradigms for vocational rehabilitation, and smartphone applications (apps) for self-management of schizophrenia (Ben-Zeev et al. 2015). Technology is used to help individuals, their families, and their support systems, and there is some evidence to show that it will be utilized. In a review of Internet-based intervention for psychosis, the authors found that 74–86 % of patients used the web-based interventions efficiently, 75–92 % perceived them as positive and useful, and 70–86 % completed or were engaged. They conclude that there is significant untapped potential for the use of Internet-based interventions for psychosis more broadly (Alvarez-Jimenez et al. 2014). One thing that can be counted on is the cost of technology reduces with time, while that of labor only increases and thus technology becomes even more affordable.

There is a novel way of looking at the workforce and efficiency of systems of care. Traditionally, health-care systems have addressed cost and quality issues by asking the workforce to work harder or become even better. However, this approach has limitations and a novel approach called building "social capital" is being looked at as a way to enhance organizations and systems to accomplish much more with available resources. Building social capital is improving ways in which people work together and take joint responsibility for the care of the client. The result is that the team is able to accomplish much more than individual members put together, for example, the entire team will take responsibility for side effects of medication and the staff who see the clients in community work as the eyes and ears of the prescribing psychiatrist in looking for medication adverse effects while the psychiatrist may identify and communicate with therapist or case manager as to what they could do to enhance their interactions. The values underlying working together are trust, teamwork, reliability, and desire to innovate and improve (Lee et al. 2015).

13.7.4 Research into Service Provision

In the USA, some recent research results and some ongoing studies are providing data and directions to improve the delivery of effective psychosocial interventions for individuals with psychosis. The Recovery After Initial Schizophrenia Episode (RAISE) was launched by NIMH in 2008 to develop, test, and deploy team-based multicomponent interventions (NAVIGATE) in the first-episode psychosis in "real-world" community settings. NAVIGATE includes four interventions: resiliency-focused individual therapy, family psychoeducation and support, supported education and employment, and personalized medication management. NIMH funded two studies: RAISE early treatment study (ETS) and RAISE implementation and evaluation study (RAISE-IES), to evaluate the feasibility of delivering these services and the outcomes from these services. The RAISE-ETS was a multisite randomized controlled trial that involved 17 settings and 404 subjects wherein NAVIGATE interventions were delivered by clinicians working in community settings. Clients in the intervention group remained in treatment longer and had significantly greater improvement in symptoms, involvement in education and work, and overall quality of life (Kane et al. 2015). The second study RAISE-IES developed several products to facilitate implementation of NAVIGATE interventions in community mental health settings. Currently, community health programs in 19 states have started such teams (Essock et al. 2015).

Another ongoing study STEP-ED is attempting to reduce the duration of untreated psychosis and evaluate if early detection can improve outcomes for individuals in first-episode treatment. The study consists of utilizing social marketing approaches to inform a public education campaign to enable rapid and effective help-seeking behavior. Professional outreach and detailing to a wide variety of care providers, including those in the health care, educational, and judicial sectors, is expected to facilitate rapid redirection of appropriate patients to STEP. The study seeks to transform pathways to care in eight towns surrounding the study area (Srihari et al. 2014).

13.8 Future Directions

While there are several effective psychosocial treatments, there is some overlap in the techniques used by some of them. Behavioral health field would benefit from a common terminology for identifying and classifying the elements across all evidence-based psychosocial interventions. A common terminology permits researchers to use the same terms so that data could be pooled from different research groups. This database can then provide optimal sequencing and dosing of elements and for whom a given element, or set of elements, is most effective. In addition, it might be possible to connect elements more precisely to purported mechanisms of change than is the case with an entire complex psychosocial intervention. Current guidelines for psychosocial treatments are provided by different entities such as professional organizations, health-care organizations, and state entities and are at odds with one another, and clinicians, consumers, providers, and health-care organizations do not have a good direction to follow. *Every country should have a process for compiling and disseminating the results of systematic reviews along with guidelines and dissemination tools.* A central organization such as the National Registry of Evidence-based Programs and Practices (NREPP) and professional organizations should disseminate guidelines, implementation tools, and methods for evaluating the impact of guidelines on practice and patient outcomes. This process should be informed by the models developed by the National Institute for Health Care and Excellence (NICE) in the UK and the US Department of Veterans Affairs.

The infrastructure for measurement and improvement of psychosocial interventions is lacking, both at the national level for measure development and at the local level for measure implementation and reporting. Current quality measures are insufficient to drive improvement in psychosocial interventions. While there is enthusiasm for incorporating performance measures based on patient-reported outcomes, there is no consensus on which outcomes should have priority and what tools are practical and feasible for use in guiding ongoing clinical care. In addition, risk adjustment methodologies need to be developed to ensure effective use of these measures for monitoring the performance of the health-care system with respect to treatment for mental health and substance use disorders.

13.8.1 Adopt a System for Quality Improvement

Purchasers, planners, and providers should adopt systems for measuring, monitoring, and improving quality for psychosocial interventions. These systems should be aligned across multiple levels. They should include structure, process, and outcome measures and a combination of financial and nonfinancial incentives to ensure accountability and encourage continuous quality improvement for providers and the organizations in which they practice. Quality improvement systems also should include measures of clinician core competencies in the delivery of evidence-based psychosocial interventions. Public reporting systems, provider profiling, pay-for-performance, and other accountability approaches that include outcome measures should account for differences in patient case mix (e.g., using risk adjustment methods) to counteract incentives for selection behavior on the part of clinicians and provider organizations, especially those operating under risk-based payment.

References

Alvarez-Jimenez M, Alcazar-Corcoles MA, Gonzalez-Blanch C, Bendall S, McGorry PD, Gleeson JF (2014) Online, social media and mobile technologies for psychosis treatment: a systematic review on novel user-led interventions. Schizophr Res 156(1):96–106. doi:10.1016/j.schres.2014.03.021

Angermeyer MC, Matschinger H (1999) Lay beliefs about mental disorders: a comparison between the western and the eastern parts of Germany. Soc Psychiatry Psychiatr Epidemiol 34(5):275–281

Barry CL, Huskamp HA, Goldman HH (2010) A political history of federal mental health and addiction insurance parity. Milbank Q 88(3):404–433. doi:10.1111/j.1468-0009.2010.00605.x

Ben-Zeev D, Drake RE, Brian RM (2015) Technologies for people with serious mental illness. In: Marsch LA, Lord SE, Dallery J, Marsch LA, Lord SE, Dallery J (eds) Behavioral healthcare and technology: using science-based innovations to transform practice. Oxford University Press, New York, pp 70–80

Bhargav H, Jagannathan A, Raghuram N, Srinivasan TM, Gangadhar BN (2015) Schizophrenia patient or spiritually advanced personality? A qualitative case analysis. J Relig Health 54(5):1901–1918. doi:10.1007/s10943-014-9994-0

Bola JR, Lehtinen K, Cullberg J, Ciompi L (2009) Psychosocial treatment, antipsychotic postponement, and low-dose medication strategies in first-episode psychosis: a review of the literature. Psychosis Psychol Soc Integr Approaches 1(1):4–18

Bradley AC, Baker A, Lewin TJ (2007) Group intervention for coexisting psychosis and substance use disorders in rural Australia: outcomes over 3 years. Aust N Z J Psychiatry 41(6):501–508

Brus M, Novakovic V, Friedberg A (2012) Psychotherapy for schizophrenia: a review of modalities and their evidence base. Psychodyn Psychiatry 40(4):609–616. doi:10.1521/pdps.2012.40.4.609

Burns JK (2015) Why searching for psychosis in diverse settings is important for global research and mental health systems development. Soc Psychiatry Psychiatr Epidemiol 50(6):895–897. doi:10.1007/s00127-015-1056-8

Centers for Medicare and Medicaid Services (2012). https://www.cms.gov/Research-Statistics-Data-and-Systems/Research-Statistics-Data-and-Systems.html accessed March 8, 2016.

Chatterjee S, Pillai A, Jain S, Cohen A, Patel V (2009) Outcomes of people with psychotic disorders in a community-based rehabilitation programme in rural India. Br J Psychiatry 195(5):433–439. doi:10.1192/bjp.bp.108.057596

Chatterjee S, Naik S, John S, Dabholkar H, Balaji M, Koschorke M, . . . Thornicroft G (2014) Effectiveness of a community-based intervention for people with schizophrenia and their caregivers in India (COPSI): a randomised controlled trial. Lancet 383(9926):1385–1394. doi:10.1016/S0140-6736(13)62629-X

Chow WS, Priebe S (2013) Understanding psychiatric institutionalization: a conceptual review. BMC Psychiatry 13:169. doi:10.1186/1471-244x-13-169

Clark RE, Samnaliev M (2005) Psychosocial treatment in the 21st century. Int J Law Psychiatry 28(5):532–544

Dietrich S, Beck M, Bujantugs B, Kenzine D, Matschinger H, Angermeyer MC (2004) The relationship between public causal beliefs and social distance toward mentally ill people. Aust N Z J Psychiatry 38(5):348–354. doi:10.1111/j.1440-1614.2004.01363.x; discussion 355–347

Drake RE, Essock SM (2009) The science-to-service gap in real-world schizophrenia treatment: the 95% problem. Schizophr Bull 35(4):677–678. doi:10.1093/schbul/sbp047

Drake R, Skinner J, Bond G, Goldman H (2009) Social security and mental illness: reducing disability with supported employment. Health Aff 28:761–770

Essock SM, Nossel IR, McNamara K, Bennett ME, Buchanan RW, Kreyenbuhl JA, . . . Dixon LB (2015) Practical monitoring of treatment fidelity: examples from a team-based intervention for people with early psychosis. Psychiatr Serv 66(7):674–676. doi:10.1176/appi.ps.201400531

Fuller Torrey E (2015) Deinstitutionalization and the rise of violence. CNS Spectr 20(3):207–214. doi:10.1017/s1092852914000753

Furnham A, Bower P (1992) A comparison of academic and lay theories of schizophrenia. Br J Psychiatry 161:201–210

Gabel JR, Whitmore H, Green M, Stromberg ST, Weinstein DS, Oran R (2015) In second year of marketplaces, new entrants, ACA 'Co-Ops', and medicaid plans restrain average premium growth rates. Health Aff (Millwood) 34(12):2020–2026. doi:10.1377/hlthaff.2015.0738

Gunn WB Jr, Blount A (2009) Primary care mental health: a new frontier for psychology. J Clin Psychol 65(3):235–252. doi:10.1002/jclp.20499

Hemmens C, Miller M, Burton VS Jr, Milner S (2002) The consequences of official labels: an examination of the rights lost by the mentally ill and mentally incompetent ten years later. Community Ment Health J 38(2):129–140. doi:10.1023/A:1014543104471

IOM (2015) Psychosocial interventions for mental and substance use disorders: a framework for establishing evidence based standards. Retrieved from http://iom.nationalacademies.org/reports/2015/Psychosocial-Interventions-Mental-Substance-Abuse-Disorders.aspx

Jablensky A, Sartorius N, Ernberg G, Anker M, Korten A, Cooper JE, . . . Bertelsen A (1992) Schizophrenia: manifestations, incidence and course in different cultures. A World Health Organization ten-country study. Psychol Med Monogr Suppl 20:1–97

Jonas KG, Markon KE (2013) A model of psychosis and its relationship with impairment. Soc Psychiatry Psychiatr Epidemiol 48(9):1367–1375. doi:10.1007/s00127-012-0642-2

Kane JM, Robinson DG, Schooler NR, Mueser KT, Penn DL, Rosenheck RA, . . . Heinssen RK (2015) Comprehensive versus usual community care for first-episode psychosis: 2-year out-comes from the NIMH RAISE early treatment program. Am J Psychiatry. appiajp201515050632. doi:10.1176/appi.ajp.2015.15050632

Kessler R, Demler O, Frank R, Olfson M, Pincus H, Walters E, Wang P, Wells K, Zaslavsky A (2005) Prevalence and treatment of mental disorders, 1990 to 2003. N Engl J Med 352(24):2515–2523

Khan S, Brabham A (2015) Preparing to implement the new access and waiting time standards for early intervention in psychosis'. Paper presented at the presentation at the north east and Cumbria and Yorkshire and Humber EIP and IAPT workshop, Leeds, 7 May, Leeds

Kigozi F, Ssebunnya J (2014) The multiplier role of psychiatrists in low income settings. Epidemiol Psychiatr Sci 23(2):123–127

Lamb HR, Bachrach LL (2001) Some perspectives on deinstitutionalization. Psychiatr Serv 52(8):1039–1045

Large M, Farooq S, Nielssen O, Slade T (2008) Relationship between gross domestic product and duration of untreated psychosis in low- and middle-income countries. Br J Psychiatry 193(4):272–278. doi:10.1192/bjp.bp.107.041863

Lee TH, Campion EW, Morrissey S, Drazen JM (2015) Leading the transformation of health care delivery – the launch of NEJM catalyst. N Engl J Med 0(0), null. doi:10.1056/NEJMe1515517

Leff J, Williams G, Huckvale M, Arbuthnot M, Leff AP (2013) Avatar therapy for persecutory auditory hallucinations: what is it and how does it work? Psychosis 6(2):166–176. doi:10.1080/17522439.2013.773457

Leucht S, Cipriani A, Spineli L, Mavridis D, Orey D, Richter F, . . . Davis JM (2013) Comparative efficacy and tolerability of 15 antipsychotic drugs in schizophrenia: a multiple-treatments meta-analysis. Lancet 382(9896):951–962. doi:10.1016/s0140-6736(13)60733-3

Lucksted A, Medoff D, Burland J, Stewart B, Fang LJ, Brown C, . . . Dixon LB (2013) Sustained outcomes of a peer-taught family education program on mental illness. Acta Psychiatr Scand 127(4):279–286. doi:10.1111/j.1600-0447.2012.01901.x

Lysaker PH, Roe D (2015) Integrative psychotherapy for schizophrenia: its potential for a central role in recovery oriented treatment. J Clin Psychol. doi:10.1002/jclp.22246

Mizrahi R (2015) Social stress and psychosis risk: common neurochemical substrates? Neuropsychopharmacology. doi:10.1038/npp.2015.274

Mosher L, Bola J (2013) Non-hospital, non-medication interventions in first-episode psychosis. In: Read J, Dillon J (eds) Models of madness: psychological, social and biological approaches to psychosis, 2nd edn. Routledge/Taylor & Francis Group, New York, pp 361–377

Mueser KT, Deavers F, Penn DL, Cassisi JE (2013) Psychosocial treatments for schizophrenia. Annu Rev Clin Psychol 9:465–497. doi:10.1146/annurev-clinpsy-050212-185620

Mueser KT, McGurk SR (2014). "Supported employment for persons with serious mental illness: current status and future directions." Encephale 40 Suppl 2: S45–56

NAMI (2009) Grading the states 2009: a report on America's health care system for adults with serious mental illnesses. Retrieved from https://www2.nami.org/gtstemplate09.cfm?section=State_by_State09

Newcomer JW, Hennekens CH (2007) Severe mental illness and risk of cardiovascular disease. JAMA 298:1794–1796

NHS Providers (2015) Funding for mental health services: moving towards parity of esteem? www.nhsproviders.org

Office of National Statistics (ONS) (2013). "Expenditure on health care in UK." 2015.

Orszag PR, Emanuel EJ (2010). "Health care reform and cost control." N Engl J Med 363(7): 601–603

Ragins M (2005) Should the CATIE study Be a wake-up call? Psychiatr Serv R 56(12):1489. doi:10.1176/appi.ps.56.12.1489

Ragins M (2012) Recovery: changing from a medial model to a psychosocial rehabilitation model. Retrieved from http://mhavillage.squarespace.com/storage/06RecoverySevereMI.pdf

Ramakrishnan P, Rane A, Dias A, Bhat J, Shukla A, Lakshmi S, . . . Koenig HG (2014) Indian health care professionals' attitude towards spiritual healing and its role in alleviating stigma of psychiatric services. J Relig Health 53(6):1800–1814. doi:10.1007/s10943-014-9822-6

Rathod S, Griffiths A, Kingdon D, Tiplady B, Jones T (2015) Pathways to recovery. Retrieved from http://imperialcollegehealthpartners.com/wp-content/uploads/2015/06/Pathways-to-recovery-ICHP-and-Wessex.pdf

Rathod S, Psychosis Pathway Steering Group (2015). TRIumPH: Psychosis Care Pathway and Narrative. Wessex Academic Health Sciences Network.

Rethink Mental Illness (2014). Lost Generation: Protecting Early Intervention in Psychosis services. London

Rubinow DR (2014) Out of sight, out of mind: mental illness behind bars. Am J Psychiatry 171(10):1041–1044. doi:10.1176/appi.ajp.2014.14060712

Sav A, McMillan SS, Kelly F, King MA, Whitty JA, Kendall E, Wheeler AJ (2015) The ideal healthcare: priorities of people with chronic conditions and their carers. BMC Health Serv Res 15(1):551. doi:10.1186/s12913-015-1215-3

Saxena S, Lora A, Morris J, Berrino A, Esparza P, Barrett T, . . . Saraceno B (2011) Mental health services in 42 low- and middle-income countries: a WHO-AIMS cross-national analysis. Psychiatr Serv 62(2):123–125

Seikkula J, Olson ME (2003) The open dialogue approach to acute psychosis: its poetics and micropolitics. Fam Process 42(3):403–418

Srihari VH, Tek C, Pollard J, Zimmet S, Keat J, Cahill JD, . . . Woods SW (2014) Reducing the duration of untreated psychosis and its impact in the U.S.: the STEP-ED study. BMC Psychiatry 14:335. doi:10.1186/s12888-014-0335-3

Srinivasan TN, Thara R (2001) Beliefs about causation of schizophrenia: do Indian families believe in supernatural causes? Soc Psychiatry Psychiatr Epidemiol 36(3):134–140

The King's Fund (2015) Mental health under pressure. Kingsfund, London, www.kingsfund.org.uk

Tyrer P (2011) Has the closure of psychiatric beds gone too far? Yes. BMJ 343:d7457. doi:10.1136/bmj.d7457

Waterreus A, Morgan V, Castle D, Galletly C, Jablensky A, Di Prinzio P, Shah S (2012) Medication for psychosis – consumption and consequences: the second Australian national survey of psychosis. Aust N Z J Psychiatry. doi:10.1177/0004867412450471, 0004867412450471 [pii]

Weil TP (2015) Insufficient dollars and qualified personnel to meet United States mental health needs. J Nerv Ment Dis 203(4):233–240. doi:10.1097/NMD.0000000000000271

Wykes T, Steel C, Everitt B, Tarrier N (2008) Cognitive behavior therapy for schizophrenia: effect sizes, clinical models, and methodological rigor. Schizophr Bull 34(3):523–537

Yang LH, Phillips MR, Li X, Yu G, Zhang J, Shi Q, . . . Susser E (2013) Employment outcome for people with schizophrenia in rural v. urban China: population-based study. Br J Psychiatry 203(4):272–279

Zipursky RB, Reilly TJ, Murray RM (2013) The myth of schizophrenia as a progressive brain disease. Schizophr Bull 39(6):1363–1372. doi:10.1093/schbul/sbs135

CPI Antony Rowe
Chippenham, UK
2017-01-09 21:26